We're Got Cancer

"I'll Start at the beginning...."

KUSHLA ROLLS

Modern Mind

Modern Mind

First published in 2020
by Modern Mind Limited
Unit 1/ 2 Rangitira Avenue, Takapuna, Auckland 0622
info@modernmind.nz
WE'VE GOT CANCER

ISBN 978-0-473-53597-1 (Amazon Paperback)

A catalogue record for this book is available from
the National Library of New Zealand.

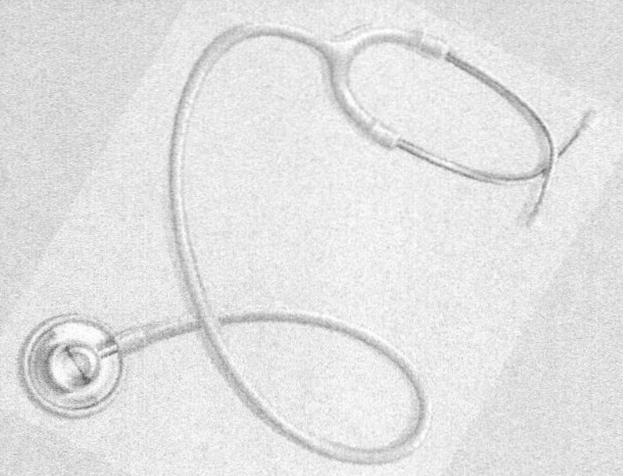

DISCLAIMER

This publication contains the information, opinions and ideas of its author. It is sold with the understanding that neither the author nor the publisher is engaged in rendering medical, health or other professional advice or services. If the reader requires such advice or services, a competent professional should be consulted. The results, consults, research, strategies and comments outlined in this book are those personal to the author's experience and are not guaranteed or warranted to be applicable otherwise.

No warranty is made with respect to the accuracy or completeness of the information contained herein, and both the author and the publisher specifically disclaim any responsibility for any liability, loss or risk, personal or otherwise, which is incurred as a consequence, directly or indirectly, of the use and application of any of the contents of this book. Some names and identifying details of some of the individuals mentioned in this book have been changed to protect their privacy.

I would like to thank Patrick for his persistent encouragement
and enduring support to write of our journey.

I would also like to thank my editors for their
professional support in helping to create a more readable story.
Janice Weston
Nicola Heath

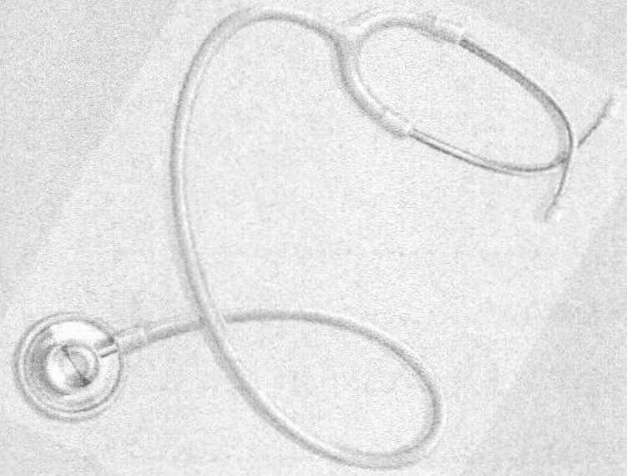

CONTENTS

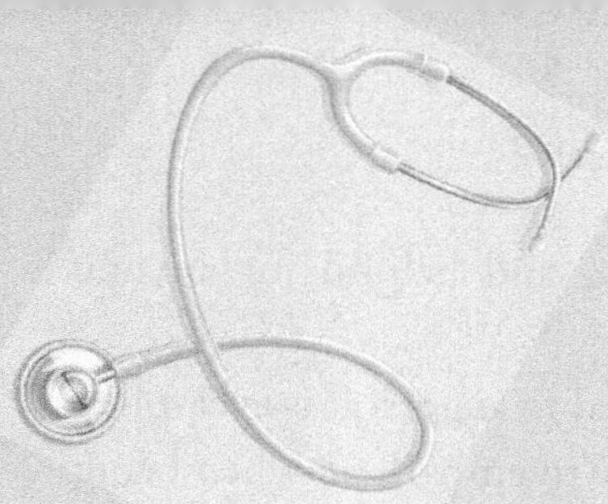

FOREWORD

Writing this story was my saviour as I became entwined in the journey with my partner and multiple myeloma. It began simply as a journal. From the warning signs to diagnosis of You've Got Cancer to We've Got Cancer. Through his treatments of chemotherapy and stem cell transplant and his incredible recovery with incredible results, my iPad became my best friend. I documented the medical aspects, their impact, incidences, trials and tribulations, together with how we were affected, throughout the 14 month journey of chemotherapy, stem cell transplant, and more chemotherapy. I also collected photos as a picture truly can 'paint a thousand words'.

My partner started with a diagnosis of 80-90% blood plasma saturation of cancer cells in his body to now being MRD (Minimal Residual Disease) - with stringent complete response (as good as it gets!). It's a great success story so I decided to take what I'd written and turn it into a read for others, hoping it may prove useful, insightful, interesting, comforting or even inspiring for others, whether they or a loved one are going through cancer, or they simply wish to understand our cancer journey. It holds all the medical and technical information we needed to know, interpreted into terms I could understand, and into a language that I could get my head around… plain English basically. And being a Counsellor myself, I share strategies that I used to help me through the darker moments.

I feel this story reaches further than just to those with multiple myeloma. Certainly it will be helpful to those who have been diagnosed with most blood disorders, but it also has a number of twists and turns that may be interesting and helpful for anyone embarking on the path of the 'C' word.

This is our story and it is not intended to suggest it is everyone's story. We all have our own unique journey to embark on when being diagnosed with cancer with our own individual diagnoses, treatment plans, and the ways we do or don't cope through it all. I only wish to honour each and every person diagnosed, their partners, their families, and their friends. This story has been told only to offer support in whatever way you may need it hence I have left it separated into 47 chapters so, should you choose to, it is easy to hop, skip and jump to wherever you personally need to go.

In many chapters I have been open and raw for a purpose - to give permission and acknowledgement to others who are either supporting someone or going through any cancer treatment, to be able to be honest to themselves and/or others about what they are going through. I'm also hoping that maybe along the way there are some stories in here that can help you plan and get on this journey a little easier than we did, with this broad insight of the entire journey.

It turned out, by the time I'd finished journaling, it was a book! So here it is, total exposure, given to you with love, in this form, in case in some way it can contribute towards being a saviour for you or a loved one.

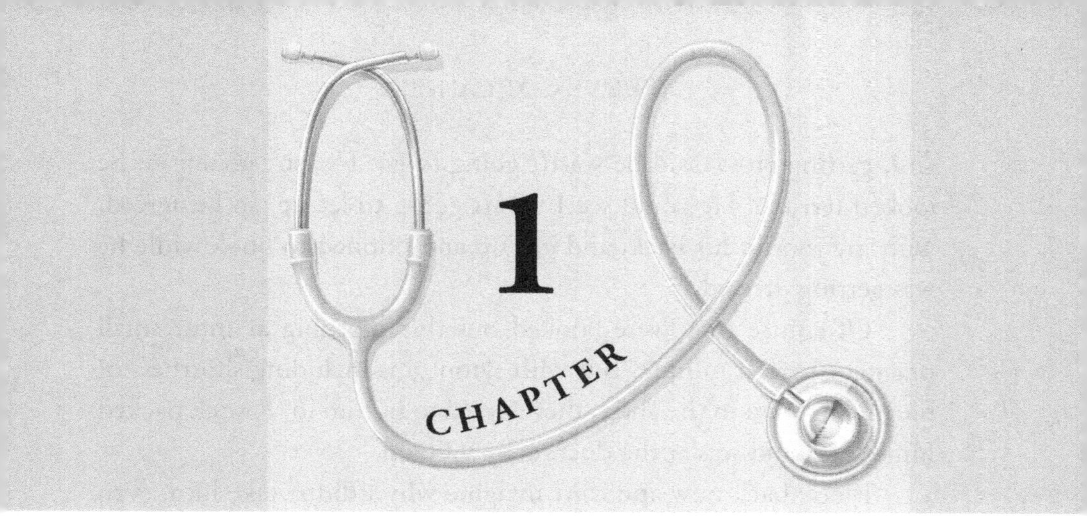

First Concerns

"What agenda does this universe have?
What game is it I am oblivious to?"
- Zubair Ahsan -

"Why is he sending you for even more tests Patrick?" The phone was pressed tightly to my ear. In the back of my mind, slight alarm bells were starting to go off. My stomach tightened and my breath started to shorten. My body and my intuition had kicked in. My intuitive voice was quietly saying to me "Something is not right and you need to get to the bottom of this!"

"I don't know," said Patrick. He sounded hesitant, unsure.

A couple of weeks earlier Patrick had caught a bit of a cold that turned into a chesty cough. A week later he was finding it difficult to breathe. He had pain in the bone across his chest area which kept him awake all night.

In the morning, he was no better and I insisted he march straight to his local GP. Honestly, Patrick's such a robust kind of guy. Rarely can I get him to a doctor although, in the same breath, he's rarely sick… but today was different. Patrick told me to stop overreacting and, getting cross, said he wasn't going to go. I wasn't giving in; he looked terrible. He could see I wasn't going to let up, so he agreed, with my foot in his back, and got up and phoned to book while he was getting dressed.

Of course they were booked out this morning as most small practices are last minute. But with symptoms including shortness of breath and pain in the chest, they agreed to fit him in. Patrick packed himself off and was at the doctors by 9.00am.

I look back now and can't imagine why I didn't take him, even the doctors were surprised he had driven himself there. Although I could see Patrick was really unwell I hadn't thought it was anything to seriously worry about, likely just a cough or chest infection that needed seeing to. I have had horrific coughs myself, once for almost two weeks of racking cough and, looking back, I think I had been subconsciously putting it down as something like that.

The doctor's practice was in Takapuna, about fifteen minutes drive from our home without peak traffic. It was some time before Patrick called me to let me know how he'd got on; I wasn't concerned about how long he'd been gone as I'd presumed he'd hit traffic on the way, or had to wait to be seen however I was surprised at the exasperation in his voice as he blurted out "I'm so bloody frustrated. They've sent me off for all these tests, it's ridiculous, they even asked me to have an echo test for my heart. I told them it's a waste of time, my heart's alright, I don't need that but they insisted. Now I've just gone and done a whole lot of blood tests and am on my way for a chest X-ray!"

It was all a bit of a surprise to me. I thought they would check his breathing, listen to his chest, prescribe an inhaler or antibiotics or something, and send him on his way. I was reeling a bit, picturing him in this short amount of time running from the doctors surgery, from one place to another getting all these tests done, when all along I thought he was sitting in the doctors practice waiting to be 'fitted in' or 'doing traffic.'

When I could get a word in, I asked why they were doing the tests? "I don't know." said Patrick. "They were concerned because I was short of breath I think, and that I had that pain across the bone under my chest. Maybe they thought I was going to have a heart attack. Bloody stupid. I told them I was fine, that it wasn't my heart, but they insisted on all these tests!"

Patrick then practically barked at me, "Look I've gotta go, I'm at the X-ray place now, I'll see you when I get home."... and he hung up, obviously very annoyed and put out, which is not a common occurrence for my kind, gentle, man. I didn't think much more of it at the time, I bought the story. They are being over cautious, of course, they have to be. It's pain around the heart, shortness of breath. Fair enough. And I got on with my day, thinking nothing more of it.

I wasn't working that day and when Patrick eventually came home we discussed the antibiotics and inhalers his GP had given him. His GP had diagnosed him with wheezy bronchitis, which seemed an obvious diagnosis, and the further tests weren't discussed again. We both had put those tests down in our minds as an over precaution by the GP.

A few days later on Friday evening, Patrick was still feeling sick from the bronchitis. The antibiotics weren't having any effect and he was feeling pretty unwell; he was tired, and drained from the coughing. Some girlfriends had asked me out for a drink but I didn't want to leave Patrick home alone, and I wanted to be with him as he had felt unwell for so long. We were watching a movie when the phone rang. It was about 9pm and I could hear Patrick talking to his GP.

I'll never forget the thoughts going on in my head at the time. "What a great GP he is calling so late at night, he must have had a really busy day and only just had a chance now to follow up on clients. How dedicated to bother at this time on a Friday night, not many GPs are that dedicated nowadays etc, etc." Subconsciously the chatter went on and not once did I think something must be wrong. I absolutely marvel at that even now. My intuition is usually so strong, yet not once did concerned thoughts or feelings come into my mind or body.

Patrick got off the phone telling me "One of the blood test results is a bit off so the doctor wants me to go back tomorrow morning and do another one."

I sat there, the movie having been paused and I, waiting to get back to it, just said "Oh what a great GP keeping an eye on the results and ringing you so late to keep on top of it." I knew this GP to be kind and caring and so automatically put it down to that. Never did it enter my mind that this could be a concern; Patrick wasn't concerned either. He clicked the remote and we settled back in to watch the rest of the movie.

In the morning Patrick went off for his blood test. We had a 50th birthday party we were supposed to be going to that night for my girlfriend Bronnie. We were having an early dinner first with Patrick's family as his brother from England was passing through Auckland for a couple of days, but by the time we were getting ready to leave for dinner Patrick started complaining of pressure in his right ear and Katelyn (Patrick's daughter) and I were laughing about man flu. A few jokes got bandied around as we were so not used to him being sick. I myself have had more than my fair share of colds and flu over the years so I guess, although I was sympathetic, I wasn't taking it too seriously.

We went to dinner but as the meal wore on Patrick was starting to feel worse and worse. Bless him, he still said he would be happy to go to the party for a bit. Here he was feeling ill, deaf in one ear as, unbeknown to us at the time, his ear drum was about to burst… and still offering to go to a noisy party of 100 people as he knew how much I'd wanted to be there to celebrate with friends.

By the time we got in the car I took one look at him and insisted we went home and he went to bed. I messaged my friends that he was ill and that we weren't coming. It is very unlike me to not show up at something I've said I will. There is a sense of integrity in me that when I say I'm going to do something I make sure I do. I really don't like letting people down or be seen as someone who is not true to their word. Another part of me also wants to respect my friends and their special occasions and make sure I honour them as a show of my love and friendship so making this decision to not go to Bronnie's 50th at the last minute was a rare thing, but not a difficult decision this night. Patrick looked terrible. Little did I know then how much his body was really battling. How much the shit was going to hit the fan when he eventually went to the GP on Monday morning!

By the next morning poor Patrick was worse, his ear drum had burst and things just got a little more serious. We pretty much worked out that the antibiotics he had been on weren't helping and I wanted him to go to our local 24 hour clinic however he insisted he could wait until Monday and go back to his normal GP. Monday morning Patrick was back at the clinic to get his antibiotic changed.

This time I was at work when Patrick phoned me to report on his appointment. "He's given me a different antibiotic. The other one wasn't working, but I'm also just off to get some more blood tests done." So this is when finally the first alarm bells started going off. Not causing too much alarm but enough for me to ask the first big question. "Why is he sending you for even more tests Patrick?" Patrick's response, so hesitant, was left hanging in the air. Simply. "I don't know."

I can still recall the silence so well, even as I write this now. It just hung there. A space of so much unknown. It was dark and foreboding and I had a sense of fear lurking, threatening to rise and take control. I jumped back "Well you need to find out! We need to know what he's worried about!"

Patrick has a scientific background. He has a science degree in chemistry and maths and I wondered where his mind had been, that he hadn't asked more by now. Then of course, looking back, he was sick and not thinking straight. When we were both home together he reassured me. "Don't worry. I have called the doctors practice and asked that I be copied into all the results that come through from now on. They have given me the name of a site where I can plug in to see all the results as they come available." Although Patrick is such a caring, sensitive man, he loves practicality and deciphering a problem, particularly where chemistry is concerned. So here he was in his element and I could see he felt good now he had a bit of control and opportunity to see possibly what his GP was so concerned about. We could all relax for a bit while we waited for the results. The worry I had been feeling was lightened just a little. Answers will come soon.

Looking back at even this small moment in time is such an indication of the power of fear, of the unknown, and the impact it has on you. Since Patrick's phone call in the morning fear had been lurking, rising into my space. All the thoughts of the mind had been coming in… "What is going on?" "What does this mean?" "Is he alright?" "Will he be alright?" All fears of the unknown for the future… I had felt it building up over the afternoon yet as soon as we had the option of finding answers soon, getting some control, the fear started to subside and the lightness was allowed to filter through a little. I found I could breathe again and I hadn't realised how much I had been holding on with the worry. In the light of the known coming through soon, it became easier to carry on, which is what we did. We carried on with our days as normal waiting for the results. Of course now with a hint of trepidation still, I can't lie!

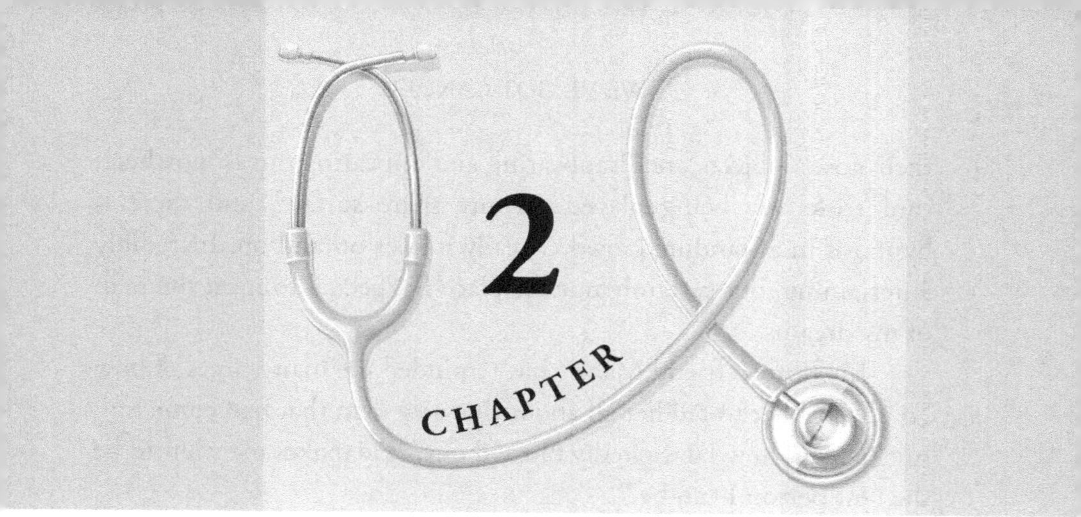

Patrick and I Met

"Love is like a river,
A never ending stream.
Love is shared by each other,
To answer someone's dream."
- John P. Read -

Patrick and I met at a magic convention. It was July 2007. He was waiting in line to buy tickets for a magic show that was about to start; I was a damsel in distress as I'd left my tickets back at the hotel room... which was about an hour's taxi ride from the convention. He looked like the perfect person to pick on to pour out my problem. Not just cute, but kind looking, and sensible. A man that could give me some good advice for my predicament.

Well that was pretty much it from there... love at first sight and all that stuff really... for both of us. Little had I known, when I had taken my son all the way to Melbourne to follow his passion of magic, that I would meet the love of my life.

It's a pretty wacky world, the world of magic. Everywhere you turn something weird is going on. People are pulling knives out of their noses, objects are disappearing and appearing out of nowhere, card tricks are being played on any spare surface, and there is hypnosis in a standing crowd… really it goes on and on. Incredibly entertaining, but certainly not the place I expected to meet the man of my dreams.

My dearest friend Mandy has reminded me many times of how I'd phoned her to tell her all about this new man that had come into my life, and how I'd excitedly blurted out, "He makes me want to be the best person I can be."

So our romance started really from that very first day. I stayed on in Melbourne a little longer with my son, and when we landed back in Auckland airport there was this most beautiful phone message from Patrick where he told me he couldn't wait to see me again… and then he sang a romantic song from sleepless in Seattle. I was pretty much hooked, line and sinkered right there! And I wish, to this day, that I'd saved that message.

It was a good few years before we actually moved in together; we both have children. I have two boys - Chase and Taylor, and Patrick has three children - Ben, Jasmine and Katelyn. Our children were our priority and, for various reasons, it worked best for us to live separately for three years and then we took the plunge, merging the two families. Patrick's son Ben didn't live with us, and Chase had started University in Otago that year. We were very lucky that there was no problem with the children getting on and the merger was relatively simple in that regard.

Chase was 14 and Taylor 11 when Patrick and I met. Patrick and Chase entered a few competitions at magic conventions over the following years as Chase was also a magician. They've had a great relationship from the start with this common passion between them.

Taylor first really got to know Patrick on the ski slopes in Queenstown. We were there for a week of skiing and Patrick came down to join us for a few days. The boys both asked me quite seriously before he came "He can ski Mum, right, you're sure he can ski?"

The last thing they wanted was their ski holiday spoiled by some novice on the ski field. "Of course," I replied, "he's skied all around the world… Canada, Japan, Europe, USA. We'll have no problem there." I put their minds at ease, reassuring them they were in for a good few days of skiing and getting to know Patrick some more.

When Patrick arrived he had to hire skis. "Make sure you get good quality skis won't you." I pressed before he went off to the ski hire store.

So off we went the next day, straight to the top. It was a beautiful day; sunny with fresh powder and we were all looking forward to a great day of skiing. We came off the chair and started down the top ridge. The boys were in front, then me, then Patrick. The boys stopped a wee way down so we could gather for our decided route down the mountain. I joined them and we turned to see Patrick just over the ridge, he'd fallen and was scrambling to get up. It was one of those 'uh oh' moments. None of us said anything and Patrick eventually got up and awkwardly skied down to us. We decided on our route and started off again but it wasn't long before Patrick fell over again so we stopped a bit further down and waited again for him to get himself up and join us. By the third consecutive time Chase politely said "I thought you said he could ski Mum." I was pretty dumbfounded myself and just simply replied "Well I thought he could." Being as polite as we are we still didn't say anything when Patrick joined us but he kindly brought it up. "I don't know what's going on," he said, "maybe it's because I haven't skied for quite some time." We were all hoping his ski-ing ability would return quickly, so we set off again but Patrick hadn't gone far before falling again, we stopped and waited for him again… and so it went all the way down the mountain.

Bless him, when we got to the bottom, he came back up to the top with us again and went through the whole process all over again… falling over I would say about ten times on the way down, again and again… and sometimes quite serious tumbles. But back up he would get and plunge forward, pretty much bracing himself for the next fall. When we finally got to the bottom we thought he'd retire, but nope, back up the chair again with us with not a word spoken about giving up.

It wasn't until the third run… we were about a quarter of the way down and we were again waiting for him to catch up after yet another fall and I was staring at his skis as he came closer, then suddenly realised the problem. He was in slalom skis! God knows what he asked for when he checked in asking for good skis but he was obviously mistaken and given skis designed for super fast skiing down seriously straight groomed paths; not at all suitable for what we were doing. So the mystery was solved, although that didn't help his predicament in getting down the mountain for the third time.

We eventually got to the bottom and we all decided it was best for Patrick to retire. We had to encourage him to go to the cafe and get himself a coffee while we did a few more quick runs before getting him home. He was pretty sore from all his falls and the worse for wear from them all. The next morning he was black and blue so we decided on a rest day and would go back up the following day. Patrick changed his skis and the following day we had an amazing day all skiing together. He was in fact an excellent skier and it was hard to believe it was the same person on the slopes.

I know a deep respect and care for Patrick formed from the boys on that holiday on the slopes. His perseverance, determination and sense of humour won them over and this has lasted through all of our years together. It is all of the above qualities in him I see now that helped him come to terms in coping with the enormity of what was ahead.

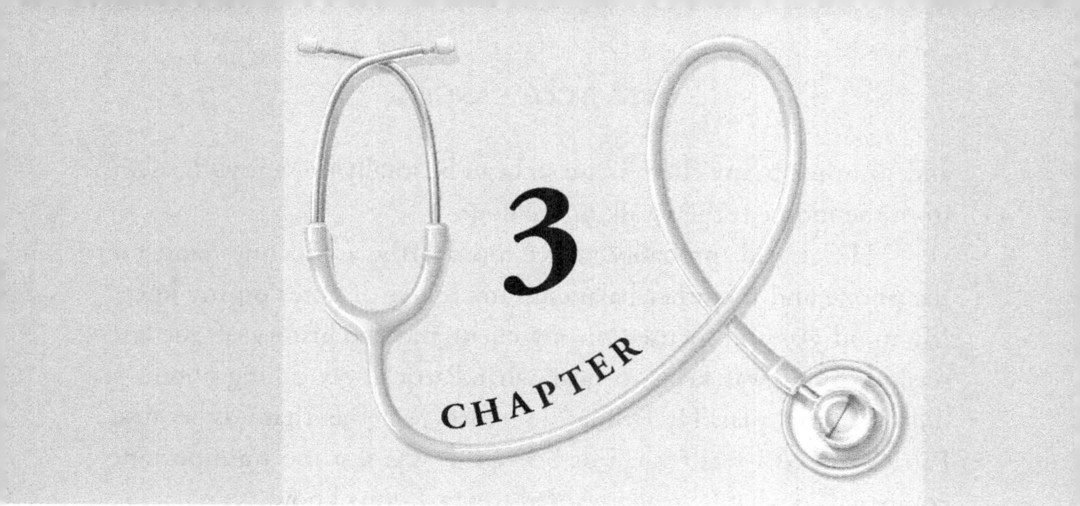

Intuition

"Someone I loved once gave me
a box full of darkness.
It took me years to understand that
this too, was a gift"
- Mary Oliver -

I was sitting in my office. It was Friday 15 September 2017. It had been days since Patrick had been sent off for more tests and we hadn't had the results. I'd only just arrived at the office and was just going through the notes for my first client, due to arrive soon. My plan was to work in the morning then drive up north to my house in Warkworth to clean for an Airbnb booking the next day.

The phone rang, the ring tone telling me it was Patrick. I wasn't going to answer as I was short on time, however since I'd only just left him about twenty minutes earlier I figured it must be important, so I picked up the call. At the back of my mind an awareness came through, that I have been on alert. I wouldn't normally have answered any calls so close to a client coming in as I like to be totally focused and absorbed in my client's case so I can be totally present with them from the moment they walk in the door.

"Hi." I said, probably rather too shortly; I had one hand on the phone and the other balancing my folder of notes on my knee. My mind was still focused on my client and the history of our last session, but I was keen to hear what Patrick was calling about. I didn't get the usual "Hi darling." in return. Whether that was because Patrick sensed I was rushed or because it was just too unimportant compared to what he really wanted to say, I don't know.

"The GP has sent me off for more tests." My stomach immediately sank as Patrick continued. "He's had the results of the last tests and he wants me to do more." I immediately demanded "What for?"

His response was quick. No hesitation or query. "One of them is a Bence-Jones test. I've googled it. It's for blood disorders."

Blood disorders, blood disorders? My brain was scrambling to make sense of what that meant. Whether Patrick knew anything more at that time, of what that could entail, I don't know but his voice was concerned. "What does that mean Patrick?" I asked. "Have you found out what the last tests were that the GP took and what the results are?" Again, he came back quickly with his answers. "I've only spoken to the nurse so far. For some reason I haven't received them myself yet but I've asked her for those test results so we can get some idea of what is going on. The results will be there later today, so we can check them out when you get home."

It felt good Patrick was now noticing this could be serious. He hadn't seemed all that concerned before now and had been just drifting along waiting for the results. I was pleased to hear he was now determined to get to the bottom of it all. My warning bells had gone off but his hadn't appeared to really, until now. He now thought to notice and search what test he was about to take and make sure he'd get access to the results. That's where my mind went. Thank you mind. It settled with the knowledge that 'we will find out more soon then, so you can let go of all this for now and get on with helping your next client.'

"OK darling, that's great." I replied. "When I get home later tonight we'll check it all out then, thanks for letting me know. Go take the blood test right now won't you?"

Patrick was silent.

"Patrick, you'll go take the tests right now, won't you?"

"Yes, yes, don't worry, I'll go this afternoon."

I really had to go as my client was going to be here any second now, so I quickly responded "Good, make sure you do and I'll call you on the way back from Warkworth to let you know when I will be home. See ya darling." and hung up.

Little did I realise while I was talking to Patrick that he was already holding on to a lot of worry. He had already started to google more on this Bence-Jones test and wasn't liking what he was reading on the possibilities of what this could mean.

I wasn't going to get home until dinner time and I felt a little anxious that I had to wait that long to see these results that were coming through but the urgency of my client arriving shortly managed to pull me away and back to the present. I parked it all, opened the client file once again, and immersed myself in my notes. It was a busy few hours with back to back clients, but I had managed to finish on time and get into the car to head to Warkworth.

I can see that moment right now. Literally, as I write this, I can see myself sitting in the car about to turn on the ignition. There was a moment of nothing happening. No action or doing. Just sitting in stillness and silence… and then BOOM! Loud and clear in my ear, I got the word booming at me, CANCER!! That was it. Just once. But so loud, so clear, so precise, I knew it was real. Every part of my being was hit with the impact of this single word.

I sat there frozen. Shock started to hit and my head started to scream NO!!!! Oh my God. NOOOOOOOOO!!! NOOOOOOOO!!! My body was overtaken with huge waves rolling through it, making me want to be sick. As the enormity of this kicked in the tears started to roll, then the sobbing kicked in. Not my darling Patrick. NO! NO! NO!!! It was too overwhelming. This can't be. How could it be? Not us. This can't be us. NO! NO! NO! I sobbed and sobbed with the helplessness of this knowing overtaking me, overwhelming me, leaving me totally defenseless. Cancer in the blood! Oh my God! How much worse could it get? How do you fight that?? It's in your whole body! NO! NO! NO! NO!!!

I have been in fear of cancer for years. My dearest friend died of melanoma 13 years ago and my stepdad died of bowel cancer 28 years ago. I had been very close to both of them through their journeys and was with each of them when they passed away. My best friend's partner died from chemotherapy treatment for bowel cancer, I was with him too when he passed away. I knew how treacherous it could be, how painful and how helpless we can be when it decides to take control. It has a force of its own that can make us powerless and left to its mercy, as it destroys our body and eventually our lives.

No, No, No!!! This can't be real. It can't be Patrick. It can't be us. No, No, No!!!

I slumped over the wheel of the car. Gripping the steering wheel the world was spinning around me; the ground opened up beneath me and I fought not to be swallowed up. My mind came to the rescue and kicked in 'Hang on, you could be wrong!' It wasn't much, but enough to help me come back. It continued, 'You could just be wrong Kushla, you could!' These words kept repeating, helping me slowly become more present. I became acutely aware of myself, and my body sitting in the car, and that I was in the carpark at work. Although I didn't really believe these words, it was enough to start to fill in the hole beneath me for now and allow me to notice my feet on the floor of the car, bringing me back, as each second went by, more to the present and awareness of what was around me.

I have very strong intuition and know I can trust it. In years gone by, another lifetime really, I used to live in such a heightened state.

I would meditate for hours every day. I stopped drinking and eating meat. I never lied and kept myself as pure as I could. The vibration I lived within led me into very easily connecting with a realm deeper than what we know from just the conscious mind. Knowledge would come simply if I asked and sometimes, as it did today, as a boom in my ear, completely out of the blue. Over the years, although I have dropped the intensity of this practice the intuition and the knowing, has remained, and I knew to trust it. However, as I sat there in the car I was thankful for my mind coming in with doubt at this moment. Just enough of a flicker to ground me and bring me back from this uncontrollable place I was heading.

I knew I had to get on the road or it would take forever to get to Warkworth so I started the ignition and the car fired up. Common sense was filtering through saving me from being swept up into the deep dark hole that had been threatening my ability to move. I reversed the car and pulled out of the car park, wiping the tears from my eyes.

My mind continued. 'You're probably just panicking… of course you've come up with cancer. Patrick mentioned blood disorders on the phone and cancer is all you really know about blood disorders. No wonder that has been your first thought, it's probably not that at all… ' Thank you, thank you again mind! It was enough to get me on the motorway and to keep moving.

Deep down, however, I knew my intuition. Although the appearance of calm was above, the waves of turmoil were still rolling deep within.

A good friend of mine, Helen, called me halfway on my journey to Warkworth. I answered the phone like nothing was going on. We chatted about various things and then somewhere along the way she asked me how I was doing. That was all it took. A kind word of enquiry and I melted down. I blurted it out. "I think Patrick has cancer!" There was total silence for a second. A second that went on forever. There it was. The words spoken out loud formed this to even stronger reality. Tears were streaming down my face again and I blurted out the recent events to her. Of course she was stunned, a reaction I have come to see with everyone we tell in the future. Dear Helen, she never stopped for a minute to question my intuition. She knew me well enough to know that when I know something, I know it.

"Oh my God!" she managed when I had finished blurting it all out. "Kushla, I don't know what to say!" And that is pretty much it. What can you say? She filled the space with "I'm so sorry to hear this. This is terrible. What can I do to help?" All the things a truly good friend would say. However none of it was sinking in, I had been swallowed into the enormousness of speaking these words and the reality of what this could mean. All I could do was sob and sob, this time gripping the phone, with words of comfort filtering through trying to ease the pain that was now forming.

The rest of that conversation is a blur. I have no idea how Helen calmed me down but somehow she did and we came back to some sense of normal conversation. Somehow we eventually got to practical matters and that really helped. The mind loves practicality and it helped to slowly bring me back to being more present once again. We talked about the further tests Patrick was taking, and how we still had to even see the blood results from the last ones.

But at the end of it all I said to Helen, "I know Helen. The way I got this message and the way it made me feel, I know it's bad. That's the message I was getting. That this is really bad."

She reassured me that she was there for me and to keep in touch with her every step of the way. I knew she meant it and I knew I would do just that. It had been good to share the burden of this knowledge. The saying 'A problem shared is a problem halved' came through for me today. We said our goodbyes and somehow I continued to Warkworth, cleaned the house for my upcoming guests and headed back home, eager to be with Patrick. I took the fast route home through the toll road and through the tunnel, I wanted to see those results and get more clarity on what was going on!

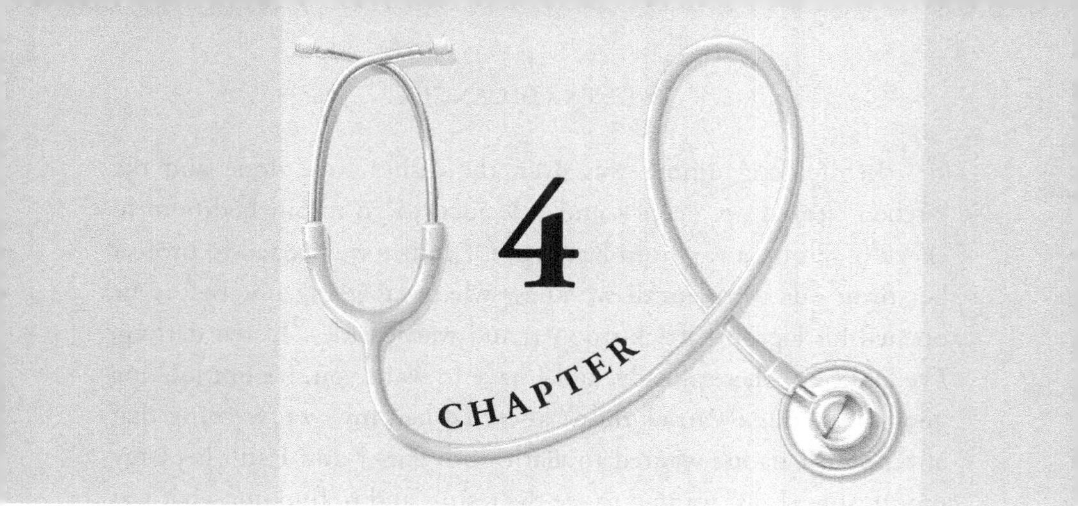

Main Test Results

"You have to conquer every obstacle
before you can reach the top of the mountain."
- Lailah Gifty Akita -

When I got home, dinner was ready. Yep. That's the kind of guy I have. Katelyn had made a lovely fresh salad and Patrick had whipped up a tofu dish. He has always had such respect for my choice of being vegetarian and embraced it with love into our home and life together.

We always eat together at the table for dinner; whether there are just the three of us or all the children home, it's our time together as a family. Part of me tonight, however, just wanted to rush and get it over with so we could sit down and check out these blood results. Patrick had already texted me earlier that he had now received them all. Another part of me though, was OK with taking time to get there. At this moment life was still relatively normal. Nothing was diagnosed officially. We were just a normal family, having a normal meal with not a lot to deal with other than day to day life.

Before long dinner was over, the dishes were done and the kitchen cleared up. Patrick and I decided to go to our bedroom to check it all out, away from Katelyn. Of course we needed to protect her from our worry until we knew what was going on. Before he opened his laptop Patrick stopped and warned me. "Listen darling, I've looked at these already, and I have to warn you, it's not looking good." Of course Patrick didn't know I'd had my own warning that afternoon. I hadn't wanted to alarm him either and I still kept my mouth shut. I just wanted to see the results and to find out what was going on.

This then became a period in time that I will never forget. There were a number of test results shown, but the following are the three that stared us alarmingly in the face. Not being doctors we had to interpret these tests in layman terms. Patrick's degree in chemistry of course was a bonus in his understanding a little of what words like proteins and immunoglobulins meant, but really it was all such a foreign language we needed to decipher.

The first thing we did was look at the numbers in the first report that listed the **Ig Test Results**. It is quite helpful the way lab reports put the norm next to results to help get a measure, it's even more helpful when they highlight in red any areas of alert. As you can see by the results following, there were quite a few of these red alerts jumping out at us on first glance. Enough to cause my stomach to tighten and to start holding my breath as we started to go through them.

L, HH, L in red blasting at us.

Immunoglobulins. To be honest I didn't even know what that was.

In my mind I was quickly scanning down, assessing the results; it didn't take a quick or great mind to see these results were seriously knocked out of the park.

"OK," I asked Patrick, "what is this Ig? What does it stand for? What does this mean?"

My forever calm, quiet and patient Patrick was in his element, stepping into practical mode and sharing his knowledge. "Immunoglobulins" he replied "are our antibodies."

Immunoglobulins, antibodies. Foreign words to me and my brain was scrambled already. "What does this mean though?!" I retorted, feeling impatient and an urgent sense to know these answers. Patrick quickly jumped in explaining further "It's our protein that is produced by plasma cells (our white blood cells). This protein is used by the immune system to neutralize bacteria and viruses."

I think I got that. Words I'm not used to and their description, trying to sink into my brain that was already, I realised, overwhelmed by emotion. Hmm, I figured it would make even more sense if I googled the actual Igs to get more specific. So out with the iPads and we started our first moments of many sleepless nights and long days googling the shit out of the internet!

IgG - our most abundant antibody found in all body fluids. Protects us against bacterial and viral infection. Found mainly in the blood and lymph fluid, it is the first antibody to fight a new infection.

Blood and lymph fluid. There it was. The first sign of something indicating a blood disorder. I knew those words. I knew they could be associated with cancer. 'Oh dear.' I thought, wishing quietly that my intuition would be wrong.

"OK Patrick," I said once we'd seen what IgG was, "what does your actual reading mean? Let's google that!" We both dived in and after a short time came up with a simple understandable answer.

IgG - 1.7 g/L (7.0 - 16.0) L

Specific hypogammaglobulinemia confers a high risk of serious bacterial infections. Suggests check full blood count and consider secondary cause.

OK, so to me this meant his immune system is low leaving it hard for him to fight infection. No wonder he couldn't get rid of his bronchitis. Of course we both knew, though didn't say out loud at the time, that a low immune system could also be a sign of cancer. It was written in the words 'consider secondary cause'!

Next result. We went to the IgA and googled all over again.

IgA measures the blood level of Immunoglobulin A which is one of the most common antibodies in the body. Antibodies are proteins made by the immune system to fight bacteria, viruses, and toxins.

Patrick's IgA Result

IgA 40.7 g/L (0.8 - 4.0) HH

Anything over 4g/L are non-specific but can be seen in pulmonary and gastrointestinal inflammatory diseases, some autoimmune conditions, liver disease, and plasma cell disorders.

We googled plasma cell disorder. This is where cancerous or malignant plasma cells overproduce and secrete into the bloodstream a myeloma protein. i.e. an abnormal monoclonal antibody or portion thereof. For the first time the word myeloma is mentioned!

Wow! This result for IgA of Patrick's was through the roof - 40.7! This explanation showed us clearly something was very wrong, but what? The list of possibilities left me clambering in the dark wanting more answers.

"OK, let's go to the next result." I said to Patrick. Our intelligent, practical minds had kicked in big time. It was not a time for emotion, or I should say, to allow ourselves to feel emotion. We both put a huge concrete wall up and focused only through the mind to find answers.

IgM. <0.2. g/l (0.4 - 2.5) L

IgM is present on B cells and its main function is the control of B cell activation. It is the primary antibody against A and B antigens on red blood cells and responsible for the blood clotting reaction during blood transfusion from wrong donors.

What the? Sorry, but this was now getting really confusing. I threw out at Patrick, "What has this got to do with anything? This is all getting too confusing, I don't get it!" Already it was getting overwhelming trying to get my head around these foreign words, to understand them and what they meant. Patrick, in his typical calm manner, softly spoke. "Lets just look at the reading to see if that explains anything more." Oh good, yes, return to something practical, find more answers. So back to the iPads to find the best answer for the last result in this test.

IgM <0.2 g/L (Low IgM levels are commonly non-specific. Significance of this result depends on the clinical presentation and other laboratory parameters.

"Ok." I said again; a word I started to notice I was commonly using. Looking back I think that simple 'OK' helped ground me as we unfolded what was really going on. In reality a whirlwind was forming around us and the word 'OK' helped to centre me in it. It perhaps was even invoking the energy of false presence that it is ok, keeping at bay the whirlwind from coming in and whisking me away.

On looking at the IgM explanation I said to Patrick, "So what we seem to be getting here is that something is really wrong, something serious but none of these tests can tell us what. Is that what you're getting Patrick?"

Patrick hesitated, thought a bit, then said "when I googled the Igs earlier in the day it seems the fact that the IgA is so high, it is suppressing the other IgG and IgM. It's not a good sign, sorry darling. But let's just look at the other tests, it shows more as we go."

I realised then of course that Patrick had already seen all the tests. He already had some understanding of what they meant by now. He just didn't know the best way to tell me. In that hesitation and thought, I realised too that he had decided the best way to tell me was to just let it open up bit by bit through the results. I felt at that moment that yes, he was right. I needed to be 'stepped' through it, anything else would be too overwhelming and hard to take in so we pulled up the next result and the same process we used for the first result started all over again.

It was with a sigh of relief that we pulled up this test result. **Complete Blood Count.** My body had a chance to relax and breathe when at first glance there was not a red indicator to be seen. We quickly scanned down the results one line at a time checking the figures and ranges more than the words. Right now we just wanted to see what was alarming and what that meant.

"Well those test results look great don't they?" I asked Patrick, looking up at him for a little reassurance.

"Yes," he replied but then he quickly pulled up the next test result and went on, "but let's look at these ones, they're not so good darling. These are perhaps the most significant of all." I huddled closer to him as we got ready to scrutinize the next result which was for **Protein Electrophoresis**. As he brought the result up on the screen I just kept staring at it blasting out at us. Two more red H letters jumping off the page. My mind seemed to be for a moment only connecting with the red letters. A flash of all the red letters I had seen tonight started jumping out at me; I felt sick, sick to my stomach.

I couldn't concentrate on what Patrick was saying as he started to explain this reading. All of a sudden I was overloaded with red letters and my brain couldn't go any further. I put my hand out and placed it on Patrick's arm and he stopped talking. Looking at me, he realised we needed a pause. "I'll make another cuppa shall I?" he asked, getting up even as he said it, knowing it was the best thing to do. I was a green tea drinker and knew it would be soothing to have a good cuppa through all of this discovery.

Patrick wasn't long bringing the tea and we sat together up on the bed, talking of other things, unimportant irrelevant things for a brief time to help regroup ourselves. It worked and we were ready to come back to the results.

I could tell Patrick was keen to get on with it. He immediately forged ahead and matter of factly stated, as we looked at the screen and this result again. "You will see where the Total Protein is high. Let's google this reading."

Total Protein - 92 g/L (66 - 84) H

On googling we started getting all sorts of weird possible conditions. Lung cancer, pulmonary tuberculosis, dehydration, or a certain type of cancer such as multiple myeloma. There again was the word myeloma. "What's this multiple myeloma?" I asked Patrick, immediately reaching for my iPad to search.

I was quietly feeling relieved that leukemia wasn't written here. To me this was the worst possible thing it could be. With all this talk of blood, leukemia had been coming up in my mind. That seemed even more serious to me, like it would be the worst diagnosis for Patrick.

Patrick remained quiet and looked over my shoulder as I typed in the search bar multiple myeloma. Many sites appeared on the page. There they were, highlighted in blue.

NZ Cancer information,

What is multiple myeloma? - American Cancer Society

Multiple myeloma - symptoms and causes - Mayo Clinic

Multiple myeloma symptoms, Prognosis, Stages, Treatment & survival rate

What is myeloma? Leukaemia & Blood Cancer NZ

Multiple myeloma - Wikipedia

I quickly scanned down the list looking for what would be the best site and my heart skipped a beat when I saw the word leukemia alongside myeloma. This was the one I immediately clicked on. Why were these two words mentioned in the same line?

It was a link to Leukaemia and Blood Cancer NZ. It read:

Every day 6 children and adults in New Zealand are diagnosed with a blood cancer like leukemia, lymphoma, myeloma or a related blood condition

There are an estimated 21,000 people living with blood cancer or a related condition in NZ

Blood cancers combined (Leukaemia, lymphoma and myeloma) are the fifth most common cause of cancer in NZ

(This is more than likely in other western cultures also)

The cause of blood cancers is unknown

I started to see the relevance as to why multiple myeloma and leukemia are mentioned in the same context. They are both blood disorders although also, it seemed, they are very separate diseases. Due to the fact that, so far, multiple myeloma had been mentioned in earlier searching I clicked on this section on the site to explore that more.

'What is myeloma?'

Myeloma, also known as multiple myeloma or plasma cell myeloma is a cancer of plasma cells (mature B-lymphocytes) that usually arises in the bone marrow.

Myeloma develops when plasma cells undergo a malignant (cancerous) change and become myeloma cells. These myeloma cells multiply without any proper order, forming collections known as tumours that accumulate in different parts of the body, most commonly in the bone marrow and on the surfaces of different bones in the body.

Myeloma cells secrete chemicals that stimulate bone marrow cells to remove calcium from the bone. As a result bones can become weaker, more brittle and break more easily.

Under normal conditions plasma cells produce immunoglobulins (antibodies) that help protect the body from infection and disease. Myeloma cells produce an abnormal type of immunoglobulin called paraprotein. This can be detected in the blood.

Little did I realise at the time, but this was going to be the simplest and best explanation I was going to get of multiple myeloma. Patrick was reading this with me and before I could put much more thought into what I had just read, said "This is where we go to the bottom of this test result darling." and he pointed to the line at the bottom of the result. I went with Patrick's direction and we viewed the last line in the test result.

Paraprotein Quantitation 43 g/L.

Patrick had obviously already researched this but I had to stick to my own process to uncover this, still step by step. I quickly changed the search bar and typed in paraprotein 43 g/L.

The first two sites that showed up didn't make any sense at all. We started scanning the third site, our eyes rolling down words like monoclonal immunoglobulin, light chain, clonal population of mature B cells, most commonly plasma cells, disproportionate proliferation of immunoglobulin-producing cells, secrete a structurally homogeneous immunoglobulin (M-component), abnormal immunoglobulin, monoclonal gammopathy. None of it was making any sense. Just words I didn't know or understand piling up in front of us, until we got to the last line in the first section, and then there it was, MGUS, through asymptomatic to symptomatic myeloma. That word myeloma that had showed up in the earlier result was here again!

As we read on:

MGUS is defined by a low level of paraprotein <30 g/L

MGUS patients are generally in good health and require no therapy, and their overall risk of progression to myeloma is 1% per year

From this, as we read on, we realised a paraprotein reading under 30 was not actually myeloma, it's called smouldering myeloma. This can more often than not never eventuate to myeloma itself and is little cause for concern, but regular observation is needed.

But Patrick's result was 43 g/L so what does that mean?

As we continued down the site, possible conditions were highlighted:

Waldenstrom's macroglobulinemia

Chronic lymphocytic leukemia

Myeloma

Non-hodgkin's lymphoma

POEMS Syndrome

However none of them highlighted paraprotein 43 g/L or discussed paraprotein >30, so we dismissed it all and went back to Google search. We needed to get specific.

"The common word showing up so far is myeloma isn't it Patrick?" I asked hesitantly, looking at him, at his face, searching for a reaction. After 10 years with Patrick I know him so well and, as he took a breath and stalled his response, it was enough to tell me this was where his research had been heading also.

"Lets type in myeloma paraprotein 43 g/L and see what comes up" he replied. I dutifully typed this in the search bar. This would be one of a million times I would put these words into Google search in various different ways in the near future.

So then it began, the endless hours of googling. What is a paraprotein?, monoclonal immunoglobulin?, immunoglobulin light chain?, proliferation of mature B cells?, plasma cells?, B-lymphocytes?, serum globulin concentration?, serum protein electrophoresis?... and on it went.

If the paraprotein is raised what does it mean? - *Symptomatic of possible infection, inflammation, or cancer.*

We couldn't find anywhere what it meant if it was at 43. All we could guess was that if it was < 30 that indicated MGUS, smouldering myeloma, Then if it was >30 could this mean it now was no longer smouldering and is then considered as actual myeloma, or could it possibly still be an infection, or inflammation?? We could find nothing to completely verify that.

Patrick pointed out though, when we were both exhausted from googling and decided to give it up for now, that if we considered these two results alone, both indicated the possibility of myeloma.

"Sorry darling," he said softly, staring directly into my eyes. "It all does turn towards myeloma. I think we have to get our heads around that I may have cancer."

I didn't know what to say. I knew my intuition had told me that earlier too. I had been hoping that this was wrong and that if I was right, maybe it wasn't serious. Cancer of the blood sounded pretty blimmin' serious to me though, hence why I had such a strong intuitive reaction in the car earlier in the day.

We just held each other tight and fell asleep eventually in each other's arms; happy to just be together right now, to be able to hold each other. Yes there was a threat lurking over us, a life threatening cloud forming above us, however, for now we still weren't sure, and this helped us to finally drop into sleep.

Unfortunately it didn't last. We ended up hardly sleeping that night. I had only slept for a couple of hours before waking with a start. I grabbed the IPad and googled some more, not only trying to find more answers to what this all meant, but also trying to find reasons it might not be something serious. About two hours flew by before, exhausted, I again dropped off into some form of sleep. I was still none the wiser. This was to become the norm over the coming nights, we were in for a real ride!

Just while I am here I want to include a result that came through a few days later. The **Bence-Jones** test. Here's the explanation of what that is:

The Bence-Jones protein urine test is used most often to diagnose and check on multiple myeloma, a type of cancer. An abnormal Bence-Jones test result may mean you have a type of malignant lymphoma which are cancers of the lymphatic system. Multiple myeloma is a type of blood cancer which affects plasma cells. These are immune system cells that make antibodies to help fight infections. Most plasma cells live in bone marrow, so multiple myeloma tumors are often found in the bone. Bone marrow is where blood cells are made and multiple myeloma takes up space and leaves less space for normal bone marrow.

Following you will see Patrick's blood result. It showed Patrick was **negative.** How confusing is that, considering all other tests showed positive towards multiple myeloma? This left us very confused. It also left us hopeful that maybe, just maybe, this wasn't as serious as we thought it was.

Date Received: 15/09/2017 6:00:36 p.m
Health Centre:
Clinician Name:
Clinician Comments: 1.7/40.7/<0.2haem

Test Results:

Patient Details

Patient Name: HENSHALL, PATRICK

NHI No:

Date of Birth: 08-Jul-1964

IgG:1.7 g/L (7.0 - 16.0) L

IgA:40.7 g/L (0.8 - 4.0) HH

IgM:< 0.2 g/L (0.4 - 2.5) L

Validated by Dr. Chemical Pathologist

Ordered by:

Laboratory:labtests

Observation date:15-Sep-2017

Ig Test Result

Name: PATRICK HENSHALL
Test: Complete Blood Count
Date Received: 15/09/2017 6:00:10 p.m.
Health Centre:
Clinician Name:
Clinician Comments: 138n

Test Results:

Patient Details

Patient Name: HENSHALL, PATRICK

NHI No:

Date of Birth: 08-Jul-1964

Haemoglobin:138 g/L (130 - 175)

RBC:4.45 x10e12/L (4.30 - 6.00)

HCT:0.41 L/L (0.40 - 0.52)

MCV:91 fL (80 - 99)

MCH:31.0 pg (27.0 - 33.0)

Platelets:226 x10e9/L (150 - 400)

WBC:8.5 x10e9/L (4.0 - 11.0)

Neutrophils:5.62 x10e9/L (1.90 - 7.50)

Lymphocytes:1.78 x10e9/L (1.00 - 4.00)

Monocytes:0.83 x10e9/L (0.20 - 1.00)

Eosinophils:0.17 x10e9/L (< 0.51)

Basophils:0.08 x10e9/L (0.00 - 0.20)

Ordered by:

Laboratory:labtests

Observation date:15-Sep-2017

Complete Blood Count

Name: PATRICK HENSHALL

Test: Protein Electrophoresis

Date Received: 15/09/2017 5:00:21 p.m.

Health Centre:

Clinician Name:

Clinician Comments: refer heamatologist

Test Results:

Patient Details

Patient Name: HENSHALL, PATRICK

NHI No:

Date of Birth: 08-Jul-1964

Total Protein:92 g/L (66 - 84) H

Albumin:34 g/L (32 - 48)

Globulin:58 g/L (25 - 41) H

Protein EPP: The previously reported paraprotein was detected (IgA lambda).

There is marked suppression of uninvolved immunoglobulins (immunoparesis).

Paraprotein Quantitation:43 g/L

Referral to a clinical haematologist is recommended.

Immunoglobulins and Calcium have been added.

The Labtests method for quantitation of paraproteins in the beta region changed on 12th June 2017 to align all regional laboratories, in consultation with haematologists. Please feel free to call and discuss with the on-call chemical pathologist.

Ordered by:

Laboratory:labtests

Observation date:15-Sep-2017

Protein Electrophoresis

Test Results:

Patient Details

Patient Name: HENSHALL, PATRICK

NHI No:

Date of Birth: 08-Jul-1964

Protein urine:0.15 g/L

Creatinine urine:9.0 mmol/L

Bence Jones: No monoclonal bands detected on urine immunofixation.

Protein/Creatinine ratio:17 mg/mmol (< 23)

Validated by Scientist.

Ordered by:

Laboratory:labtests

Observation date:20-Sep-2017

Bence-Jones Test

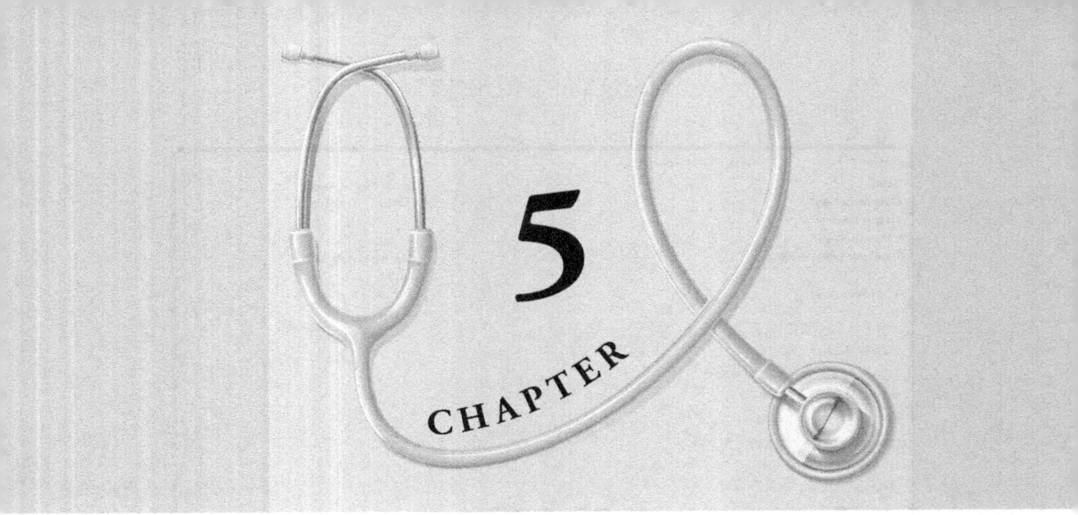

Missed Diagnosis

"Cancer is a word,
not a sentence."
- John Diamond -

Last week of September - 2017 - Dr X[1]

I was so over trying to work out what all these blood results meant. The hours spent over the past few days pouring through Google searches, was getting exhausting. It was all so incredibly scary reading the possible prognosis and still being hopeful none of it was real.

On Monday morning I woke and insisted we go and see Patrick's GP again. His GP had already sent his results to the Specialist Department of Haematology at North Shore Hospital and requested an urgent assessment. Very quickly they had come back requesting to see Patrick.

That should have been enough warning to us, but at the time we didn't know you only get that appointment so quickly if there

---

1 Name has been changed to protect the identity of the individual.

is a real problem. The specialist appointment however was not for another nine days and I just couldn't wait that long. The sleepless nights and uncertainty was horrid.

We called the surgery to book in to see Patrick's GP but unfortunately he was away so we booked an appointment with another doctor. Any doctor would do thanks, just to try and get these questions answered. What does it look like Patrick has?! We made a booking for the next day to see Dr X. We let go of googling over the next 24 hours which was a nice reprieve. I was looking forward though, with of course trepidation, to the appointment.

Well what a lovely surprise it was to see Dr X. We presented all the blood results to him and he took some time going through them. He almost laughed at our concern and said he didn't see anything alarming here. These were the same blood results that Patrick's GP had forwarded to the haematologist, and the same results I mentioned earlier. He suggested that the haematologist would probably just advise Patrick to keep an eye on his bloods, in fact he implied that Patrick's GP was being over cautious and that we were silly worrying so much.

He commented that Patrick's white and red blood counts were good. The fact that his red blood count was down a little was nothing alarming so because of those results he could see nothing serious was wrong. If there was anything serious these results would be a lot worse. He joked that Patrick needn't worry, he would live to get his pension. He said that rheumatoid arthritis (one of the milder possibilities of what it could be) would be serious compared to anything Patrick had to worry about.

I can still see it now. I walked out of there feeling so much better and as we neared the car I put my arm around Patrick and with a sigh of relief said "Thank God we have nothing to worry about!" Patrick responded with a wry smile and said "sorry darlin' but I'm not convinced. That paraprotein level is a worry but I'm glad his comments have made you feel better for now, we can relax until the appointment next week." I don't have a great memory, but I will not forget this snap in time. The doctors' comments really did help and I was back to sleeping again, with Patrick and I just having the occasional google; mostly I decided to wait now.

Finally Tuesday arrived, 3 October 2017 - 9.00am. Patrick and I arrived at the hospital for his specialist appointment to see Dr Ross Henderson, a week after we had seen Dr X.

We had already researched Dr Henderson and knew he was the Clinical Director for the Haematology Department at the North Shore Hospital and was one of the best in his field in New Zealand. Patrick and I both felt very blessed we were seeing a top specialist and this was all provided through New Zealand's public health system. We didn't have to wait long before we were sitting in Dr Henderson's office. A very tall and confident man, he had welcomed us warmly.

Once we had sat down he pulled Patrick's results up on his computer. He took some time to read them all before he spoke and first asked how Patrick was. By now Patrick's chest and bronchitis were a lot better and it had all pretty much cleared up. He asked if Patrick had any other problems, which was a definite 'no', other than being probably more tired than perhaps he should be. This had been an ongoing problem we had noticed in Patrick over the last year, that he didn't seem to have the same energy.

After Patrick spoke Dr Henderson continued scanning his results then he started speaking out loud confirming some of the test results. It was the next moment that rocked our world, our core, our lives, our existence, pretty much forever, when he said, "Well I'm sorry to say that looking at your bloods, there are strong indicators that tell me you most certainly have multiple myeloma." Wow, what, back it up, what!! We both sat there stunned.

"I'm sorry," he said, "this is obviously not good news I'm giving you today. It's uncommon for someone your age to get multiple myeloma as it usually presents in people over 60, more commonly even around 70." Patrick is 53. We knew this age association with myeloma already from googling and it was something we had been clinging to that could mean Patrick didn't have it.

He went on to explain a little about multiple myeloma; that it develops from the cells in the bone marrow called plasma cells and that it can be anywhere there is bone marrow, basically wherever we have bones. As it can occur in several places of the body it is called multiple myeloma. That was a bit of a blur for me. I had read up on it but wasn't really paying attention. I was still stuck in the diagnosis and how odd it was for Patrick to get this, given his age, and so shocked this was positive considering what the doctor had said the other day.

I tuned in as Dr Henderson continued, he was saying that this was also not a common form of cancer. He turned to Patrick. "Tell me," he asked "have you been around chemicals at some stage in your life?" Patrick calmly replied, "Well yes, I worked for a petroleum company for 10 years from around 1988-1998 but I'm not sure what my exposure would have been through that time. At times, I used to go into paint factories and also would inspect chemical tanks occasionally. That would have been only about a dozen times though. I also would visit BP production factories, where they made all their chemicals, once every couple of months." Patrick let that sink in, then continued, "I also worked for De Witt and Company, global petrochemical consultants, from 1998-2000 then I joined Methanex in 2000 to mid 2001."

I'll just stop here and tell you a little about Methanex. Methanex produces methanol and they were the global number one user of methanol in Patrick's time there. Methanol is a chemical product that goes into making things like acetic acid, formaldehyde etc, which in turn is then applied into products for paint, glue, inks, dyes, wood preservation products. It's a carcinogen that has been classified by the Food and Drug Administration of the US as a cancer causing substance. It is an odorless compound that if you are exposed to it, even a minute amount, it causes death.

Interesting story: Apparently in the old days, before Patrick's time, chemical companies using methanol used to have live birds in their factories to monitor any methanol leaks. If the birds stopped tweeting, they were about to die. It was a sign that there was a leak and everyone was to evacuate immediately. Really, I don't know if this is fact, to be honest it seems too incredulous to be, but that's what I've been told. Nowadays they put a product into the methanol that has an odor to warn of exposure which gives the alarm for people to evacuate. I'm sure the birds are very thankful for that!

In saying this right now, Patrick, who has a Bachelor of Science majoring in Chemistry and Maths, says you can't really single out just methanol as all chemicals have a certain degree of risks. (One of the reasons I use only plant based cleaning products etc now.)

Patrick went on telling the specialist "As a sales person I frequently went to the factory to check on products where I would occasionally tour the factory, and in some areas the smells were very strong. Although methanol is virtually odorless, it was being combined with benzine and other related compounds to produce the paints, glue, dyes, inks, wood preservation products etc." Patrick paused again letting that sink in. Then asked "Do you think this could be a cause?"

Dr Henderson gave the response you would expect, I mean how would he really know? It's impossible. But a very reasonable question was hanging there. He replied "That's very interesting. Of course it's very hard to know however there have been studies that have shown chemical exposure as a possible cause for multiple myeloma."

That's it, it was left there. What else could be said? It was unknown although it was another shock to the system. Gosh, could Patrick have exposed himself enough to get cancer? My mind went to Patrick's dear magician friend Wayne Rogers, "The amazing Chicane". Wayne had lung cancer that appeared to have originated from asbestos. He never understood where he picked this up from. Quite unbelievable how even though asbestos building materials were banned from being produced in New Zealand from 1987, the damage of it was showing up some 30 years later.

Though really this was going on in the back of my mind at the time. Shock upon shock of words being said that I was trying to absorb. I couldn't speak as my brain struggled to get to grips with it all. Patrick, still so calm and collected asked, "Can you tell what stage it is at?"

We had both googled enough by now to have at least a little understanding of the different possibilities of what his results could have meant. We also had googled myeloma and suitable treatments. So although we were shocked we were not complete novices and had a few pertinent questions at the ready. Luckily Patrick was calm at the time and could think of them.

Dr Henderson went back to his computer and scanned the results again. Patrick took this opportunity to pull out some blood results from an earlier Doctor he had seen back in September 2013. These showed his paraprotein at <1.0g/L. He handed them to Dr Henderson saying, "It appears the paraprotein level started going up in September 2013, if that helps."

Patrick had taken it upon himself over the last week to go back through all his blood results from the last few years to see if there was a clue anywhere on a lead up to what might be wrong with him. He fell upon a set of bloods taken by a holistic doctor, Dr Z[2], in 2013. Right there was a blood test taken showing:

Paraprotein Quantification <1.0g/L, with the comment: The monoclonal protein is modest in size and may be a monoclonal gammopathy of undetermined significance (MGUS). Suggest follow up four monthly in the first year (clinical review, serum electrophoresis, Immunoglobulins, blood count, calcium and creatinine). If stable, annual follow up is recommended.

---

2 Name has been changed to protect the identity of the individual.

At the time Patrick hadn't even googled it as it didn't seem serious and the doctor hadn't mentioned it. The focus was on the fact that the glandular fever blood test, taken also at the same time, had shown positive. A few months later the doctor moved overseas. No one from the practice had followed up since then but we now knew that was MGUS right there. Smouldering myeloma. We also now knew this should have had a close watch on it with constant blood tests taken and it hadn't, Dr Z had totally ignored it!

Dr Henderson took this from Patrick, looked at the results, and then went back to his own computer. It seemed like ages before he spoke again, but of course it probably wasn't. In that short time we pretty much held our breath. How bad is this? What does this mean? All the horror stories you hear of people getting diagnosed who are too late for treatment. Who are at stage IV and there is little they can do. The fear was palpable in the room.

It was with a little, just a teeny weeny little bit of relief when Dr Henderson finally said "Looking at your results I would say you are probably in Stage 1, but it's too early to confirm without further tests at this point." I looked at Patrick. By now we were holding hands, tight as! Well that's not so bad, I thought... though I still hadn't spoken.

Dr Henderson then went on to say, "Though looking at where your paraprotein was at in 2013 it seems to have progressed very fast which means we should really get on to treatment very soon." (So if Patrick had received the regular blood checks he was supposed to, with its fast progression this would have shown up for action a lot earlier) "How soon?" asked Patrick.

Dr Henderson replied "Within the next two to three months, probably within two months would be good. You see," he continued, "your blood results showing your paraprotein at <1.0gl is what we call smouldering multiple myeloma. The reading can go up to <30 over time and we just keep an eye on it up to that stage. It is not until it goes over 30 that we would consider treatment however this usually takes quite some years, if at all. For most people it stays smouldering for the rest of their lives and they don't require treatment however you have increased to <42 in what we consider a short time period being four years. It's better we start treatment as soon as possible."

The next obvious question, again asked by Patrick, "So what are we talking? What sort of treatment will I need?"

So here it all started. Dr Henderson started rattling it all off. "We recommend for multiple myeloma that you have what we call induction therapy, which is five months of chemotherapy, then a stem cell transplant, and then further chemotherapy for another four months. Basically you are looking at about 14 month's worth of treatment."

Amongst all that he rattled off names of drugs etc, but none of that sank in, it was a whole new language. That part was gobbledygook to me so I chose to pick out the important things I needed to hear right now and concentrate on them. I was still floored. I still hadn't spoken. Not like me at all.

The Specialist went on to say "Unfortunately there is no cure for multiple myeloma however they are coming out with new treatments all the time that are having great success in helping people live longer. There is a lot of research going on around it and we are finding people are living for longer and longer with the new treatments, so it's hopeful for the future."

It was pretty hard to think straight right now I must say. Patrick was amazing. He seemed to be keeping up, I was stuck on cancer. Chemotherapy. No cure. The rest really didn't register.

Chemotherapy, chemotherapy, chemotherapy. Oh my God, the initial message I received coming out of my office that day, when Patrick called two weeks ago about needing to take more blood tests, that booming 'he's got cancer' was right after all. Oh my God, oh my God. I was once again frozen in shock.

Dr Henderson continued saying "some people with multiple myeloma are living seven plus years now, some reaching ten years or longer, and we expect that to increase as time goes on with new treatments coming out. But unfortunately it's not good news for you today, I'm sorry." Patrick got up. As the Specialist looked up at him he said he needed to go to the toilet. He seemed to be so calm and accepting, I still hadn't spoken.

When Patrick left the room Dr Henderson turned to me. He was so kind as he said to me "I'm sorry to give you this news, it's obviously a big shock. Are you alright?" I finally spoke. "Well," I said, "it is a big shock". I had to choke back tears as I went on. "When we first got the results we were very worried, but we visited a doctor last week to get an opinion of the blood results, and he didn't seem to think there was anything to worry about so I'm staggered to hear this now."

Dr Henderson stopped in his tracks for a brief second, pausing, then looked to his computer, then back at me. "No sorry, this definitely is multiple myeloma. The combination of results that I see in front of me indicate that."

These are the exact same results that Dr X was looking at last week.

Wow! On finally speaking, it seemed to have kicked my mind into action. I recalled all that I had read on cancers and my first thought was that Patrick needed to get the best of treatments and the best of treatments I'd read came through getting on the latest trial programs. So I finally said something useful. "What about Patrick getting on a trial program for his treatment?"

I think Dr Henderson was surprised I had come out with this. My silence may have been interpreted as ignorance very easily. "Yes, yes", he said. "Patrick could well be eligible for a trial program." Just at that point Patrick came back into the room and he continued to both of us. "There is a trial program we are running at the moment called the 'Kiwi Trial'. We can take some further tests to see if you are eligible, but looking at your blood results and seeing you in person, so far I think you would be. It does however involve you having three forms of therapy at once, as opposed to just two, using an extra chemotherapy drug called Carfilzomib. A patient of mine calls it a car full of zombies, he smiled, to try and lighten the mood a little. It worked and we managed a slight laugh. This drug is proving to have good results overseas where it has been used for a number of years now so yes, we can definitely look at getting you on that trial program if you want to. It does mean you have to come in twice a week for chemotherapy instead of just once a week though. It consists of coming in two days a week for chemo, one day after the other, then a week's break after three weeks. Then repeating that same cycle each month.

I jumped in "That's no problem, Patrick works for himself so he can get the time off to do that." I wanted nothing to get in the way of his receiving the best treatment. Little did I think at the time of the effect it would have on him having the drugs in his system twice a week rather than just the once. In fact I didn't consider any of the consequences, I just wanted him to get the best possible treatment. Dr Henderson turned to Patrick. "What do you think Patrick?"

Patrick too of course had read enough to know that getting on a trial program would be his best possible option. Amazingly he was still so calm as he replied so nicely, "Yes, I'd be very grateful to get on the trial program if that's possible." Really at this point there were only two things going on in both of our heads. You have cancer. You need the best treatment. Nothing else really entered our minds. At that stage it was black and white.

"OK then," continued Dr Henderson, "the first thing we need to do is send you off for a few more detailed tests to further assess the extent of the multiple myeloma and how this has affected your body. I had a wee panic here and blurted out, "So is there a possibility the tests may show something up that would mean Patrick can't go on the trial program?"

Dr Henderson was back at his computer by then tapping away, putting in requests of tests to be done. He turned to me for a moment, then went back to his screen and did some scrolling. He then turned back to me and said, "Looking at what I see here I see no reason why Patrick won't qualify. He's young, relatively, by multiple myeloma standards, and appears in good health otherwise. I feel quite confident he will get in ok but cannot confirm that, sorry, until the results are all in."

We were silent while he finished his typing. He turned and spoke to us both when it was complete. "Dr David Simpson is in charge of the Kiwi Trial and he is a colleague of mine. I will be putting you forward as a candidate and will also speak to him personally. Try not to worry. Unless something major comes up, which it doesn't appear at this stage that it will, I will be highly recommending you for the trial."

I now was the first to speak. "That's so great to hear Ross." Already I felt on first name terms with this man who was offering the best possible opportunity to help Patrick. "Thank you so much. It means a lot to us to know Patrick will be having the best treatment possible. We are so very appreciative of the opportunity." Oops here come the tears. I let them flow. Silently.

Dr Henderson picked it up from there, bringing our meeting to a close saying "OK let's get all the tests done. I have booked you in to come back on Monday 9 October for your tests. I'll see you again once we have the results."

We walked out with Patrick holding a bunch of material on multiple myeloma from the Leukaemia and Blood Cancer NZ in one hand, and the other hand once again gripping onto mine. Once we were clear of the office, walking down the hospital corridor to the lift, I heaved out a big sigh.

Bless Patrick. He put his arm around me and apologised! "I'm sorry darling," he said. "I know you were hoping this wouldn't be such bad news. This is a big shock for you, and I am sorry we now have to go through this." Right there. How sweet and caring is that. "Me!" I exclaimed. "Patrick it's you that will be going through this.

Darling I'm so sorry for you. Gosh I can't believe how calm you are, how calm you were in the meeting."

We had arrived at the lift and were waiting for it to get to our floor. Patrick gave me a tight squeeze around my shoulders as he replied "Darling to be honest, I knew it was going to be bad news, I've known since I got the paraprotein results. There is no way the paraprotein could have been at that level and it not be serious." "Then that doctor last week should have known too." I blurted. starting to feel angry.

"Yes, said Patrick. "I told you I wasn't convinced at the time, but felt it was best to leave you feeling hopeful. At least it stopped you worrying for a time." So here was me finally getting some sleep this past week, not discussing or googling any further thinking all is probably well, and poor Patrick had been carrying this load on his own.

The lift arrived, we went to the ground floor and left the hospital. The car park is only a short distance away so we paid for our parking at the machine and walked to the car pretty much in silence. We were both obviously still trying to absorb it all and I cried quietly most of the way home. Patrick drove one handed, his right hand on the wheel and his left hand holding mine all the way home, giving us both a modicum of comfort. We arrived home pretty much dumb founded. Thankfully the house was empty as Katelyn was at school so we had the day to get ourselves together, I thought, although I had no idea really what that meant or what that would look like.

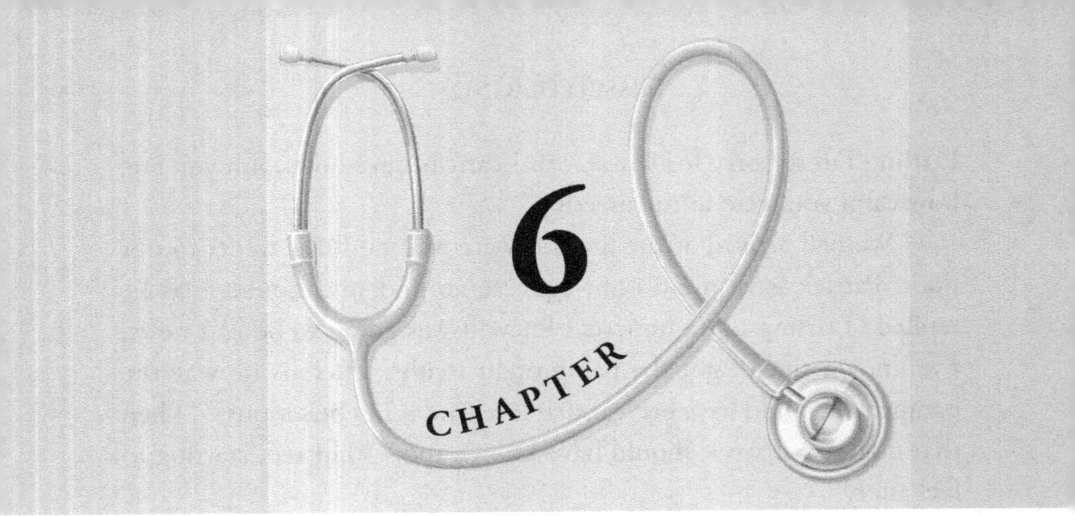

Diagnosed With Multiple Myeloma

"What lies behind us and what lies
ahead of us are tiny matters
compared to what lives within us."
- Henry David Thoreau -

I made a cup of tea and we cuddled up on the couch together. We talked about the fact Patrick was now diagnosed with multiple myeloma. After everything that doctor had said last week, that Patrick's blood results showed nothing serious, yet here we were. I didn't want to harp on about it, now wasn't the time, but gosh I was angry. As I said to Patrick, wow, he actually misdiagnosed you!

We were so rocked by the confirmed diagnosis of multiple myeloma though right now and were feeling so very thankful that Patrick's actual GP, had picked up on Patrick's blood results showing something unusual in the first place and continuously followed through.

We started reflecting together on the past few weeks. We went back to that Friday night when his GP had rung to ask Patrick to go and do more blood tests on the Saturday. We had just thought he was busy and only just now had time to call. I recall how I'd thought he was a great GP to be so conscientious working late, catching up. Looking back I find it hard to see how I hadn't seen the warning signs then.

We talked about how fortunate it was that Patrick had his chest infection in the first place. Goodness, if it weren't for that he would never have seen his GP. Then, more fortunate, that he had such a good GP. It was only because Patrick was so ill by the time he got to the doctors with coughing, chest pain, and the pain he felt in the bone around his chest area, that his GP must have noticed warning signs to do a couple of extra tests just in case.

We also talked about the tests Patrick had coming up: blood tests, ECG, MRI and a bone marrow test. The bone marrow test was the scariest. It sounded pretty awful. I had googled it recently and it involved screwing into your bone to get bone marrow while you are still conscious, albeit slightly anaesthetised. Patrick had a couple of friends who had done it in the past so he decided he would ring them in the next few days to find out how it was all to be done. Honestly, I was staggered how lucky we were that all of this medical help was available for Patrick so quickly, and at no cost! Gotta love New Zealand!❤

We were thankful too that we had done so much googling and weren't totally caught by surprise. That we at least had our head around what multiple myeloma was, what the typical treatments were for it, and in that knowledge, chemotherapy was no surprise. As much as it was a shock, we were prepared. Funny. Here we were with this horrid diagnosis and we were sitting there being thankful. It's a funny thing being fearful, it creates so much worry and anxiety for us when it presents with the unknown. Once we know, the fear seems to dissipate so quickly, and now that we knew what we were dealing with, a whole new host of emotions were rising.

We decided that now wasn't the time to tell the children or family. Patrick thought we should know everything first, including what the next lot of tests show up, and whether we are on the trial program so they can have the full picture instead of worrying. That meant friends too. I came clean and told Patrick that I'd already told my girlfriend Helen. I told him about the day I got that blaring message that it was cancer and asked if I could just keep confiding in her so I had at least someone to talk to. He was OK with that. A girl's gotta share, right? Patrick seemed quite happy keeping it between just him and me. Men are from Mars, women from Venus!

And then we did what we thought we were pretty good at, googling. We spent the afternoon, and in fact any spare time, over the next week googling the crap out of multiple myeloma, life expectancy, remissions, secondary cancer, chemotherapy, studies done on what drugs have had good success, the latest successful trial programs around the world, stem cell harvesting, stem cell transplants, and pretty much started learning another new language surrounding specifically the treatment for multiple myeloma.

I started waking in the night again. I'd get online, lying there in the dark with further questions, rechecking something I'd learnt earlier, often googling the same thing again and again, and reading the same sites, reports, and trials (which can be quite lengthy) until I was spent on it all.

By Friday 6 October 2017, three days after we had seen the specialist, I decided to do something about one thing that was really bothering me - Dr X's misdiagnosis. I had woken in the night often, bothered by this misrepresentation. I kept feeling his attitude towards us in his surgery, like we were being over reactive. I'd see him almost chuckle as he told Patrick not to worry, he'd get his pension. The specialist Dr Ross Henderson had said multiple myeloma patients can survive seven years, and sometimes up to ten years now. Patrick was 53. 53 + 10 = 63. You get the pension in NZ at 65. Even with the best odds, it didn't look promising at all that Patrick would live to get his pension.

I decided to write to him to let him know the outcome, mainly to create awareness that he needs 'to brush up on his assessing of blood results' (as I put it), 'as this could be very detrimental to future patients.' I didn't have his personal email address so I addressed it to the clinic to be forwarded to him. I received a letter very soon after I sent the email, from the doctors' practice, advising me that the clinical leadership team had taken this up for investigation.

Unbeknownst to me at the time, any complaints addressed to the practice were sent not only to the doctor but to a clinical leadership team and they are then opened as an investigation. They then contact the Doctor involved to respond to them directly, rather than to the patient. Pretty much the leadership team picks up the complaint and deals with it. Apparently once the Doctor responded it would be discussed with the clinical leadership team where learning outcomes will be acknowledged and any necessary new practice policies implemented.

I felt pretty pleased with that actually. Although it had not been my intention to have Doctor X 'investigated', I was pleased my complaint had been taken seriously, and it seemed appropriate steps would be taken. It's amazing how much of a load drops off when you don't have to hold on to injustice. They asked me if I wanted to be informed of the outcome of the discussions but I declined. I told them I had enough on my plate to deal with ahead of me, but that I was grateful that I had not been ignored and that my letter was getting heard and appropriate action would be taken.

Interestingly, when quietly enquiring some months later, it appeared Dr X didn't practice at that surgery any more. We didn't ask, we didn't want to know. We trusted the correct course of action had taken place and whatever the consequences, it was OK by us.

We had let it go, we had bigger fish to fry. Just such an important learning though huh?

Dr X screwed up, and so it seems did Dr Z. They both missed fundamentally life threatening results. Thank goodness Patrick's GP had picked up on what the blood results were indicating, investigated further, and had referred Patrick to the specialist. We will always be forever grateful to him.

An important note though. We think we can rely on doctors like their word is gospel or God. We often don't second guess or question them or what they say. So many people go blindly through the system not even knowing how to assess their blood test results, not even knowing what they mean, let alone be able to question them. My advice…get informed! Check everything yourself. Everyone knows someone who at least knows someone who has been misdiagnosed at some stage in their lives, whether it is for minor or major things.

Doctors are human, they can make mistakes. Get second opinions and if you feel your Doctor doesn't care enough, isn't checking enough, whatever, change your doctor. Loyalty to one doctor all your life is the old way. It's just like we used to be loyal to the same bank and not switch due to the benefits you would receive being a good local customer. Now we shop around for the best option for us based on what we need now and don't think twice about it. Your health is paramount. Don't leave it in someone else's hands. Take charge. You are the only person who truly cares about yourself and the only person who suffers the consequences.

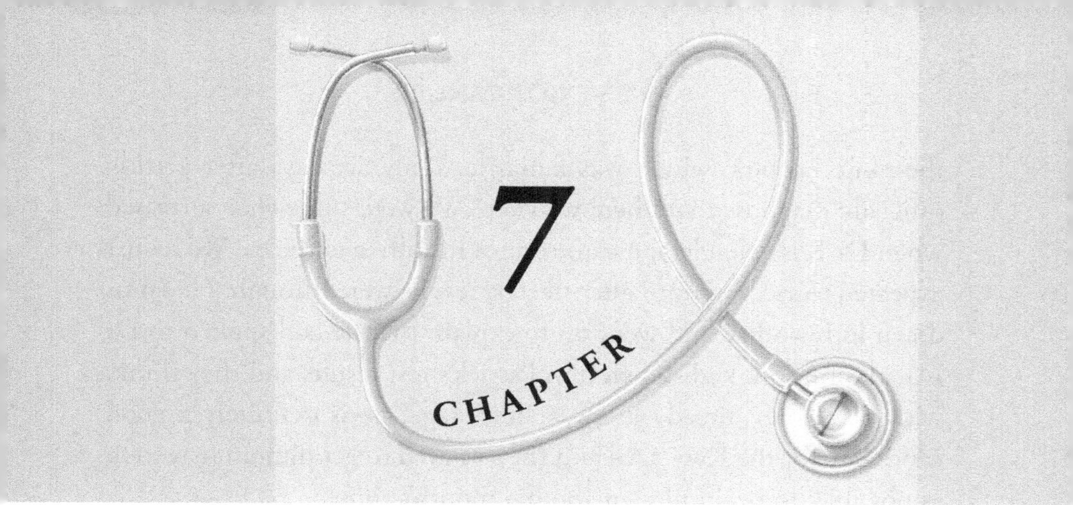

Kiwi Trial program – Bone Marrow Test

"If you only say one
Prayer in a day, make it
'Thank You'."
- Rumi -

By the time Patrick went in for his tests on Monday 9 October 2017 we were feeling reasonably informed. Our time on Google was paying off! We felt very confident and happy that if Patrick could get on the Kiwi Trial he would be receiving the best treatment possible, right here in little old NZ! We were pretty exhausted. We were only getting about five hours of sleep at night and I guess we were in a heightened state of awareness; on alert. It was good to finally start our visits to the hospital for tests, to be doing something productive… and we felt prepared.

We had been told to go to the main haematology office for the first lot of tests. They were all getting done on the same day at the same hospital which was fantastic. Only six days after getting officially diagnosed and here we were. We were somewhat surprised when Dr Ross Henderson came out of his office to see us. We hadn't expected to see him until after the test results were through. He sat us down in his office and went on to explain that he had spoken to Dr David Simpson, had shown him Patrick's test results and they think, with what they already know at this stage, he is definitely a good candidate for the Kiwi Trial and they wanted to get him on it as soon as possible; to begin now in about a month's time!

He then went on to explain that the tests Patrick was about to do today were through the general North Shore Hospital system however once Patrick signed up to the Kiwi Trial he would need to do the tests all over again. The trial insists on doing its own tests under its own supervision and analysis etc. They were concerned particularly about the bone marrow test Patrick was to do today. They didn't feel it very fair on Patrick to have to do two bone marrow tests unnecessarily in one month therefore wondered how Patrick would feel about signing up for the Kiwi Trial today, like right now, and then his tests can be done under the Kiwi Trial program today, meaning he won't need to do them twice. Dr Henderson went on to say he and Dr Simpson both agreed it would be highly unlikely Patrick wouldn't qualify for the Kiwi Trial after the tests, so they decided to go ahead and sign him up now, if he was willing.

Are you kidding? Hell yes!! Wow this was amazing. I was buzzing... so was Patrick; obviously he agreed. Within minutes the room was filled with people we were being introduced to, all were staff of the Kiwi Trial. It was quite incredible and we felt like royalty. One nurse had the forms Patrick needed to sign to be a part of the program. Patrick read them carefully while Dr Henderson was giving instruction to the others in the room as to what needed to take place. Patrick signed the forms and dated them; Dr Henderson also signed them and then we were whisked away. It all happened so fast it was amazing. One nurse took us first for blood tests; she apparently was one of the head nurses for the trial programs, however not specifically for the Kiwi Trial. She had been called in to help out with this unexpected sign up today.

After the blood tests she took us to the ECG department of the hospital and left us for Patrick to have the ECG.

We were then picked up by the same nurse again and taken for an MRI. Another nurse picked us up from there and took us for the bone marrow test which was to be taken in the chemotherapy ward.

As we entered the nurse pointed out that this was where Patrick's weekly chemotherapy would take place. We stood at reception waiting and I was quite shocked. It consisted of a row of chairs - lazyboys, all sitting against a wall facing out into the room. There must have been about a dozen of them, maybe more and around each chair was all the medical paraphernalia; stands for drip lines, blood pressure gear, etc. A curtain rail surrounded each section to be pulled if required. None of the curtains were pulled however, and the chairs were full of people sitting there just staring out into the room, sitting through their treatments, most with drip lines attached; the ward was very quiet.

It seemed so exposed and morbid, I thought it was awful and insensitive to have no privacy from each other, and those coming and going. Tears started to well as I stood there picturing poor Patrick being subjected to this environment in the very near future - mental note to make sure he didn't come on his own. Pretty much a vow formed right there that I would make sure he wasn't left to feel alone and scared in this environment which was the way I felt right now seeing it for the first time. I didn't have long to linger on this however as we were shortly whisked away to the one private room they had on the ward which is where the bone marrow tests were done.

A bone marrow test is done to investigate or confirm the cause for an abnormal blood count. It assesses the extent of the saturation of cancer, and also assesses the involvement of lymphoma or other types of blood cancers.

We had been informed that while they were doing the bone marrow test they were also going to do a FISH test on Patrick. A FISH test 'maps' the genetic material in a person's cells. It can be used to visualize specific genes or portions of genes and we knew from our googling that this was quite common to do in the initial stages of diagnosis. It was done through the same process as a bone marrow test, so basically, while they are at it, they take an extra sample.

To be honest I really hadn't gotten my head around what a FISH test was. It was a bit too complicated and too much to absorb when there was already so much going on. I just knew it needed to be done and was going with it.

A doctor and two nurses greeted us in the room. The doctor introduced herself and went on to explain how she was very used to doing bone marrow tests, and that Patrick was in safe hands. She was really lovely, and kind to me also. They all were and we immediately felt quite relaxed.

As they were prepping the instruments for the bone marrow test she started to explain the procedure that they were about to do. She explained where she was taking the sample from, which was around the back, the top right of Patrick's hip joint, and that they were going to inject a local anaesthetic into the area. She pointed out the nitrous oxide gas (laughing gas) on supply also, that Patrick was to use during the procedure.

Patrick interrupted her at this point. By now Patrick had spoken to one of his friends who had had a number of bone marrow tests. He told him that the first one he'd had was so painful and he highly recommended that Patrick also ask for Midazolam to help with the pain during the procedure. He had said that once he had that for his second and consequent bone marrow tests it was a breeze. A good tip right!

"I'd also like to have Midazolam as well if that's OK?" Patrick piped in.

"Oh yes, of course." replied the doctor. "We can do that for you." and one of the nurses left to get this for him. Whew, it was no problem. We had our minds at ease since Patrick spoke to his friend on what to do, but it was still a relief seeing this would be OK, no problem at all. The doctor turned to me and warned me with a laugh, "Midazolam is like a truth serum. Pay attention when Patrick takes it, he might let out a few secrets. It also makes them forget what has happened and what was said throughout the procedure." I looked forward to seeing what would take place however Patrick was so high on the laughing gas through the procedure he pretty much just cracked silly jokes or dozed on and off to sleep.

I sat close to him through most of it, holding his hand, I think more for my own security than his. I talked to him, trying to distract him a little, and kept a light banter going, stopping only when he would doze a little. It's quite incredible how they do this bone marrow test, it seems quite antiquated really. They make a small incision and actually do use a hollow needle that looks like a thin screw that they screw down manually into the bone, and it's quite hard work for the doctor doing it. Patrick winced a few times as they screwed through the bone, but with the combination of drugs he seemed OK.

Then, once they know they are through the bone and into the actual marrow, they use a syringe and withdraw a sample of it which is then put in a container and sent off for analysis; we were only in the room for about half an hour. A bandage is put on the area and no stitches are required. You can't shower for a day or so and that's it. We had to sit around outside for some time for all the drugs to wear out of Patrick's system, to be sure he was OK, before being allowed to go home. It was our last test of the day and we were going home straight after.

Patrick was tender after the bone marrow test for a couple of days and didn't sit or lie on that side for a while. Otherwise though, he was fine. Thanks to his friend's advice it was so much easier than we thought it might have been. That afternoon we left the hospital quite exhausted from it all, but also exhilarated that Patrick was signed up on the Kiwi Trial!

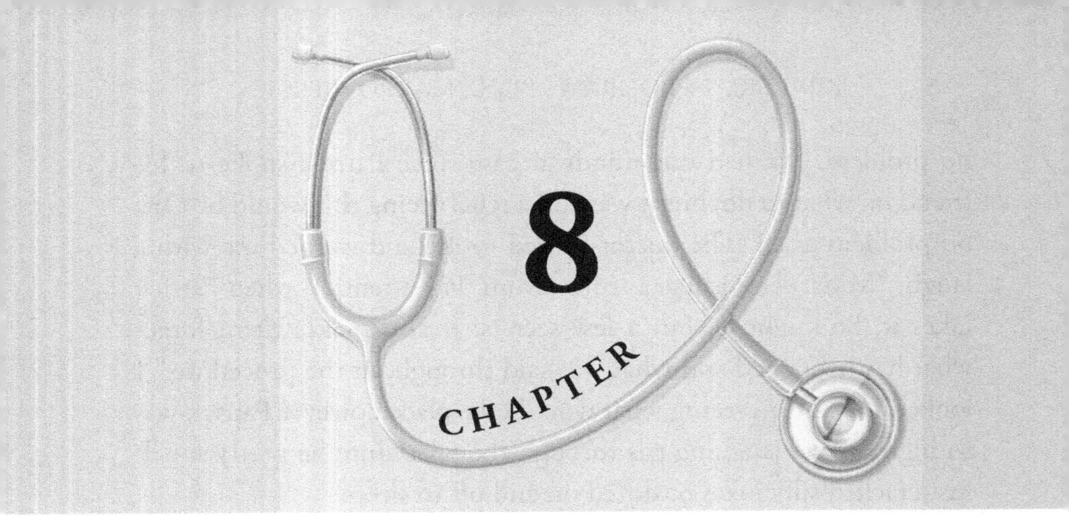

Stage 2 Multiple Myeloma

"Life shrinks or expands in
proportion to one's courage"
- Anaïs Nin -

So now we were waiting. Waiting for the results of the tests and waiting to find out when the Kiwi Trial was going to start exactly.

We didn't have to wait long. We were called back to see Dr Henderson within a few days but unfortunately he didn't have good news for us. He was again looking at the computer after all the formalities and we had sat down. He was scanning Patrick's results then turned to him and said "Looking at all your results we now have a much fuller picture of what is going on. Your bone marrow test shows 80-90% plasma cell burden (that means 80-90% of Patrick's blood was saturated with cancer!) and unfortunately," he continued, "it means you are actually in Stage 2, not Stage 1, as it initially appeared. The good news is that none of your organs have been damaged. At your stage you could have well expected some vital organ damage, but surprisingly you are relatively healthy considering your saturation."

Oh shoot! That stopped us short. We hadn't been googling Stage 2. What did this mean?

"How will this affect Patrick getting on the Kiwi Trial program then?" I quickly asked. The right treatment for him was at the forefront of my mind.

"Well," Dr Henderson replied "actually to be honest, I know this doesn't sound great, but with the type of treatment we use for multiple myeloma the saturation quantity isn't really too important. The chemotherapy blasts the cells very well and the majority of cancerous cells get killed off quite quickly. It's the last percentage that is the hardest to budge so it doesn't affect you getting on the program at all. We can still proceed with that." That was a relief. My main question of the day had been answered! I blurted out, probably too quickly and loudly, "Brilliant! Thanks Ross very much, we so appreciate this opportunity."

Patrick had been a little quiet. Dr Henderson turned to him and carried on. "It does however mean that we really do need to get into starting the treatments as soon as possible. He let that sink in for a moment. Patrick then piped up, "How soon?"

This had obviously already been decided between Dr Henderson and Dr Simpson, the Kiwi Trial specialist. Dr Henderson promptly responded " We would like you to start in two weeks."

Wow. What could we say? Hang on a minute, we're not ready for that. We'd planned for it being at least a month away. Or - how can you expect us to sort our lives out in just two weeks to start treatment? Or - hey wait on, there's too much to do to be ready by then. Or - shoot, we need a breather to catch up on ourselves with all of this before starting treatment. All of that of course was true.

But what did we say? Patrick and I, both almost in unison "OK." That was it. Nothing else. It was all we could say. All we really should say. All we wanted to say at the end of the day.

Patrick was in Stage 2. Patrick had 80-90% saturation of cancer in his body. Patrick needed treatment now! There was no problem today for either of us having any of this sink in, we knew this was serious. We knew we needed to act now. And we were thankful. So grateful and thankful. Patrick had no medical insurance so this was the public health system at its best coming through for him with the best treatments available in the country, in fact in the world. We weren't going to argue. We weren't going to complain. We would do exactly as we were told on the advice of the experts and start treatment whenever they said. If they had asked Patrick to do a handstand right there and then he would have done that too… and so would I.

Dr Henderson again ran through the planned chemotherapy course. The possible side effects were discussed at length and how they would be managed. This time I was taking it all in. I'd done my research so the words were now familiar. I was over the shock of 'cancer' and was now ready to hear it all. It was really good to learn that the chemotherapy Patrick would be taking was quite well tolerated. It didn't induce vomiting for starters which I was so relieved about. I really had been dreading him going through that, as I had seen a dear friend of mine go through it some 15 years earlier.

I brought up how relieved I was. Dr Henderson said people were starting to reject having chemotherapy because of those types of side effects being too hard to tolerate hence they had to get that perfected better so it is more easily tolerated. He talked about peripheral neuropathy being a potential problem, in which case they adjust the doses if they need to, to help cope with that. Peripheral neuropathy is nerve damage which can happen mainly in the hands, fingers and feet. It can appear in many different ways; tingling or numbness, pain on touching things, feelings of cold, or burning, making you lose balance or coordination. That didn't sound too great. Obviously tiredness was a side effect, especially in the days after treatment. There can also be mood swings with the steroids Patrick would be taking. Otherwise, he said, it is generally well tolerated.

These are the ones I remember coming out of the meeting. There was a lot said, but this is what stood out. I remember I kind of calculated it all and came to an - OK, that's OK, we can handle that - position!

Patrick went on to ask how many were in the Kiwi Trial in New Zealand so far and we were quite surprised to hear that he was to be the third person. There was a man who was at stem cell transplant stage right now, being seven months into the Kiwi Trial, and another lady who was a month ahead of Patrick.

Dr Henderson jumped in quite quickly at this stage to reassure us that although it is new here the treatment plan has been running for years overseas, it is well documented and helps patients tremendously. He didn't need to do that, we had already done our research. We knew this was a proven best option through the past trials and papers we had read on its success, however it was still reassuring to hear it from him too.

Dr Henderson also went on, reiterating to us, "There is so much research going on for multiple myeloma. New treatments are being discovered that are having great results so try not to be too discouraged. I fully expect you to do well on the Kiwi Trial and to get you into remission. Then, by the time you relapse again, new and better therapies will be available." We drank it all in, they were words we wanted to hear.

Patrick couldn't help himself, he wanted to discuss life expectancy again. Well, how could you blame him? It was his life on the line. He knew it had been discussed with us broadly before but that was around our expectation he was at stage 1. He needed to ask again, more specifically this time. Fair enough, it was the elephant in the room as far as we were concerned.

"So," he asked, "if I am at stage 2 now, from what I have read, the average survival rate period becomes less. What are your thoughts around that?"

Dr Henderson turned in his chair and placed himself looking directly at Patrick. "Look," he said, "when you read life expectancy in published articles they are talking an average, so try not to read too much into it. As I've said to you before, people with multiple myeloma are living a lot longer with many up to ten years plus now with the new treatments on offer. There is also so much research being done on multiple myeloma that new drugs are coming out all the time helping people to live longer and longer." He turned back to his desk and his computer and scrolled a little looking at Patrick's results again, then said "You are very lucky, even at Stage 2 you have no organ damage. You are relatively otherwise healthy and I have no reason not to expect a good outcome for you."

OK. Thanks. That was good enough for me, I'll take that thank you. Patrick also decided to accept this explanation and let it be. He simply replied, "That's great to hear then."

Dr Henderson then turned back to us and continued "The treatment plan you are about to go on is all designed towards getting you the best remission possible. The better the remission, the harder it is for the cancer to come back. The longer it takes to come back, the easier it is to fight it the second time round. We would also expect better treatments will be available by then. Try not to worry, multiple myeloma treatment has come a long way even in just the last few years. I feel very happy with the Kiwi Trial for you and expect you to do well on it."

He turned back to his desk again, and started typing into the computer. I could tell we needed to finish up now. Gosh, we'd been there long enough. I got my last ten cents worth in adding "That's good to hear Ross, thanks for explaining that. We're pretty much just keen to get started now!"

We just wanted to get on with it. We were ready to go and nothing was going to get in the way from our end. The world stops when you get diagnosed with cancer. Nothing, as in NOTHING else matters, but getting into treatment and getting well again. Dr Henderson brought the meeting to a close, advising someone from the Kiwi Trial team would be in touch with us with the start dates for chemotherapy and the full day and time schedule for the month.

We had all stood up by then and were walking to the door. My usual alert around people following up on things kicked in. It comes from my days as a Project Manager in the building industry, making sure tradesmen commit to dates and times, constantly following up and checking and rechecking they will be there to ensure deadlines are met. I knew you shouldn't just rely on 'we will be in touch' as it is too vague and left open to no urgency or accountability to contact or perform in a timely fashion. The importance now was on a whole other level, involving life and death.

"Oh," I said, as we got to the door, "who should we contact if we don't hear from anyone?" Dr Henderson smiled at me with kindness again, "You don't need to worry about that, we are watching everything closely and someone will be in touch."

Oh really? Ouch! That hurt having to let go and trust him. Eek, I'd better not push it as I normally would. I decided then and there, I shouldn't stand and question the word of a man with whom we were entrusting Patrick's life; that just didn't seem right. I needed to trust him, so I let it go. I did secretly have a mental note that last week we were given phone numbers of some of the staff of the Kiwi Trial team. I grabbed that in my mind as a bit of reassurance, as my insurance policy on where to go if we didn't hear from the hospital.

Patrick and I of course were blown away it was all coming up so soon. We left the hospital and decided to go for coffee and cake, something that became a bit of a ritual after hospital visits. We discussed the appointment and the first thing that came up was of course the fact that he is in Stage 2. We both talked about how damn lucky he was to be at this stage and have no organ damage. In fact he had no signs at all other than a level of tiredness running through him day to day. The bronchitis he had suffered from when he went to the doctors had nothing to do with multiple myeloma, it was just the catalyst that had got him to his GP who fortunately started taking blood tests.

Today it was so very hard to believe Patrick was so sick. Sitting across from him at the cafe, he looked gorgeous, healthy and well. Yet his blood is 80-90% saturated in cancer cells. What the?! As we talked about it we both got pretty emotional. This was some serious shit but hey, treatment was only two weeks away. We didn't talk about the possible side effects, what was there to say really? We had no idea what Patrick would experience. We knew we would just have to roll with it and deal with it as we went. That's all we could do, be present with it.

We did talk however about finally telling people. Who should we tell when, how, etc? These became quite big decisions. Did Patrick want to keep it private? Do we tell people everything? Who do we tell in person? Who do we phone? It all got a bit too much so we decided to start with family and we'd work out the rest later. Patrick sent a message out to our children asking if they could all make it over for dinner tonight, we had some news to share; thankfully they could all make it. Although it was going to be hard telling the children, I was relieved that the time had come; I didn't like holding it from them and they needed to know. We now had the full story for them and it couldn't be delayed any longer.

Patrick's brothers had already been told. They both live overseas - one in England and one in the USA. Patrick had decided to ring them both after our first visit to Dr Henderson when he had thought he was at Grade I. They, at this stage, other than Helen, were the only people who knew. They apparently had been amazing, so kind and supportive. Obviously they were very shocked and keen to do whatever they could to support Patrick. In fact one of his brothers immediately transferred a very sizable sum of money over and told him to use it to take the kids on a holiday before treatment; he suggested Japan as Patrick had lived there for a time in the past, or wherever took his fancy. How seriously kind was that? That was when Patrick had thought he had a couple of months before treatment was to start. Of course now we would have to call them and update them on the latest prognosis and that the treatment was now starting soon.

Driving home we chatted about the children and how nice it would be to have a break away of some sorts with them before treatment started as Patrick's brother had suggested but now, with treatment starting so soon, an overseas trip seemed out of the question. We knew the following weekend was Labour Weekend. This meant a public holiday was on the Monday for everyone so we decided, if the children could make it, we'd have a nice time away for those three days at least.

We also talked on the way home that no matter what, Patrick's brothers' money would be put aside for other small holidays for us to have a break through the treatments. If he was up to it, every week off, being once a month, we'd go for a break for a couple of days at least and we would use this money for it.

Then there was silence, unsaid words hung in the air. Patrick and I had googled enough to know that patients with Stage 2 multiple myeloma have statistically a shorter lifespan overall than patients with Stage 1. We knew Stage 2 wasn't good news and we knew the consequences. Even though he was going into treatment we wanted to still make the most of life during this time of treatment as much as we could together.

According to the American Cancer Society (ACS), these are the average survival rates by stage:

Stage 1: 62 months, approx 5 years

Stage 2: 44 months, approx 3-4 years

Stage 3: 29 months, approx 2-3 years

I'm just going to add in here that another site added to this: **'However significant medical advances are helping to increase survival rates.'**

Driving home my thoughts then moved to silently offering so much gratitude to Patrick's brother. With this money assigned to holidays we will definitely go and have some good times, enjoy what time we have together through all of this. Without this money I knew we wouldn't take this time away. We hadn't discussed it yet, but gosh, how were we going to survive? Patrick won't be working full time and I'll be cutting my part time job down even more. I decided right there that the financial side was the least of my worries for now. Somehow I could park it, it didn't matter. Financial survival seemed insignificant compared to actual physical survival so making this pact in what to do with his brothers' gift was to me a very important decision.

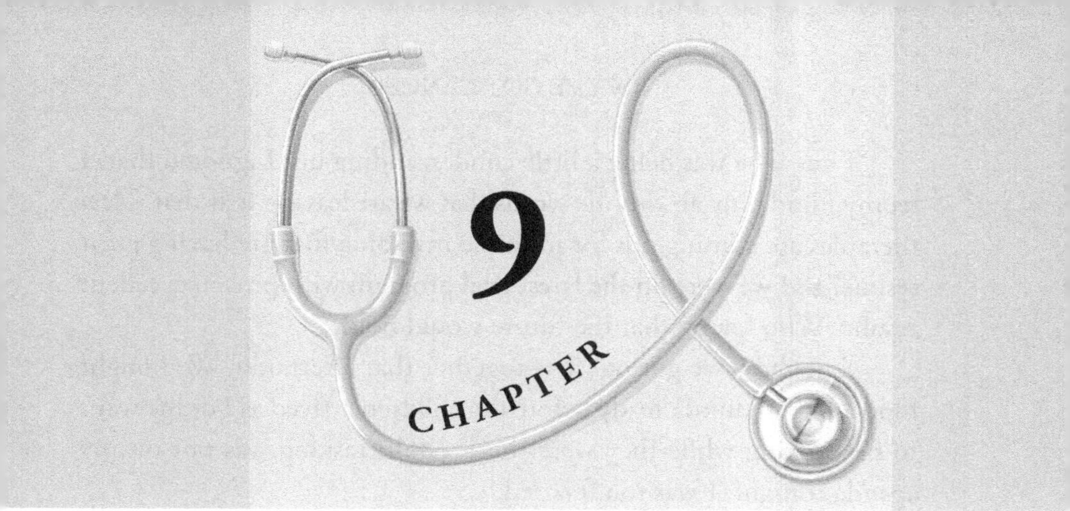

Telling the family

"Love doesn't need reason.
It speaks from the irrational
wisdom of the heart."
- Deepak Chopra -

When we got home we sat huddled on the couch together again. A pot of green tea had been poured and we finally brought up the dreaded Stage 2 diagnosis to discuss.

"Gosh," I said, "just when we thought we were getting our heads around everything, now this!" "I know," Patrick replied. "It seems to have gone from bad to worse."

I jumped in on this straight away with the words of hope from the specialist. "I know what we have read Patrick, but I think it's important to remember what Dr Henderson said about the amount of research that is going on now, and the new therapies." I didn't want to hear any doom and gloom talk right now. Patrick looked me in the eyes. He could feel every fibre of my being desperate for hope right now. He softly spoke. "OK darling, let's leave it at that for now."

I knew he was being a little condescending but I ignored that. I let my mind only absorb the words that we are leaving it at that. New therapies are coming out for multiple myeloma that are having great results, and we were on the latest trial program with proven excellent results. Who knew what the future would hold.

Somehow we got our acts together that afternoon. We bought food and had dinner ready before the children arrived as I didn't want to be cooking while they were there. Multi tasking was not on my agenda tonight, I was too frazzled.

We told the children after dinner; I can't remember the dinner itself. My mind and vision of that night can only see us sitting in the lounge telling the children, the rest is blank.

Patrick told them. He did it so beautifully. He is such a soft spoken person anyhow, but how he delivered the news was very special.

Once he told the children of his diagnosis he then went on to explain what multiple myeloma was. The children were all so shocked they said nothing, they didn't even move, they just froze as it all sank in. Then the devastating news that multiple myeloma is not curable; he had to stop at that point. Everyone of course reacted to that, it was heartbreaking to have to shatter their happy lives with such tragic news.

Patrick, as soon as he could, went on to tell them about the Kiwi Trial program. He tried to give them some reassurance, hope, that this was the best possible outcome for him. That he was very thankful, and that he felt confident he would get good results with it. One of the children spoke up, "Wait, what do you mean good results? Could it then cure it?"

How do you tell your children that good results don't mean a cure, you just don't die as early. Sorry, but that's it. He continued as diplomatic as he could be. "As I said earlier," he replied, speaking as he had been, to everyone, as he answered this question, "there is no cure." He had to be real. He didn't want to mislead them though he also wasn't going to give them the Stage 2 3-4 year life span figure either. He went more for the 'new treatments are coming out all the time' version, and explained almost word for word what Dr Henderson had told us.

Patrick then continued with the most perfect comment. I don't think I'll ever forget it. Speaking more softly now he said to them all, "But you know what kids, we can look at this another way. This could have been Kushla sitting here, telling you all I had been hit by a bus today and had died. Seriously. That sort of thing happens, whereas, here I am, still here, and we still have lots of time together, and I feel very grateful for that."

Nice speech, right there. My heart swelled. What a perfect thing to say. What a perfect way to look at this. What a perfect way to ground this news. What a perfect way to give the children a slice of peace in all of this. It was so true, and it worked, it helped us all touch into gratitude which I think helped with the shock for everyone. There weren't many questions. Of course not, what did they know to ask? This had just been sprung on them. We didn't want them to have to know everything anyhow so we were pleased to leave it there for now.

Patrick then went on to ask who was free Labour Weekend to go on holiday. Unbelievably they all were, or if they weren't they didn't say. They all made themselves available so we planned we would go away on the Friday after work and come back late on Monday. We also decided together that it was to not be too far away. We planned transport etc and it was a good distraction from the news.

It was a week night and we needed to wrap up. We all confirmed we'd keep in touch on Messenger with plans. As we were all starting to move from the lounge I piped up. "We do need to accept life is going to change for a while though for everyone once Patrick starts treatment." This hadn't been discussed and I felt that was wrong, it needed to be acknowledged. This shouldn't be something that everyone thought was just Patrick's thing to go through. No one had asked what they could do, or how could they help yet, and this just blurted out of me. Everyone stopped and one of them asked, "What do you mean?"

"Well I don't really know what it is going to mean but for starters Patrick is going to have to go to the hospital for chemotherapy twice a week and I don't want him to go on his own." Chase, my eldest, then spoke. "Well I certainly could come to the hospital with you occasionally Patrick. We could maybe set up a roster each month so every month one of us goes with you."

The conversation became bubbly around this. I joined in and said I would be happy to do one day a week, if they could take turns doing the other day, it would only be one day a month for them each… and even then it's just for a few hours that day. Half a day off school a month for Katelyn. Chase and Taylor weren't sure how to arrange it with work, but they said they would definitely look into it.

I had no idea what we were in for in the coming months nor how much support we would need, so I decided to stay present, not suggest anything else and deal with it all when I needed to. To be honest, I really didn't want to disrupt the children's lives if possible. This is such new territory for all of us. It was great some suggestions were made and the children were clear that I expected this to be a team effort of some form, so we'll see where it goes.

That night the googling was picked up again. Stage 2, multiple myeloma. We had thought we were done with googling. Friday night, 15 September 2017 was when all the googling had started; that was just over a month ago now. First it was trying to understand all the results… gosh that was huge. Then to understand multiple myeloma Stage 1 and its prognosis and treatments. Now Stage 2 multiple myeloma. Again, its prognosis, best treatments etc, again and again!

We were up until the small hours. It's incredible how quickly time can go when you are so absorbed, searching from one site to another to another. We were both coming to the same conclusions; the treatment plan Patrick was about to undertake was still the best treatment for him. Even with Stage 2 there was nothing better. Everywhere we googled the life expectancy would hit us in the face… 44 months… 3-4 years. It was horrid. We put down our iPads finally and snuggled up with at least some comfort we were on the right track for treatment, and we knew that these treatments were proving to achieve great results for patients with multiple myeloma.

One thing we had seen constantly though through our googling was what Patrick needed to achieve through his treatments to have the best chance possible. MRD-!!

Minimal residual disease - or ***MRD-*** *is a highly sensitive* ***measure of the effectiveness of therapy for multiple myeloma****, a cancer of the plasma cells of the bone marrow. A patient who tests 'MRD negative' after treatment for multiple myeloma has less than one million cells per million bone marrow cells. Data from recent clinical trials suggest that* ***patients with such a low level of disease may be less likely to experience a relapse of their condition than patients with higher levels.***

We went to sleep that night both acutely aware of the importance of achieving MRD-. We had made a pact right there and then before going to sleep that this was our goal, this is what Patrick was going for. We both put it out there that with all the treatment he was having, this is what he would achieve. The portal had been opened to the universe to allow Patrick to achieve this result, to allow his body to be rid of this cancer to such a deep positive and clear response. We just had to get on now to achieve that.

The next few days were spent either working or going to visit family to tell them the news. There was Patrick's dad, his sisters, my mother, my brother and his family and we wanted to make sure they were told as soon as possible. We had made it our goal to do that over the next few days as we didn't want one knowing without the other.

To be honest it was really awful having to do that; I can see why some people make the choice to not tell people. For example, walking into Patrick's dad's apartment for what his dad had supposedly thought was to have a nice cuppa and chat with him and his new partner Betty. Patrick's mum had sadly passed away a few years ago. Here they were looking forward to a nice catch up until we came along and dropped the bomb shell.

They were, of course, traumatized by it. We obviously stayed for some time, but no time is the right time to go after telling an 88 year old man that his son has terminal cancer… because that is what it is. Terminal, right! How can you prepare them for it? We hadn't wanted to say anything over the phone, as we felt that would have been worse. It's just an awful thing to have to do. We didn't want to leave them after such horrid news, yet you have to go at some stage.

However, what blew me away was Patrick speaking again once all the questions were answered. "I want to say this though Dad and Betty, I really don't want this to spoil your day. I am OK with this now, it is what it is and I'm OK with it… honestly. I want you to go out for lunch like you were going to do together today, and have a lovely lunch and a lovely afternoon, I really do. It may sound crazy but I feel grateful. I could have been run over by a bus and not had the opportunities I do now to make the most of my time here, to spend time with the people I love, to say things I want to say, do things I want to do. I'm incredibly grateful for that, so I'm OK. Truly," he said, "it's OK. I really want you to not worry and have a lovely day, it's going to be OK."

What a man! I sat there, so proud of this wonderful, caring, sensitive man, who showed me clearly just now how he was finding his way to acceptance of this new diagnosis… through gratitude. One of the biggest secrets to a happy, joyful life and he found it right here amongst this devastation, so simple yet so profound. When we look for what we can be grateful for we find happiness. We see what we can be thankful for, not what we can be regretful or resentful for. The mind once again to be used as a savior to take you to the highest of knowings. A place of peace, and where harmony can lie within all chaos.

We left his dad's with hugs and smiles. I know we had just rocked his father's world, however Patrick had given him full permission to be OK with this news, to carry on and be happy, and you could see and feel they were taking this precious gift he had given them and were going to use it. Patrick's dad, his whole life, had been a very optimistic man. He has achieved many great unprecedented things in his life and this approach of positivity was second nature to him, so at least, outwardly, we left them to go and enjoy a nice lunch.

I marveled again at the way he had handled this. I felt blessed I had experienced this today as I really got where he was coming from, firstly acceptance which had then so beautifully taken him to gratitude.

People talk so much about fighting cancer, beating cancer, not accepting it, not owning it. However, what does this create in return? Underlying all that fierceness and blocking is fear. How good is that for your mind, body and soul? How good is that for your healing process? To be holding on with such intense fear. Once we move through the fear we open into acceptance. It's a natural progression that allows us to come to peace, calm, softness, and kindness to ourselves. If we then allow ourselves to open further, we come to gratitude and love. Imagine starting your healing process from this place. It doesn't mean you accept that you are sick and will do nothing about it, it means you are coming from a place your body can truly begin healing from. This then can allow it to heal easier as it does not have barriers in its way.

For some reason, in the car on the way home, I didn't say anything to Patrick about how proud I was of him, and how truly thankful I was too that he was showing us all this way, it didn't seem the right time. He needed to just be this, without accolades or ego getting in the way. For it to be just his truth there in the space for now, being passed on through his energy, words, and actions to those he shared with along the way.

Patrick went on his own later to tell his sisters; together we told my mother, my brother and his son. Unfortunately my brother's wife couldn't join us at the time but we didn't want to leave them without knowing any longer. It had by now been two days since we had told the children.

By the end of the weekend we were done with it... to be honest we were still grappling with the news ourselves. We still were very sensitive to it and struggling to come to terms with it. Each time we told someone we felt we were taking that burden on too, their worry and pain. The good old saying, a problem shared is a problem halved didn't quite equate on this occasion.

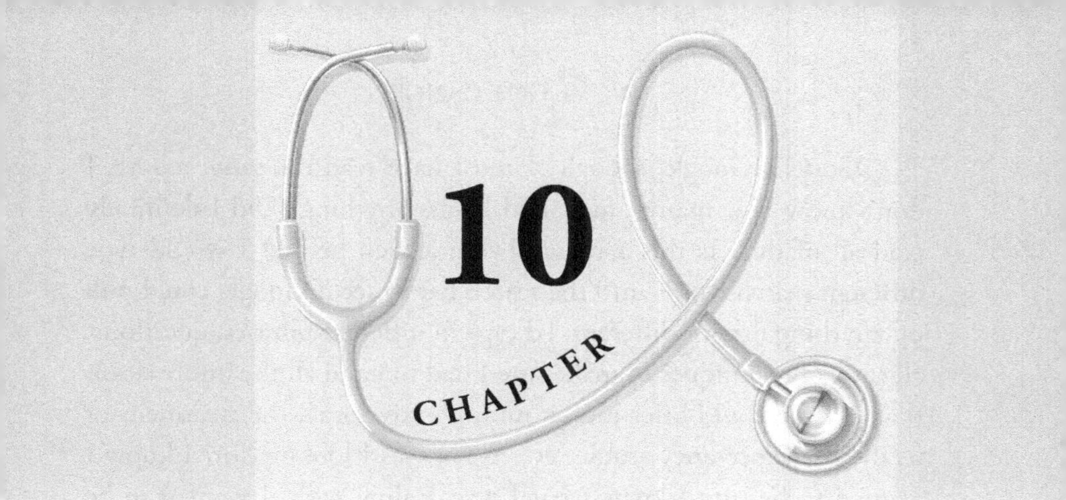

FISH Test

"Happiness is a continuation
of happenings which are not resisted."
- Deepak Chopra -

The following week we spent racing around trying to get things accomplished. Work, jobs around the house, preparing for being away this coming long weekend… and then starting chemotherapy. We seemed to have now fallen into such a heightened state of worry, fear, anxiety; yep, pick any and all of those, that I'm not sure how much we were really achieving, but it was good to keep busy. We were still awake late into the night, googling together, still searching for answers, information, treatments etc for multiple myeloma. We couldn't help ourselves.

I, unfortunately, was also experiencing the 2.30am wake up and would pull out my iPad and google some more. What else could I do at that hour of the morning? It felt like I was at least doing something useful however I was surviving on only about five hours of sleep a night if I was lucky.

Google, Google, Google. I must have read the same reports I don't know how many times. Did I miss anything? Did I definitely read all of this? Is this a report I've not seen before? I would type different search words into the search bar to see if Google could pull up anything new or different. I'd type in different phrases, questions, all sorts of techniques to make sure I had to hand all the information that Google could offer me on multiple myeloma, the treatment of it, the life expectancy studies etc. What was I looking for? I know I wanted to be sure I knew what I was dealing with. I wanted to be sure Patrick was having the right treatment. I wanted to be sure I knew what we were in for in the coming months. Most importantly, I wanted to be sure he was going to be OK.... and nothing yet could tell me that.

One thing I haven't mentioned. When we were with Dr Henderson, Patrick asked him if he could write a letter for his life insurance company acknowledging his medical status. Patrick had notified them of his health and position, as you are supposed to, and they needed an official medical letter from his specialist stating his condition. I mention this now as the result of that request opened into the next bombshell which arrived by email. We received Dr Henderson's letter on 19 October 2017, the day before we were going away with the children.

Patrick was going through his emails as he regularly does throughout the day, when he saw an email from North Shore Hospital. When he clicked on it he quickly scrolled down to see it was from Dr Henderson. He was pleased as it looked like it was the letter for the insurance company that he had been waiting for. It appeared to be just what he needed, the first paragraph stating his diagnosis with all the blood, bone marrow and scan results.

As he started to read the second paragraph, poor Patrick, apparently his heart took a leap. He was very disturbed by what he saw.

"FISH analysis from his bone marrow has shown 1p32 which is a recognized finding in myeloma associated with a less favourable prognosis."

At this stage Patrick had no idea what 1p32 was but he certainly knew what 'less favourable prognosis' was. He was so shocked to see this. This was the first he had heard of the FISH test result, he hadn't even known the result was in yet. As he told me later, he of course started googling to find out what 1p32 was, and what this meant. Very quickly he discovered it was a chromosome abnormality and he figured it must be something he was born with. (Although later he discovered this wasn't in fact true). Of course the next thing he needed to google was what this meant for him. He couldn't find much about it at this stage and it was very frustrating for him that there was so little written about it. There seemed to be a lot of information on other chromosome deletions but 1p32 was difficult to find, however what he did discover explained Dr Henderson's comment of 'less favourable result'. The life expectancy with this deletion and multiple myeloma seemed to be not much more than a couple of years. This was a significant difference.

By the time I arrived home Patrick was in a bit of a state and I could immediately tell something was wrong. He told me he had received the insurance letter from Dr Henderson and that there was news he needed to tell me. He insisted on making us a cup of tea before sitting me down to tell me what was going on; I knew that wasn't a good sign from the start!

As we were making the tea I looked at the clock, it was mid afternoon so we had a good couple of hours before Katelyn was due home from school. Whew! We were trying so hard to protect the children from things until we knew fully what we were dealing with, and until we had adjusted to it ourselves. When we were settled on the couch together he gave me Dr Henderson's letter.

To be honest with you I skimmed the 1p32 bit, I didn't know what it was or understand it. Less favourable prognosis didn't mean much to me at the time. I already knew he had a bad prognosis. It was the last paragraph, however, that had me gasping.

'Patrick has asked what his prognosis would be if he has no treatment for his myeloma; untreated and unsupported in my opinion his prognosis would be around 6-10 months on the current available information.'

I looked at him in disbelief as I blurted "Oh my God Patrick, 6-10 months with no treatment!!" We had no idea it was this serious! "Patrick, thank God for your GP! You had no symptoms, it could have so easily gone undetected until too late!"

My heart went fully out to my dear man as I sat there looking at him. He looked so gorgeous. So normal. He had lots of colour, his body looked perfect, he looked absolutely fine, yet all the while his poor body was going through this torment of ill health; struggling to survive. It felt almost unbearable to think of what he was going through. My mind kicked in with logic and I grabbed it! "Shoot!" I blurted, "Well we are just so lucky you are on the Kiwi Trial darlin'. I am even more thankful now. You're going to knock this out of the park with this new therapy!" Thank you mind.

Patrick took the lead. "Yep," he said. Then he voiced his other thoughts around this shocking news. "This will also sort out the life insurance company too though won't it? They won't be able to dispute my request now." Apparently the Life Insurance policy Patrick had stated that if you only had a prognosis of under a year to live you could access the policy funds immediately.

I felt a twang at this comment of Patrick's. Patrick had an existing life insurance policy stating that if he died I would get the funds. It wasn't a lot, but enough to help keep me financially stable. Patrick was trying to have it released early due to his having a terminal condition of multiple myeloma. As much as I knew this would be great for him, in the back of my mind, to be honest, I felt a little concerned for myself.

Eek! Sorry, just being honest. I was torn between the two. I wanted Patrick to be able to have the funds, to have peace of mind, but it would be at the expense of my peace of mind later. I really wanted to put myself aside for him, which outwardly I was doing, but honesty here, inwardly I was struggling. Right now however, this seemed inconsequential to the issue of life and death for Patrick so I left these thoughts in the back of my mind.

The true reality of what poor Patrick was facing was right here on this piece of paper… staring at us now. What he was trying to fight! He deserved to get that insurance money now. If this wasn't enough reason to award it to him early, what would be? A large part of me was pleased he now had something solid to give the insurance company.

Those words in black and white stayed with me over the coming months as an underlying threat and knowing… 6-10 months if untreated and unsupported. Actually I think they'll stay with me forever. That's some pretty serious shit right there!

Patrick entertained the conversation around this prognosis for a bit as we drank our tea. We both came to the conclusion that, wow, at least he was to start treatment now, as early as next week, and we were so, so, very thankful. No wonder the treatment start date kept getting brought forward and they wanted to start so soon, we sure got that now. The shock was again filled with gratitude.

I had still ignored the second paragraph; Patrick finally came to it. He pointed to the letter and said "What we really need to worry about darling is this 1p32." I picked up the letter and started to read again the paragraph he was pointing to on the FISH analysis:

'FISH analysis from his bone marrow has shown 1p32 which is a recognised finding in myeloma associated with a less favourable prognosis.'

As I read the paragraph I looked over at Patrick and said "What is this 1p32? Sorry, I don't get it." Patrick quickly responded, "It's a chromosome deletion I have and it's not good darling. You need to prepare yourself for this news."

I got a bit agitated. "Patrick I don't even know what a chromosome is, what are you talking about? What does this mean? Gosh tell me the short version, you're scaring me!" By now it was sinking in, feeling his manner, his words, his tension. I could feel my world was about to rock even further and I needed to know now. What's going on? That's my way. I want to be able to know a problem, fix it or deal with it, rather than carry the unknown and the underlying fear it causes in us.

"I've been googling it," Patrick replied. "To be honest it's quite new to me. I don't know much about this sort of thing but it seems that with this deletion with multiple myeloma it can give an even shorter life span. I think it's part of your DNA that you are missing and it makes it harder to fight the cancer"

This in fact didn't turn out to be true. A chromosome deletion is a particular chromosome that should be there, but was missing from every cell in Patrick's body that was cancerous. It is not missing in the cells that are healthy. However to be honest, what it was really didn't matter much at the time. What its consequences were was more important.

Remember Patrick's diagnosis was 80-90% plasma cell burden. That means up to 80-90% of his entire blood cells are cancerous and this chromosome is missing in them all. What he had discovered on searching the internet later on is that a 1p32 chromosome deletion is not common. This was why there was so little material or data on it for Patrick to find online. He could find a lot on the other deletions, del (17p), t(4;14), t(11;14), t(14;16), t(14;20),t(6;14). There were many reports relating specifically to del(17p) and t(11;14) because these were much more common deletions, therefore it was researched more so they could advise more on that condition.

Trust Patrick. Firstly, multiple myeloma is **not a common** cancer; it's only 1% of all cancers. Secondly it's **not common** to get multiple myeloma at Patrick's age, also it is **not common** for it to develop as quickly as it did for him, and now it is **not common** to have this deletion. None of this was helping.

"This is all I have found at this stage." Patrick said as he handed me a single piece of paper of an article he had printed off. It was headed **'Deletion of the 1p32 region is a major independent prognostic factor in young patients with myeloma: the IFM experience on 1195 patients'**.

I was anxious. All the old feelings rose from when, just a few weeks ago we had been googling his initial results. Oh my God what were we in for now? Patrick put his arm around me as I started to read it. There were a few words in there I didn't know, but I skipped through them just trying to get to the point of the survey to get some idea what this was all about.

Standing out were the words **overall survival 1p32: 26.7 months.**

I turned to Patrick. "Seriously?!" I asked. "I'm sorry," he said. "I'm so sorry, it's actually terrible news. It's all I could find on it but it doesn't look good for me at all."

Slowly it was sinking in. My man. My beautiful man. Two years! No, I didn't want to believe this. It was too much. Too much! I decided I needed to see more. Know more. What was behind what Patrick had just shown me!?

Although I was shocked at what I saw, my mind went into rescue mode. Thank you again mind. "Are you sure you can't find anything else on this Patrick?" I asked. "This is just one report, and look how old it is." I had noticed the report was published first in 2013. Patrick declared he hadn't found anything else, despite his best efforts. Because it was so rare, so little had been investigated around it.

"Well, I don't know darling." I said to Patrick as my mind started down what was shown to me a very clear path. "I keep coming back to what Dr Henderson said the other day, treatments for multiple myeloma have come such a long way, even in recent years and this report is already at least four years old. The chemotherapy you are going to be on probably wasn't even available back then. In fact what you have here doesn't even say what treatments were used for these patients. "Don't forget also," I quickly continued, "you are young, which is in your favour, and you have no organ damage."

I hadn't studied the article properly otherwise I would have noticed the whole study was actually done on 'young patients'.

"The other thing," I pointed out, "is that two and a bit years overall survival is an average, as five or six years is the average for multiple myeloma, or as is the average years overall survival with the different stages of multiple myeloma, whereas we know people can often survive up to ten years now with multiple myeloma. Honestly," I said dismissively, "I wouldn't worry about it too much. It's old data and you are on the latest and greatest of treatments. Dr Henderson himself said he expected you to have a good outcome, so let's just go with that for now."

What I hadn't factored into the equation of course was that Dr Henderson didn't know about the FISH test when we saw him; it seemed it had come out only yesterday. Still, if it was really that bad a news, surely Dr Henderson would have rung Patrick to discuss it with him before sending this letter.

"True," said Patrick " it's quite frustrating there is so little to be found on it." "I hear you darling," I replied softly now. "Hey, don't forget also what Dr Henderson said about how, with all the research going on, great new treatments are coming up all the time, so when the time comes that you relapse, who knows what will be around to help you."

I reached out to Patrick holding his hand, stroking it as I spoke on. "We have such a nice time away planned for this weekend with the children. How about we just forget about it all for now and enjoy the weekend. No googling. We can talk to the Specialist when we see him next week about it. How's that for a pact?"

Patrick looked at me deeply, very deeply. Too deeply when I look back. I'd forgotten he had a chemistry background. Even though he didn't have much of an idea on chromosomes, he knew this was serious. Apparently he chose not to alarm me anymore. He agreed with me. I'd said enough that gave us both permission to drop it for today anyhow and just look forward to our long weekend away with the family.

For the first time I was happy to make a decision to not google. Actually I couldn't deal with any more, this new test result seemed too much. I needed time to get used to what we had ahead of us in the coming weeks, to get used to the fact Patrick even had cancer let alone all this chromosome stuff. I stayed vigilant that night and the next day keeping away from googling and I didn't pick up my iPad once. I thought he was doing the same but, unbeknown to me, already he was googling every chance he got. Well you can't blame him can you? He wanted to know more and was perhaps also looking for a glimmer that this could not be as serious as it seemed.

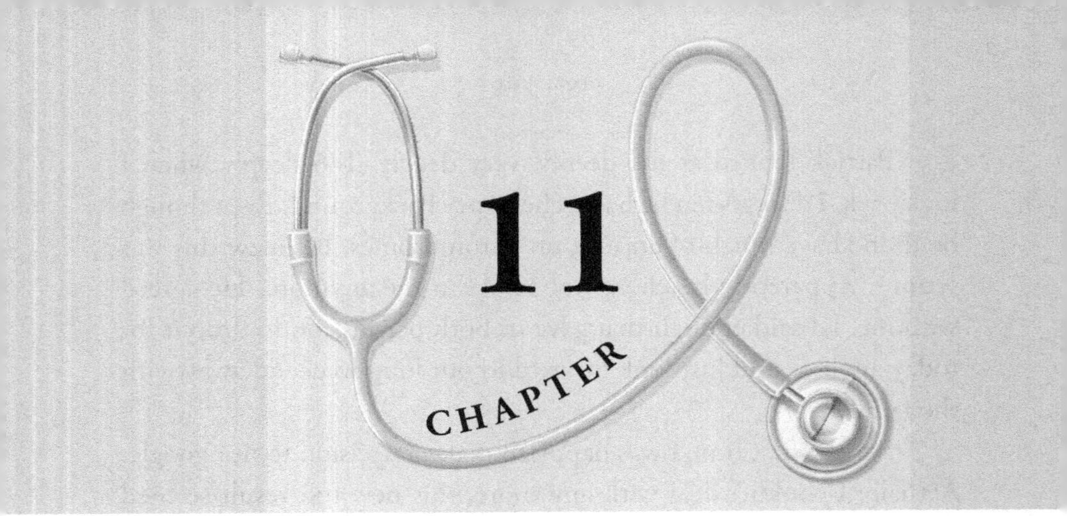

Family Holiday

"A man travels the world over in search of what he needs,
and returns home to find it."
- George A. Moore -

It hadn't been easy finding, at the last minute, a three bedroom plus home in a nice holiday area for Labor Weekend. We got lucky, we found a house at Mangawhai, a lovely small seaside resort town up north that was perfect for us; it was close to the beach with a nice big deck. It had beautiful views, a table tennis table, fireplace and spacious living areas, and was only an hour and a half from home! It wasn't cheap but with Patrick's brother's money it didn't matter, we could do it.

Despite the dreadful news that hung over us all everyone was determined to have a great weekend. It wasn't often we all got together for a weekend away, so it was a real treat. Patrick and I kept the latest findings close to our chests, in fact over the whole weekend we didn't discuss it once. For a change I put my head in the sand, this time was too precious and I wanted as few spoilers as possible.

It was such a lovely relaxing fun weekend. We didn't do a lot, just hung out together for meals and walks, played games, and had a lot of laughs. It's a beachside town so the vibe was slow and just what we needed. It was really nice to be out of town away from the reality of it all and having time with our precious babies.

Patrick had been given the schedule for his chemotherapy. He was starting the coming week, actually the day after we got back from holiday - Tuesday 24 October 2017!

On one of the nights the children all decided who was best to spend what day at hospital, supporting Patrick for his first month of treatments. It was decided that I was doing the first day in the first week as I wanted to be there to see how it all works and Katelyn was going to do the second day. The others would take turns the following weeks. I was very proud of them all and I know Patrick was thrilled too that they were so supportive. He insisted he didn't need us all to go with him, but none of us would have a bar of it. No way was he doing this journey alone!

One thing to note here, this is a blended family. Although Patrick and I had by now been together for 10 years, their difference in age gaps and maturity didn't lend towards the children being that close. They got on, that wasn't a problem, but they didn't usually hang out together outside of home.

We had the odd family holiday but with Chase having been away at university for the past five years and Taylor also away a lot, due to his interest in extreme sports, and the children often staying with their other parents, they hadn't spent a lot of time together at all. So something good comes out of everything. I could feel this tragedy bringing a common bond between them which I was very grateful for.

It ended all too soon. We had such a fabulous time together and it was a special weekend to always remember and cherish. We headed home in convoy back to Auckland City. Back to real life; back to a new life and a new beginning. Chemotherapy.

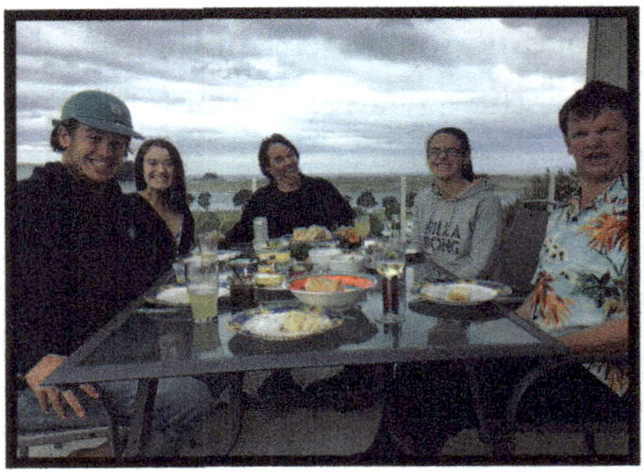

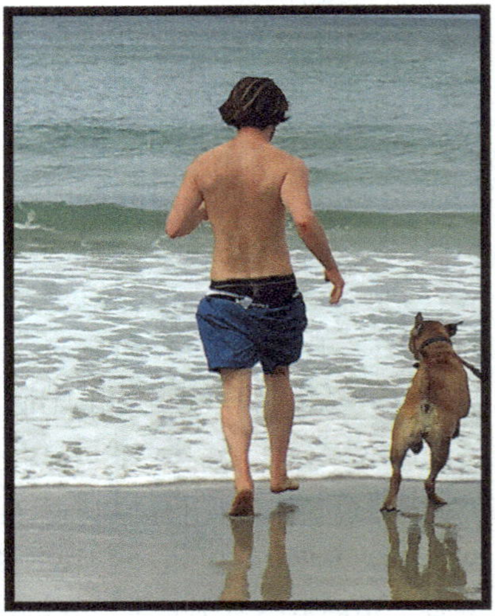

It is hard to get a serious photo with this lot, but I thought you might like to see our gorgeous children and gorgeous New Zealand. The photo of the three dogs has our girl Indi in the middle enjoying her time away too. It's not a family holiday without her, and she made some great friends on the beach that day.

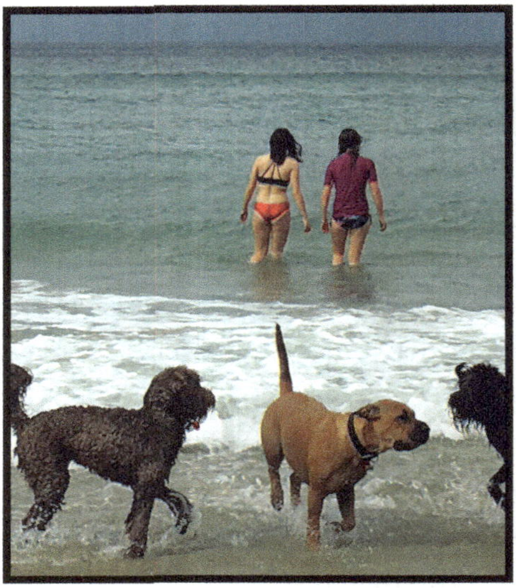

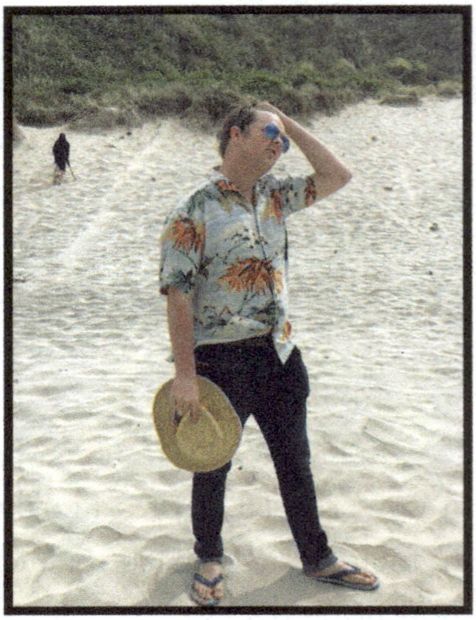

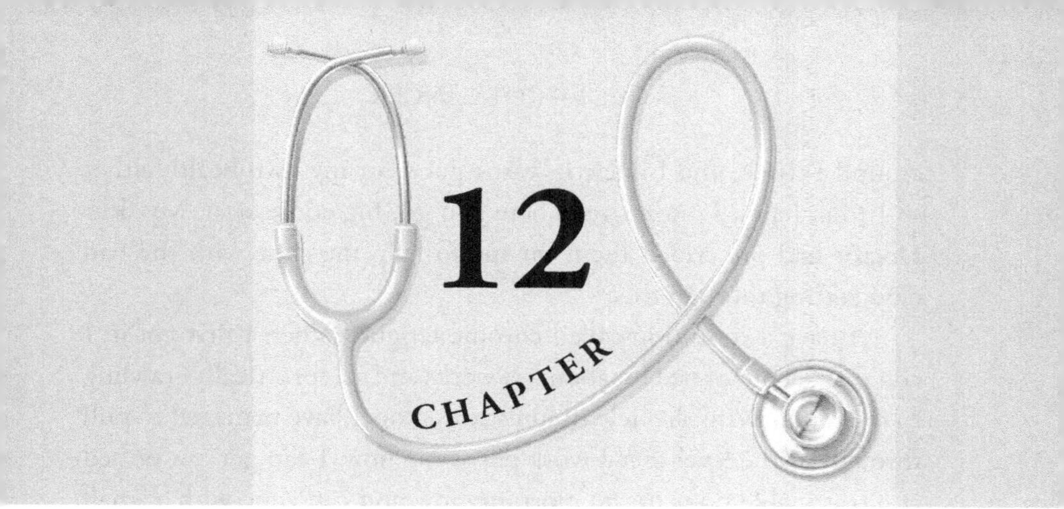

Induction Therapy Treatment

"The way to get started
is to quit talking
and begin doing."
- Walt Disney -

24 October 2017

Precisely three weeks after Patrick's official diagnosis of multiple myeloma, he began his first day of chemotherapy! We have a pretty impressive health system right? Just reiterating, the whole treatment plan is free. Patrick doesn't have medical insurance, but even if he had, he wouldn't have used it. The Kiwi Trial is a Government funded trial, so good old NZ, we are very thankful.

We are about to embark on the journey of a lifetime. Not exactly one we are looking forward to in one way, but very much so in another. Perfect yin and yang right there.

I woke up anxious. Gotta say it, sorry, but I was. After half an hour of being up, the anxiety was building up further and further; and I had to do something about it. I didn't want to be this way around Patrick, and I knew it wasn't good for my own health either so I took half a Lorazepam. There you go, big confession. My dear Doctor had prescribed them for me to help me cope with the bad days getting through this.

I have a condition called chronic fatigue. When I first got it, I couldn't get out of bed for about six weeks and was practically crawling to the toilet. With the help of holistic doctors I have managed to pull through to the level that I work part time now. I can get out of bed at a reasonable hour in the morning now and can cope with a small level of exercise. Although I am not yet 'cured' I am now living a reasonable life however I do still, at times, 'crash', as I call it, with fatigue, when I overdo things or if there is too much stress in my life. I also have a mild level of fibromyalgia where my body can really ache when I do too much.

So when Patrick was diagnosed one of the first things I did was have a full blood checkup to make sure my body was as up to speed as it could be. As a chronic fatigue sufferer, if your levels drop, life is just that much harder to cope with. Thankfully all was looking good. I also requested something to help keep me calm on the really bad days as I knew how much I needed to keep the stress under control. Knowing that stress contributes majorly to causing relapses of fatigue my doctor prescribed me Lorazepam.

I'd been saving them like hens teeth for any possible 'really bad days' in the future. Today when I woke, I knew it was one of those 'really bad days.' We had no idea what we were in for with the treatment process, the consequences of side effects for him, or the effectiveness of the treatment. Let's just say I was overwhelmed with the enormity of it all and not present at all. Just quietly, not only did I take half of one in the morning, but I also took a spare Lorazepam with me to the hospital... just in case I needed a top up. That little pill gave me a sense of security and I knew I'd be alright with one of these up my sleeve.

Patrick on the other hand seemed cool, calm and collected. I decided to take a functional approach for the morning; getting ready, organizing the house, walking the dog, and staying away from the emotional stuff. He didn't seem bothered and I didn't want to invoke emotional distress for him, so after I secretly took my Lorazepam away we went with the morning. It certainly seemed to do the trick.

Just saying here, looking back again nearly two years later I should never have felt guilty about being stressed or for taking a drug to help me through. Honestly, whatever you need to do to get through these times as best you can, to get through with as little stress or anxiety as possible is key. It's not just about the person getting treatment, those that care and are supporting the patient need to be helped too. You know I didn't use all the Lorazepams I was given, and looking back, I wish I had. I also should have given myself, and/or accepted from colleagues, more therapy to deal with how I was feeling. Everything was just happening so fast, I felt I didn't have time to breathe, let alone deal appropriately with my feelings.

We were on the way to the hospital, totally unprepared (in my view), but I was now ready to be present and open to whatever the day would bring. We had been told to go to haematology reception and that someone from the Kiwi Trial team would meet us there, which they did… two of them actually. We were escorted into the chemotherapy ward where Patrick had gone to have his bone marrow tests done.

There they were, all the chairs lined up, with about three quarters of them filled by patients. We were immediately greeted by one of the nurses who took us over to one of the beds; Along with the lazy boy chairs, at the back of the ward they also had two hospital beds. Patrick was getting a treat on his first day it seemed.

Amongst all the medical paraphernalia, there was also a chair next to the bed for me. Patrick was in high spirits, seemingly enjoying the new experience and possibly enjoying being the centre of attention with all these lovely women around him. This was the first thing I noticed, we were having a lot more attention given to us than the rest of the people on chemotherapy that day. I came to learn that this would be the norm for the next five months of therapy. The reason for this was simply that we were on a trial program.

With a trial program everything is recorded. Every week your blood results are recorded, the treatments given are recorded, any side effects are recorded, and progress is recorded. The hospital nurses and doctors cannot do anything without permission or instruction from the Kiwi Trial Program team. Everything has to be checked, monitored and recorded by someone in the Kiwi Trial team.

Blood tests had to be done today first before any treatment could begin and this was to be standard practice at the start of every week's treatment. The blood would be taken to another area of the hospital immediately and checked, and we'd all wait for the results which could take half an hour to an hour.

We met a lovely ward nurse who was part of our team. We were, in future months, to discover she was one of the many angels on this ward. The first thing she did was to put in the IV line; a vein is found and the line is inserted and this we were told would not be removed today. Every week Patrick was on chemotherapy, the line was to stay in for 24 hours for the administration of his chemotherapy that day, and the next day also.

As the morning went on we discovered the line had multiple purposes. Patrick's veins were great and the nurse had the line in, in no time. She then took blood samples through it with the Kiwi Trial nurses at her side advising what they wanted to test for. While the bloods were getting tested the nurse was so lovely and showed me where I could find tea and coffee and where the toilets were located etc. She made me feel very welcome and was so kind and reassuring to Patrick. I fell in love with her straight away.

There was a small kitchen on the ward where the tea and coffee was, and usually a couple of packs of biscuits. While we waited for the blood results to come through, Patrick took the opportunity to be taken pity of, asking for a cuppa and a couple of biscuits; I dutifully fell for it and got them for him. Biscuits are usually a no no for us, we never have them in the house, but this became regular practice as a treat for him on chemotherapy days, one I willingly and lovingly bought into for him.

Once the blood results came through, the Kiwi Trial nurses checked and recorded the information. The bloods were apparently all looking good for him to have chemotherapy today so they then administered the first lot of drugs to Patrick.

Cyclophosphamide - 13 small tablets! This is a chemotherapy drug used to treat multiple myeloma and other cancers like lymphoma, leukemia, breast cancer, ovarian cancer, and small cell lung cancer.

After this drug is taken you need to wait an hour before anything else can be administered. Once the hour was up the nurse attached to the IV line a **saline bag.** She explained this was done to flush the line before the Carfilzomib was administered. This is needed to ensure the line is clear and clean to prevent blockages. The saline can be administered through the line at different rates and it can take anything from half an hour to an hour, the rate depends on what your body can handle. Being Patrick's first time, we decided to take an hour to check he was coping with it all OK.

During this time the nurse suggested Patrick take anti-nausea tablets before his chemotherapy but he wasn't sure if he would need them. As a fisherman he had quite a good tolerance for the sea unless it was really rough, so he was thinking he might be OK without them. I on the other hand was desperate he wouldn't end up vomiting and so jumped in encouraging him to take them… just in case. Patrick agreed and I am so grateful he did as he did feel a little nauseous later even with the tablets.

The **Carfilzomib chemotherapy** fluid is then administered. This is done by intravenous infusion through the IV line so the chemotherapy is delivered directly into a vein and it flows through to all areas of the body.

Following you will see the picture that we sent to the family on the day. Patrick has his line in and is awaiting his first dose of chemotherapy; you can see it lying on the side table next to the bed. Everything to do with chemotherapy in the hospital is purple.

The bag of chemotherapy for Patrick, Carfilzomib, had been delivered that morning to the hospital and had been kept refrigerated at a certain temperature until it was sent to the actual ward for administration.

Believe it or not the Carfilzomib is not just a standard product off the shelf. It gets made up specifically for each patient each time it is administered; the strength is dependent on his last weight reading and blood results and each dose apparently costs about NZ$7,000.

The nurse hooked the bag of chemotherapy up to the IV line. Notice in the picture all the protection that she is wearing when working with Patrick and administering Carfilzomib. Purple everything again, signifying chemotherapy drugs are being used. Purple gloves, purple apron, purple chemotherapy bag.

I sat and watched as the first drips of Carfilzomib started to fall through the line. We had been at the hospital for some time by then and I could feel the Lorazepam I'd taken that morning was wearing off... either that or it just wasn't coping with the emotion that was rising in me right now. My past experience of chemotherapy was certainly influencing me right now and my fear and dread of it was rising as each drip fell through the line. I started to feel overwhelmed and knew I was about to break down.

Patrick on the other hand was handling it so beautifully. As the chemotherapy started flowing into his body he commented that he could feel it. He said he could feel it starting to disperse through his body. At that point he opened his arms outward, palms facing up, in a way of opening his whole body to the treatment that was flowing through. "I welcome this." he stated, looking down at his body. "I welcome all chemotherapy into my body from now on, to flow through and kill off all the cancer cells that are not welcome here." He stayed with his arms out and open for some time, concentrating on his body as if he was encouraging the drug to flow through and wipe away this 80-90% filtration of cancer. At that moment he gave full permission for it to do its thing.

"Absolutely Patrick." was all I could say. I wanted it too, most definitely but I was struggling with the fear of what this would bring. As soon as I felt it acceptable to leave I told Patrick I needed to go get myself a latte from downstairs, and quickly left the ward with my hand bag and Lorazepam in tow. As soon as I was out of the ward walking down the corridor I let the tears out. Oh dear, I became a bit of a mess. I took the back stairs to go down to the cafe so I couldn't be seen. With tears streaming down my face I could hardly see where I was going so I stopped half way down, sat on the stairs, and just let it all out. Oh my God. What was my poor Patrick in for? So much fear of the unknown was welling up in me. I gave myself some time to feel what was here. To allow these emotions to be seen, felt, known, and opened into the pain, the worry, the fear.

Thankfully it didn't take long. The more I opened the more the intensity of what I was feeling thankfully released. Soon I was feeling a lot better but didn't want to take any chances. Patrick was handling this so well I certainly didn't want to go back and break down in front of him.

I so desperately wanted to be there for him. I needed to be positive and at his side right now. I reached into my bag for the Lorazepam I had brought with me… extra precaution coming up. This time, no halvsies! I took the whole tablet, pulled my socks up, wiped my eyes, and proceeded down to the cafe. By the time I had got my coffee and was heading back up I was ready. I could do this.

Patrick was none the wiser of my wee melt down. I hadn't told him how I felt about chemotherapy, of my experiences and fears related to it, there had been no point. He was doing this and I just needed to get on board as positively as I could. We sat together just chatting about general things throughout the rest of his treatment; I made him another cup of tea and really the time went by quite fast.

Patrick seemed to be coping and having no problem with the treatment, not physically or emotionally. This whole process today was proving to be a walk in the park for him. He remained positive throughout the treatment process as if he had just had a simple blood test done that day… but then, this is pretty much how he was over the next 14 months. Truly he was incredible, he had a job to do - to survive - and that was that!

Once the bag of Carfilzomib was empty an alarm rang. We got used to this sound as the weeks and months went on, ringing through the ward whenever anyone's treatment was complete. The same lovely nurse returned and replaced the chemotherapy bag with yet another saline bag. This was now needed to flush the line again, this time to ensure there is no medicine left in the line.

Patrick was told he now needed to drink as much water as he could for the next 24 hours to help flush out from his body all the chemotherapy he had just received. Amazing huh! It only needs to be in the body for such a short time to do its work. It shows how powerful it is! No wonder the nurses wear all that protective gear right?

Patrick was pretty much done after that. He could go home with his IV line in to return the next day. We walked out of the ward with a script of drugs to collect as part of the Kiwi Trial. These were to become Patrick's regime over the next five months. There is a chemist on the ground floor of the hospital where we went to pick up his medications and I'm going to list here all the drugs he was now to take as he started on the Kiwi Trial.

Allopurinol - 1 tablet daily. Taken to prevent high Uric acid levels that can occur with chemotherapy

Vaclovir - 1 tablet daily. To treat infections and to help prevent shingles, a side effect of chemotherapy

Aspirin - 1 daily in the evening to help blood thinning

Ondansetron - take 1-2 tablets three times a day as required for nausea

Metoclopramide - to be taken 15-30 minutes prior to administration of chemotherapy

Cyclophosphamide - 13 tablets on the 1st day of each week of chemotherapy treatment. Chemotherapy drug

Dexamethasone - 5 tablets on each day of chemotherapy treatment. Steroid

Co-trimoxazole - 2 tablets on Monday, Wednesday, and Friday

Carfilzomib of course was the other chemotherapy he was to take but that was administered through the IV line only

On one particular day of each week Patrick was to take 25 tablets, and in total approximately 60 tablets a week, not including the intravenous Carfilzomib he'd received that day, and was to receive tomorrow also!

Check out the picture following of the handful of drugs Patrick was to take in one day. It's a bit blurry sorry, as it's off a video. Can you believe he could down all of these in one go, with one of his big beer glasses of water. I have a video to prove it, but just as well he could! Gosh if it was me it would have taken me an hour to get all of that lot down me.

To be honest I was pretty overwhelmed at the list of drugs he was given to take home. I didn't say anything, again, there wasn't any point. He needed to do this and that was that. We walked out of the hospital with Patrick cradling this huge bag of his month's supply.

I drove home that day. He said he felt OK to drive which was good news, but I insisted. When we got to the car we checked the time… we had been at the hospital for five hours.

When we got home Patrick felt a bit nauseous despite having had the anti-nausea tablet at the hospital. He didn't want to eat and just wanted water. He went and lay on the bed and ended up resting for the afternoon. I encouraged him to continue to take the anti-nausea tablets as the day went on, which helped him a lot. We both agreed at that time that he would always take the anti-nausea tablets before chemotherapy as he obviously needed them. He said his body felt heavy and wiped out as well and I was pleased he just took it easy,

I was wiped out too. The day had been exhausting for me in the end and I hadn't even taken one drug. Oops maybe one!

I made a light dinner that night which Patrick managed to eat… and he didn't throw up. This thrilled me no end. I had been so dreading he may end up going through that horrific experience, even though the specialist had said it wasn't a likely side effect of his drug regime… However he couldn't sleep… well at 4.00am he apparently finally climbed into bed. He said he didn't mind that much as he was wide awake and got lots done. He was happy, so I wasn't bothered by it either. Of course we were just present at the time, not realizing as time would go on that this would have a huge consequence on him.

I, however, had slept like a baby. I hadn't noticed he wasn't even there, nor did I hear him come in at 4.00am. It was quite amazing how I slept so well that night. You could say it was the Lorazepam that helped me sleep, I knew it was more than that though as the week went on, it seemed I finally had started to relax.

The last month's many nights spent waking at 2.30am in the pitch dark with my brain shouting 'google this', or 'you haven't checked that', had stopped this past week. We had searched all we could on multiple myeloma by now. We knew what this multiple myeloma was, knew the meaning of Patrick's results, knew the only real avenue for treatment, and knew we had the best treatment available. Patrick had started treatment. There was no need to google right now, we just had to get on and get him through the first lot of treatments. That was the primary focus.

I knew we still had so much we needed to know on the 1p32 chromosome deletion, but somehow I had very successfully managed to park it. I realised with Patrick now being in treatment, it seemed to be more a sigh of relief, not what I had expected at all. It's such a clear example how anxiety and fear is so much about worrying about the future yet, when you are finally there it dissipates.

My heart was swelling with pride for Patrick in the way he was dealing with this. He was not concerned, worried, anxious or stressed about the upcoming treatments. I'd like to think that was because I was doing all of that for him! However, it really was just because he was so present, he seemed to know he would handle everything just as it was presented to him. So I slept. For the next few weeks actually, I slept. I did wake every day at 5.30am which wasn't so great, but so much better than 2.30am.

For this first week of treatment we weren't due at the hospital until 11.00am the next day. This was great for Patrick. He had the opportunity to sleep in a little after being awake half the night. We were pleasantly surprised that our time at the hospital on our second day turned out to be much shorter than the first. Patrick had already taken **five Dexamethasone tablets** before going to the hospital and this he continued to do each day he was to receive a treatment of Carfilzomib.

Dexamethasone is a steroid. Patrick had been advised to take this as early as possible on the day as this is what keeps you awake at night; this is what had kept him awake until 4am the previous night. We were told that taking it early may help it to wear off more by evening. He had taken the **Valaciclovir** and **Allopurinol** in the morning with the Dexamethasone and just before we left he took the **Metoclopramide** for nausea. The hospital was only about fifteen minutes from our home so this was perfect timing.

The **Aspirin** was to be taken at night so he'd had that the previous night.

The **Cyclophosphamide** was only to be taken on the first day of treatment each week, which he had done yesterday. Patrick had arranged with the Kiwi Trial team to have the Cyclophosphamide prescribed for him so he could take it in the following weeks **before coming into hospital**, that way we wouldn't have to sit at the hospital for an hour waiting before further treatment could begin. They agreed that this would be OK, which was great, as this would save us considerable time at the hospital in the future. Already I was more relaxed about coming in today and there was no need for my secret supply of Lorazepam. Of course I now knew what the day would be like, so fear was a lot less present.

We were greeted again at haematology reception, this time by only one person from the Kiwi Trial team. We were taken straight through again to the chemotherapy ward and Patrick was shown to a La-Z-Boy chair which was at the back of the room amongst the beds. The nurse we'd had the day before greeted us again and it was nice to have a familiar face. We were to discover as time went on that it was very random which nurse was to be administered to which patient each day. It just depended on workloads and schedule. We also learnt as the weeks went on that it didn't matter much to us as all of them were so efficient, lovely, kind, positive and encouraging.

Before treatment started there was a checklist that needed to be ticked off for the Kiwi Trial by the Kiwi Trial assistant. Patrick was asked a lot of questions in regards to how he had been since the treatment yesterday. They also checked that he had taken all the drugs he was supposed to before coming to the hospital. Once the checklist was complete, it was all good to proceed.

The nurse then started into action setting up the saline to be flushed again through his existing IV line. Due to the fact that the line had been put in already and the blood tests had been done the day before, all that was needed was for the flush of saline to take place, then the chemotherapy, and then the flush of saline again. In less than three hours we were out of there which was a nice surprise. As we walked down the corridor on the way to the lift I high fived Patrick. "Done and dusted." I exclaimed! "Two down Patrick, we're kicking that cancer's butt!" This became a ritual of ours after each week's treatment. We'd have a laugh around it and it felt good to have that wee celebratory moment.

A small note here, as we left the hospital building we paid our parking ticket at the booth. Two visits to the hospital this week for eight hours total. Cost NZ$4 an hour = NZ$32 for this week's parking costs! We were quite shocked.

Fortunately, the following week, we mentioned this cost to the nurses. They kindly suggested we contact the Leukaemia and Blood Cancer NZ saying they sometimes can give out parking vouchers, which they did. A handful of them that we saved and used for the times we would be at the hospital for longer visits. It may not seem like a lot of money but it adds up, plus it felt nice to be supported by the Foundation in some way. It was nice for them to acknowledge they knew we existed, that Patrick was in treatment, and that they were there for us.

I drove us home again and it was pretty much a repeat of the day before when we got home. Patrick packed himself off to bed for the afternoon feeling heavy and tired, though he didn't sleep. By late evening I was in bed and he was still up and about again. The Dexamethasone was still very active and he had another sleepless night.

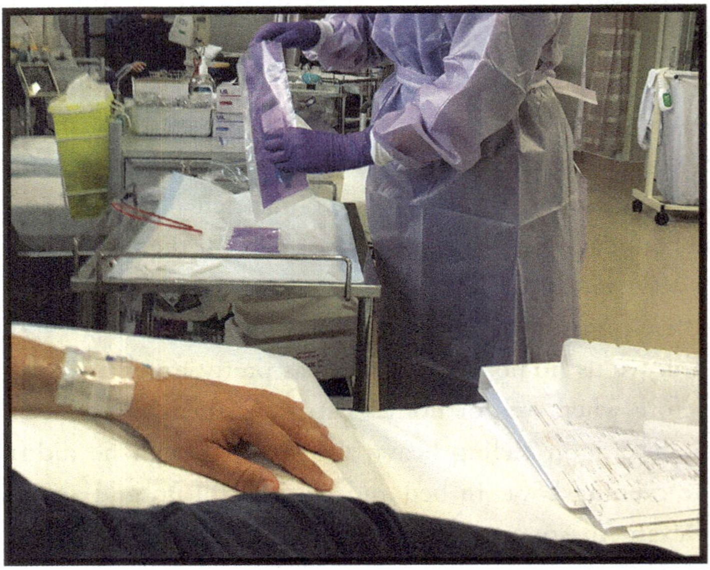

Purple For Chemotherapy

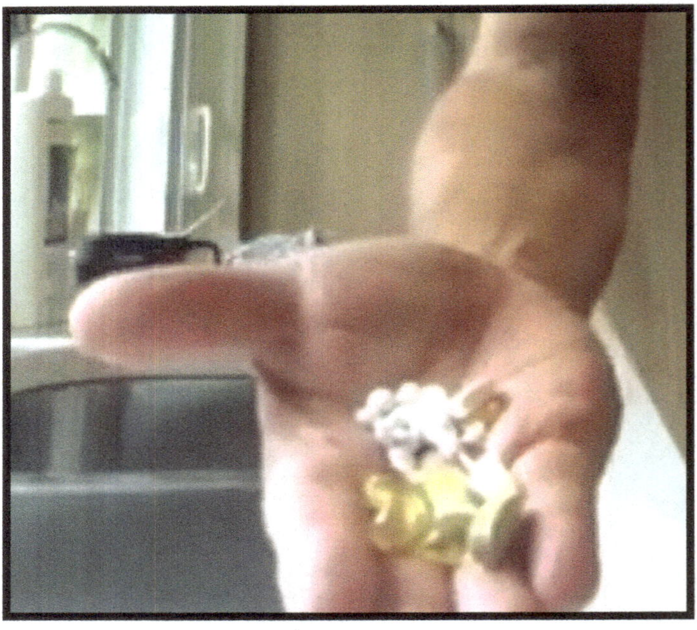

25 Tablets In A Day

Chemotherapy and Heart Attacks

"I have decided to stick with love.
Hate is too great a burden to bear."
- Martin Luther King, Jr. -

I had arranged a chat on the phone with my dearest friend Nikki who was on holiday in Europe. She had been gone for a few months already and was to be away another month still. I knew she was going to be one of the hardest people to tell about Patrick's diagnosis as Nikki had lost her husband to cancer seven years earlier. Well, I say it was cancer, but in reality it was a side effect caused by the chemotherapy!

I knew she would be rocked by the news and I didn't want to worry her while she was away. I was also concerned it may bring up and heighten her own past experiences and her loss while she was away having a well deserved break. For these reasons I hadn't told her of Patrick's diagnosis, and I didn't intend to until she was back in New Zealand.

Nikki's husband Darryl was diagnosed out of the blue, with bowel cancer on 22 February 2011. He had been feeling low in energy and finally went to the doctor about it some six months after he had started feeling this way. From what seemed like the day of diagnosis, Darryl quickly started to lose weight. A week later, at his follow up appointment it was urgently arranged for Darryl to have an operation the very next week as he was declining rapidly. This all took place quickly, thanks to NZ's Government funded medical system. Within two weeks of diagnosis he was in hospital for his operation which went very well and he was home within a few days.

Darryl was a really lovely man, a gentle, kind soul. He had a lot of friends and loved the outdoors. Being a keen kiwi surfer, he enjoyed many holidays up at Ahipara which is an area of some of the best of the rugged west coast of NZ. A good friend of theirs had a section there where Darryl and Nikki would camp out on the land, and surfing was the order of the day. Apparently it was quite gradual when they both noticed him starting to lack energy, but once it became more regular, it was time to see the doc.

It's incredible how life can change so drastically, so quickly. During the operation, the doctors discovered the tumour was very large, but they managed to get it all out. Unfortunately though, it had spread to Darryl's lymph nodes so as a precautionary measure, Darryl was advised to undertake chemotherapy. Nikki struggled with this deeply as she is an incredibly holistic person. Drugs and chemicals were not on her radar so she searched and searched for more holistic options for Darryl. They opted for a high alkaline diet and powder drinks to begin with. Providing Darryl's body with the right environment that makes cancer hard to form or grow is a popular theory for fighting cancer cells.

As the weeks went on Darryl came to the decision that he wanted to be on the 'safe side' opting to undergo chemotherapy as well as an extra precaution. It's so hard when you are faced with a life threatening condition. We are just laymen who know so little about the disease, how it generates, how it spreads, and how to stop it. At the end of the day we often come to the conclusion that you just have to do all you can.

When it came the day to discuss the chemotherapy, Nikki and Darryl saw the oncologist's assistant (an oncologist trainee who fully qualified a short time later). She talked about the treatment and what Darryl could expect as side effects; things like sensitivity to the cold, tingling in the fingers, feeling tired, but on a positive note, he wouldn't lose his hair. She then presented Darryl with a consent form and suggested that Darryl and Nikki have a read of it before signing.

Nikki took this time to voice her concerns about Darryl's need for chemotherapy. The scans Darryl had before the operation showed that the only tumour he had was in the bowel and this had been removed completely and successfully in the operation; of course it had spread to the lymph nodes, but was chemotherapy really necessary? The trainee oncologist responded to Nikki using the expression that the chemotherapy was to 'spray the weeds' so to speak which made a lot of sense to her. She felt yes, there could be little seeds still in the body, so if they are spraying the weeds, it can kill those seeds too. She understood why they felt it was necessary.

Nikki and Darryl proceeded to read the consent form together right there and then. Towards the end of the form under the section on 'side effects' there were written the words that Nikki recalls went something like - although rare, there is the chance of 'ventricular fibrillation'. She had never heard of this before so she asked the trainee oncologist what this meant. Being concerned about chemotherapy already, Nikki was on alert to ensure they were totally aware of what the treatment involved and possible consequences for Darryl.

The trainee oncologist was quite dismissive about this side effect explaining to Nikki that it's a type of heart attack. Nikki came up short. "Wow, hang on a minute!" she exclaimed. "As far as we are concerned Darryl doesn't have cancer at the moment. Sure you found it in the lymph nodes and you explained this treatment is to 'spray the weeds', so why should he risk a heart attack just to spray the weeds?"

The trainee oncologist quickly went on from Nikki's outburst to reassure her, almost eradicating this possibility, saying it is extremely rare. She also commented that Darryl is a fit and healthy person, if it was to happen we would expect it would happen to an older person who already has a pre-existing heart condition. That's why we always say to people if you ever get a tightness in the chest, or a pain in the chest, you phone 111 immediately.

This put Nikki at ease. She considered that Darryl was only 49, very healthy, never had a pre-existing heart condition, and was extremely fit. She also felt, with what she was told, that even if in the rare instance that it did happen, he would have warning of a tightness or pain in the chest and have time to call for medical assistance, even an ambulance in the worst case scenario. In fact, the doctors' dismissiveness also left her feeling she really didn't need to worry much about it at all so she didn't think more of it. She certainly didn't investigate CPR, learn about how to access local defibrillators, or even think about getting a defibrillator for their own possible use.

What Nikki wasn't told, and didn't know, is that ventricular fibrillation is not just a standard heart attack. It can be triggered by a heart attack, which then causes the heart to beat with rapid, erratic electrical impulses. This causes the pumping chambers in your heart (the ventricles) to quiver uselessly, rather than actually beat, meaning little or no blood is pumping through to the heart. This then can cause complete collapse and cardiac arrest within seconds of onset. **Immediate** cardiopulmonary resuscitation (CPR) is necessary, and defibrillation with an automated external defibrillator (AED). If treatment is not provided or is not delivered in time, death can result.

Nikki insists to this day that if they had known this and thought there was any real chance of this happening Darryl would definitely not have gone ahead with the treatment; they certainly wouldn't have wanted it with this risk involved. Even **if** Darryl had himself ended up insisting on going ahead with chemotherapy, knowing the full effects and risk of a ventricular fibrillation, Nikki knows that also, without a doubt, she would have at least learnt CPR and also would have bought or hired a defibrillator to have with them at all times. Knowing Nikki I'm sure she would have too!

Darryl was two months into his chemotherapy treatment when they decided to go for a walk up North Head in Devonport, a place they often visited for a good bit of exercise and to enjoy some of New Zealand's beautiful nature. It's called North Head as it's right on the edge of the land where the ocean runs into our harbour on one side and on the other side the harbour begins. It is basically a historical hill that has been made into a beautiful park. During the Second World War bunkers were built into the hill for our army to base themselves with machine guns. It was the perfect place, up high, with a clear view of any enemy ships coming into the bay.

Today, children and adults alike, love exploring the bunkers and as you wander up and over the hill, the views are spectacular. On one side you can see the eastern beaches running up the coast and the harbour opening out to the sea, and on the other Auckland city sits in all its glory, shining out on a sunny day.

Auckland is known as 'the city of sails'. We have more boats per head of population than any other city in the world and it's a spectacular sight on a sunny day from North Head, watching all the boats coming and going through the harbour. Sail boats, ski boats, launches, all shapes and sizes, enjoying a day out on the water. Fishing, visiting islands, water skiing, or just a cruise with friends, it's all on the back door of this city and we kiwis know how to get out there and enjoy it!

This day was one of those spectacular days. Nikki and Darryl started with a coffee at a cafe in the quaint town of Devonport, before driving to the base car park and heading off for their walk.

They had done this walk many times, so they knew their way around and where they were going. Taking their time they slowly made their way around the mountain, taking in all the beauty. As you come around, a pathway of approximately 500 metres takes you up to the top. At the peak there are a few historic army buildings which have been preserved by the council, kept for the public to view.

As they were about three quarters of the way up Darryl started to get a little breathless and not far from the top he stopped for a bit. Nikki stopped with him and asked if he was OK. He assured her he was fine but was a bit short of breath. He joked a little that he must be getting a bit unfit now with all this treatment and little capacity to surf, and they continued on. They got to the top and, as Darryl was still a little breathless, he decided to sit down on a concrete ledge. He commented to Nikki, "Is it alright here darling, I hope it's not too sunny for you?" He then leaned forward, putting his head in his hands… and within a matter of seconds, his body jerked, he flung backwards, his body arched, and he started twitching with his eyes rolled back in his head. Nikki screamed in shock! She looked out for help and screamed to a lady walking by not far from them to call 111. While the lady was talking to the ambulance operator Nikki was with Darryl wondering what on earth she could do. She noticed he wasn't breathing at all and all she could think of in that split second was to breathe into his mouth. She did this a few times, noticing his lungs inflate a little as she did, and then they stopped; Nikki knew something more serious was needed.

If you have ever been in an emergency situation like this before you will know the time spent talking to an emergency phone operator, giving them all the information they want to know seems endless as you worry for the person who is suffering, and feel you should be doing more quickly. This was going on for Nikki. The only advice she was getting right now from the lady on the phone was to stay calm. Apparently the lady that had called the ambulance operator had told her Nikki was doing CPR on Darryl so the operator did not realise more should be done immediately while waiting for the ambulance to arrive!

What a place to be to have a heart attack! And not just a heart attack, an acute heart attack causing ventricular fibrillation. Darryl had completely, suddenly stopped breathing with so little warning. And on top of the hill they were so far away from an ambulance. Nikki felt so helpless and panic set in. Here was her dear man lying in front of her not breathing and there was nothing she could do. She tried to get immediate help running to the edge of the hill screaming out to the people down in the car park below, “Is anyone a doctor, please is there a doctor, we need help up here?” As she talks about it now she says it was like it was in slow motion, as they all looked at each other and called out or shook their heads slowly saying no. She ran to the other side of the hill screaming out again “Is anyone a doctor, please is there a doctor, we need help up here?” again to no avail. Nikki was totally beside herself as she ran back to Darryl. Another woman was there when she got back who was already doing CPR on Darryl and Nikki felt such huge relief that something at least was being done for him, but he was still not responding. She knew he needed more and felt frozen in time waiting for the ambulance to arrive.

Nikki finally heard the sirens in the distance and then suddenly a guy came running up over the hill in some kind of uniform carrying a machine she learnt later was a defibrillator, another person was right behind him. To this day Nikki has no idea who those men were or where they had come from. They were so out of breath from getting up the hill as quickly as they could but wasted no time in getting to Darryl's side. They quickly cut through his jacket, immediately put the defibrillator on his chest and started giving him electric shocks. Defibrillators are used to restore the heart's beating if it suddenly stops. Nikki watched on as each shock sent Darryl's chest heaving into the air and after three shocks Darryl finally started to breathe. The St Johns Ambulance officers had by then finally arrived and quickly took over. For Nikki It had seemed such an endless time before they had arrived, but in fact she found out later it had been only exactly 13 minutes from the time of the call for them to drive to the mountaintop car park and get up the hill… however it wasn't over. Darryl stopped breathing a number of times right there on top of the hill! The St Johns Ambulance Officers didn't give up, shocking Darryl each time to get his heart going and to get him stabilised.

It was unbearable for Nikki watching Darryl going through this. At one point she had to turn away and it was then she frantically called me. Being a beautiful Sunday I was off on my own family jaunt for the day and hadn't taken my phone; something I will always regret, so I missed her call. I still can remember it like it was yesterday, the message on my phone. I haven't a clue where we went that day, I only remember coming home and picking up my phone and seeing a message was there. When I played it I couldn't work out who it was, there was just this screaming stream of desperation, I couldn't even understand what was being said. The voice was so loud and so strained I couldn't even pick out it was my dear friend Nikki. I played it again and again, then slowly deciphered it was her, but still could not understand a word. I knew though of course that something terrible had gone wrong.

Poor Nikki was so alone, however she was incredibly thankful for the ladies who had stopped to help. They held her and comforted her throughout the entire time as Darryl was again and again defibrillated to try and get his normal heart rhythm to resume.

It is important to note here that the success rate of defibrillation decreases about 5% - 10% for each minute after the onset of ventricular fibrillation. Of course Nikki didn't know this at the time, and it was maybe just as well. Finally Darryl's breathing had resumed and stabilised so they could carry him by stretcher down the hill to the car park where the ambulance was waiting and he was raced to the hospital with Nikki at his side.

Nikki is a seriously kind soul. She is always saving some poor stray kitten or dog, or feeding the hedgehog in her backyard. She is incredibly sensitive and was not coping at all with her gorgeous Darryl going through this, and there being nothing she could do.

The first thing they did when they got him to the hospital was to lower Darryl's body temperature with what is called mild therapeutic hypothermia (MTH). This is to help improve neurological outcomes. They also put Darryl on a ventilator to help him breathe - life support! When someone's heart has stopped beating suddenly for a period of time as Darryl's had, there is a real concern of irreparable brain damage. The best result after stopping breathing from ventricular fibrillation is to be revived within seven minutes; it was worked out later that Darryl had gone at least ten minutes before his heart was revived even the first time, let alone the amount of times it stopped after that and the time it took to finally get him stabilised. The ambulance officers, as you know, took 13 minutes just to get there, so the outlook was grim.

By now I had phoned Nikki and had heard what had happened. Darryl had been taken to North Shore hospital, and, as I lived not far from there, I rushed over to be with her. Of course she was a mess... and poor Darryl; I wasn't leaving. I got in camper beds from home and we stayed at the hospital for three days hoping he would pull through. Family and friends came and went, doctors came and went, it was all a big blur.

The only thing that stands out now was the meeting with the family and the doctors telling us his brain damage was so severe that they did not believe he would survive off life support. They did not think it appropriate to continue him on life support, as by now he should have had improvement and this was not happening. Of course you never forget a time like that. The family were all incredible the way they coped with this news... but then again what is there? Acceptance is all there is when there is nothing else you can do.

I was so sad for Nikki who was about to face losing her life partner. She was still reeling from the fact this had even happened, trying to absorb and find the reality in that, let alone that they were now being asked to let him go!!

This is such a difficult thing to go through when it is your loved one. There he was lying there. You could see his chest moving, breathing in and out. His blood was flowing through his body. He appeared normal, fine, alive… I myself found it incredibly difficult to comprehend letting him go. The stark reality was brought to the fore though when you consider all the tubes and machines attached to him; the mask on his face and the hospital bed he is on; the plain white walls and the tears and sadness on everyone's faces, bringing the reality that you are in the Intensive Care Unit (ICU).

Of course Nikki drilled the staff as to the certainty of their prognosis. They had to go on and tell her that even if Darryl did survive, he would have such poor quality of life due to the brain damage that had occurred. As horrible and tragic as that was it somehow helped to come to terms with releasing him from this now badly damaged body. Nikki knew how much Darryl would hate life if he couldn't be active, if he couldn't surf or ride his bike, let alone if his disabilities were more severe.

The hospital gave the family a lot of time to be with Darryl, and when the life support was removed we were all with him. He managed to breathe for a time, a few hours. He never regained consciousness but we were all there at his side talking, sharing, singing him away until he took his last breath. So tragic, so sad, and also possibly avoidable!

What happened to Darryl still remains with me so vividly, and now facing Patrick on chemotherapy, I recognised the huge risk of the potential life threatening side effects from chemotherapy. In telling Nikki of Patrick's diagnosis and treatment plan I knew that this also would be a huge concern for her.

Well when we finally spoke, the theory of not telling her didn't work. We had occasionally caught up by phone for a chat while she was in Europe when the timing worked. This day though, as the good friend that she is, she picked up that something was wrong. In the end I blurted it all out and we were both sobbing our hearts out. Such a sad but truly beautiful outpouring to someone who really cared and understood, and who truly knew what we were going through. This of course was coupled with what we both knew and others didn't, the risk of chemotherapy and heart attacks.

Nikki had felt begrudged, resentful, and angry about the fact that she and Darryl had not been correctly informed about the extremely life threatening potential of ventricular fibrillation from the chemotherapy he was on. Sure it had been in writing in the contract, but the trainee oncologist had clearly dismissed it as a real possibility. Nikki was also disturbed that the warning signs she had been told to look out for were limited. Nothing had been said about watching for shortness of breath, just this pain or tightness in the chest, so when Darryl was short of breath on their walk up the mountain they didn't consider for a minute the possibility he was heading towards ventricular fibrillation.

Some months after Darryl passed away Nikki decided to put in a formal complaint to the hospital and I became her support person for this. The hospital arranged a meeting for Nikki with one of the heads of Oncology at Auckland Hospital. Darryl's actual oncologist was away so she wasn't attending. I went with Nikki as well as Darryl's mother and one of his brothers.

The oncologist was very sympathetic and appeared understanding. An autopsy had been done on Darryl and the oncologist now had the report, and felt it was appropriate during this initial complaint hearing to discuss this. He told us, it was his personal opinion on reviewing the autopsy, that it was the chemotherapy that caused Darryl to have the ventricular fibrillation. He then went on to say that the autopsy discovered Darryl had cancer in another part of his body; secondary cancer in the stomach. He commented that this would have given Darryl a poor prognosis anyhow.

Sorry, but the cheek of it! Talk about trying to transfer the seriousness of the situation. 'Oh well he was probably going to die anyhow, so it's not that big a deal he went early.'

Poor Nikki was shocked at this news of course, and so was I. We went very quiet at this point trying to absorb this, and, sorry again, but I feel the oncologist got what he was hoping for… it shut us up. It took the wind out of our sails. However, it was irrelevant to our argument of course, which was that Darryl should have been alive with us right now and wasn't, because he and Nikki hadn't been well enough informed.

I'm still pissed off about this. That was so inappropriate and I consider even now that it was a real hit below the belt. Nikki should never have been told this news in that context in the middle of an enquiry. I felt it was a dirty tactic, in fact it was irrelevant to the point of the complaint… and who was he to imply that it wasn't so bad this happened as Darryl was going to die anyhow? Not that way, he wouldn't have; suddenly, without warning. He would have had more time with Nikki, his family and friends. He would have had time for goodbyes when the time eventually came near, which could have been goodness knows how much later. No, that was seriously unprofessional and inappropriate.

In saying that, something good did come of the meeting. He asked Nikki what she hoped to achieve by this complaint, what she wanted from it. Nikki being the sweetest person she is, said she didn't want this to happen to anyone else. She wanted people to be well informed that this is definitely a possible consequence for everyone before embarking on this type of chemotherapy. Her main concern was that the possibility of ventricular fibrillation happening is very real, and people should be well informed of the risks, not in the dismissive way she was told.

The need for this was even more pronounced following my query in the meeting, as to whether anything similar had happened to anyone else in the same way it had happened to Darryl, with so little warning. There had been a big pause before the doctor almost sheepishly replied, admitting there had been a case earlier in the year of another young male passing away in the same way as a result of ventricular fibrillation from the same chemotherapy.

Nikki reiterated to the specialist that patients should be entitled to know in detail about this side effect, even if it is a small possibility, so they can make informed decisions whether to proceed and be better prepared if they choose to go ahead with it. She firmly told the specialist that it was so wrong that they had been led to believe it was of little concern for Darryl.

As mentioned Darryl and Nikki were in two minds whether to even have chemotherapy since Darryl had already had the operation and was on a more holistic approach of prevention. Quite emotionally, Nikki adamantly said to the oncologist that if they had known this possibility was more real and so life threatening, she felt certain that she would not have gone ahead with it, and more importantly she felt certain Darryl would not have wanted to either.

So the specialist agreed that this should be made clearer to patients. He said that in the next oncology meeting with all the doctors, as Head of Department of Oncology, he would discuss this and ensure that in future this is more appropriately addressed, doctor to patient. He agreed that this should be implemented as standard for the future. Two people in one year, well the stats are getting up there, and I'd like to think they probably would have felt obliged to ensure patients understood the risks more whether we'd met with them or not.

This concern of Nikki's showed during our phone conversation as she asked a lot of questions about Patrick's condition. I knew by the line of questioning what she was quietly thinking. Would alternative therapy be better or be able to help? I quickly assured her that we felt we had no choice. With 80-90% saturation of cancer in Patrick's blood and bone and 6-10 months life expectancy we weren't mucking around. We had to blast this cancer out of his body as soon as we could, there was no choice in our minds.

Bless her she totally got it, she just wanted to support us however she could, and gave her assurance she was with us all the way for the ride; she reminded me she was to be home in about a month's time. I felt so dreadful I had dropped this bomb while she was overseas, but in the same breath, glad I did. She was so upset she hadn't known and that I had been hiding it from her. It was better she knew, and I wasn't holding on to the stress of keeping it from her. It was such a relief to have it out.

It's funny, even things like that you don't realise are affecting you. I think there is so much stress going on it's hard to break it down into chunks, it just becomes one big stress. I'm a therapist and you'd think I would have known better than to not have stopped and addressed STRESS. Like I said though, we were in a whirlwind and there seemed no time!

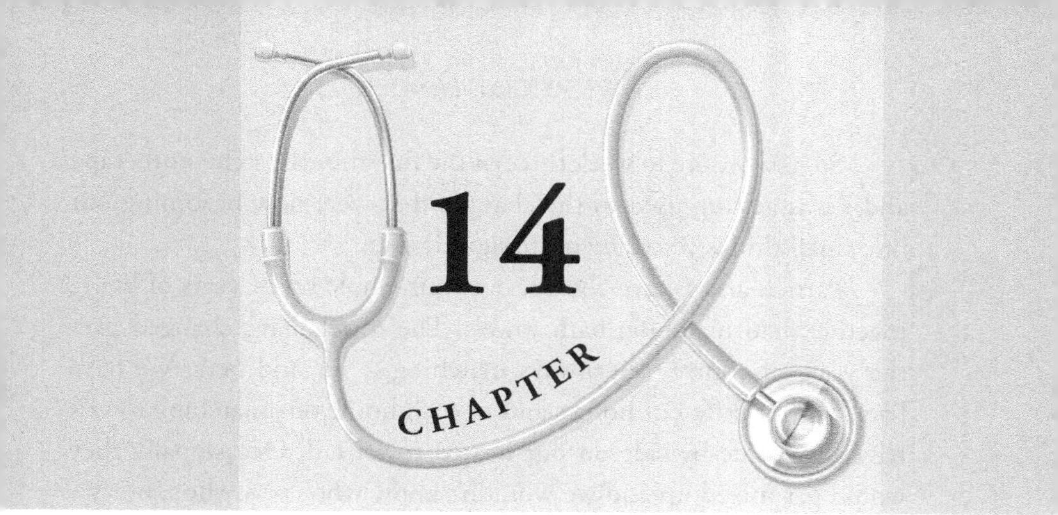

First Month Of Chemotherapy

"Start by doing what's necessary;
Then do what's possible;
And suddenly you are doing the
Impossible."
- St Francis of Assisi -

As I was still doing the 5.30am wake ups I decided to take up writing, it was better than just lying there letting my mind go crazy, and I was over googling. Writing was healing too as it often gave me the time to really think and feel what I had been through that day, that week, or that past month and how it was affecting me. At times I would find myself in tears, actually often in tears, but it was a good release and I always felt better afterwards.

Writing was helping me to acknowledge, accept, and move through built up emotion. It gave me a sounding board to work through what I was feeling or experiencing. It was giving me a record of everything Patrick was going through and giving me a good reason to keep track of the medical side of things. It seemed to help clear my head too… and it created this… what you are reading now!

So now we are in week three of the first month of chemotherapy and I was getting used to the changes that were now becoming our life, small things yet really quite significant.

Patrick and I have always, over our whole seven years of living together, had matching bath towels. The towels have changed over the years of course, but always matching… his and hers. We have lived in four different homes and in each home our matching towels have hung side by side on our heated towel rail. Occasionally they would get mixed up and we wouldn't know who's was who's, but we didn't care, that was the point of them matching. It was symbolic in that it didn't matter if they got mixed up, we were together through thick and thin, warts and all, and mixing up towels occasionally and not caring was one of the symbols of that.

However, on the first Saturday after chemotherapy, when Patrick learned he had to be so cautious of bacteria, he cleaned out the fridge but he also changed his towel and hand towel to a totally different set of towels. Different color, shape, size, fabric, everything. It's crazy, as I write this I am in tears. Patrick had also learned of the toxicity of chemotherapy and was concerned about it leaving his body each week so he decided to have different towels to protect me from it.

Now every day when I go to the bathroom, I'm reminded just by the towels, of the danger that now looms between us, and that my gorgeous man is in danger, and that the love we share between us is now in danger. It also reminds me of the enormity of what he's going through. It breaks my heart to see the different towels now permanently hanging… such a small thing yet so profoundly significant.

On this same day, Patrick then proceeded to wash all the bed clothes thoroughly, stating that dogs were full of bacteria and Indi couldn't sleep on the bed anymore. I was devastated but said nothing. I knew it was too important to him at the time to stand in his way but I also secretly hoped it would be a five minute wonder, which thankfully by the way, it was. Patrick was too much of a softy when it came to his little girl, and we both loved her sleeping on the bed with us. She is a comfort to us with her unconditional love, her innocence and her need for our comfort too.

Indi was a rescue dog from the Chained Dog Awareness Association - CDANZ. We were only supposed to foster her until they found her a good home but there you go… two years later here she is still on the bed.

Then there's the beer glasses. Patrick has a few of those really large beer glasses that rarely came out of the cupboard. Now they are constantly present - on the kitchen bench, by the bedside, in his office, or the lounge. Wherever Patrick is, a beer glass sits, and wherever he has been, a beer glass sits. Being the largest glass in the house, this was Patrick's preferred choice for filling with water to drink constantly throughout the day and night to flush his body of the chemotherapy toxins. He became obsessed with that, as he had been told to drink up to four litres every day.

I think about how strong the chemotherapy must be. When they say you are getting blasted with chemotherapy it seems to literally be true. The body is blasted with chemicals, the cancer cells receive that blast, and then as quickly as possible, you need to get rid of the residing toxins, like, now! Like fly spray killing a fly. You zap him and he dies almost instantly then you open the windows to rid the unneeded residue!

So now, no matter which room you're in you're bound to find a glass beer mug sitting on a surface somewhere. This type of mug will now always be a reminder of chemotherapy. As a consequence of this vast volume of water, another subtle change to our life has arisen; we always need to be near a toilet. Poor Patrick can't hold on for too long so there have been many holdups while he rushes to the toilet, or we search frantically in some mall or street for one. So toilet hunting has become a part of our life too now.

Something else very significant… honestly, again, it's even the subtlest things that matter… Patrick shouldn't pick up our dog's poop now when we go walking as he has to be careful of bacteria. It's quite funny really, we used to always banter on who would pick it up when we walked our gorgeous dog Indi. Neither of us really minded but preferred not to of course. Now that he has to be so conscious of bacteria, I carry the plastic bag and it's my job alone… and although that has a bit of a laugh with it, it's also very sad that we don't have that banter anymore. These are the small things. Not to mention the expected and obvious like Patrick being so tired and needing to rest or sleep a lot during the day. Fortunately Patrick works for himself so was able to adjust his schedules to accommodate sufficient rest periods.

Patrick has a business performing magic shows for mainly corporate events however this was really a side business, more a hobby that paid him a bit of money, which I'd say he used to help him keep purchasing more magic materials. His main business is a private investigation company… he's a pretty interesting guy right! A large part of Patrick's business was finding people and serving documents to them. Patrick now started to find that sometimes he was too tired to drive for work, and so one of the family, or extended family would drive him to do a serve, an investigative job, or other necessary errands.

Our life was already getting smaller and we found we were venturing out less on the weekends. Saturday night seemed to be a night in now and our weekends seemed to be spent recovering…for both of us. It has been tough giving up almost two weekdays each week going to hospital. We are always shattered after being there and really not much has been getting done those days, so then of course we have got behind on our day to day life, things to do, and our work. And me, well I was on high alert. Patrick just needed to move in the night, or groan, or get up to the toilet, and I was checking in. Was he alright? How was he feeling? Watching and listening with an eagle eye and pointed ears! Was he about to be sick? Was he dizzy? How was his heart? So unlike me as I am definitely not a 'safety' personality type however I'd had enough experience with chemotherapy in past years to feel I had reason to be concerned.

I now sported two new apps on my phone, one for St John Ambulance to tell me how to do CPR on the spot if I needed to, and another 'AED' which can check my location and tell me where the closest defibrillator is.

Another thing I was becoming aware of was the impact of running into people, for the first time since diagnosis, when we were out. When they would ask how you were… well what do you say? If it's someone you know casually we'd just say good, good then transfer it straight back asking after them. If it was someone we knew more intimately, we felt compelled to tell them of Patrick's diagnosis. I know for me that was for two reasons. One, because I didn't want to lie. Two, because I didn't want them to find out from someone else and think we didn't care enough about our friendship to tell them. Even if we weren't close friends I still value every friendship I have on any level. Patrick was very open with telling people himself. He seemed to work on the same philosophy.

Patrick's home is in a small seaside town so we could often get stopped on a trip to the shops, a walk on the beach, or coffee at a local cafe. Trips out could become quite lengthy if we ran into people we knew. The other side was running into people we hadn't previously seen who had heard through the grapevine. The first time that happened was one evening when we were in the supermarket. It was meant to be a quick trip while our Italian takeout was getting made. Patrick ran into a squash buddy who had obviously been told. We were in the vege section and I was some distance away when his buddy came up to him. I could hear their conversation as he asked Patrick how he was doing. He came straight out and told him he had heard he had cancer and asked how he was getting on.

I was quite shocked, I don't know, it just made it all so real. Patrick had only just finished his first week of chemotherapy at that stage and we had only known ourselves for a few weeks and here was, to me, a complete stranger, coming out of the blue discussing his condition in the middle of a public place. It was clear the word was out.

The feeling of everyone knowing seemed to bring the reality so much more to light. I slowly, quietly walked out of the vege section hoping not to be seen by Patrick and be called back to meet his friend. I was in tears, I was overwhelmed. So this was part of adjusting to life with cancer. News like this spreads like wildfire and I felt like that's how people will see us now. The couple with this life threatening illness over them. I felt separate and alone and I wished at that moment we hadn't told anyone, I wished we'd kept it close. But how could we? It would have been virtually impossible. People needed to know for various reasons. I went backwards and forwards with it in my mind as I wandered aimlessly through the aisles waiting for Patrick to catch me up, calming down, pulling myself together as time went on.

Eventually I realised I needed to go back. This conversation had really gone on long enough. I rallied up and went back to meet his lovely squash buddy. I could see he only wanted to be caring towards Patrick and I could see Patrick was really enjoying the support, camaraderie and friendship extended towards him. It meant a lot to him, and I knew at that moment, for Patrick, we had done the right thing. He needed his friends, the community even, to be there for him. Their support helped prop him up.

We quickly finished the last of our shopping and went back to get our takeaway meal only to find we had been away so long the shop was closed. Ha ha, luckily someone was still inside who opened up to give us our food. Living life with cancer!

I'm just going to say here, as time went on and we told more and more people it got really interesting. We began discovering a lot about people and friendships in the way people were responding to Patrick's diagnosis.

Look at this lovely friend of Patrick's that he ran into in the supermarket. I don't think Patrick knew him terribly well but he was so genuinely interested and caring. He took so much time out to stand there and talk to Patrick for as long as he wanted. He genuinely wanted to know how he was, and was caring. The conversation was all about Patrick and you know what? For once it should be. This was a big deal, he deserved it to be all about him. We never heard from that friend again throughout his treatment, but neither did we expect to. He was, I suppose, an acquaintance but that sort of contact and concern and support, even as I write this piece now nearly two years later, meant a lot.

As time went by we noticed there came to be almost categories in the way people reacted towards Patrick having cancer and being in treatment. It seemed the true friends and family were simply devastated. They cry with you, offer help, follow up with messages and phone calls. They invite you to things, want to do things for you to make life easier, bring food. There's a handful of those, if you're lucky it seems. One of those friends was Patrick's best friend Mark. Patrick had told him about his diagnosis soon after he'd told his family. As well as being shocked and sympathetic, Mark was one of the ones that offered to help out in whatever way he could, however he not only just said this, he followed it up with real action. It was the week before chemotherapy was to start that he phoned Patrick out of the blue to tell him he was going to be in Auckland next weekend. Mark lives in Palmerston North and he stated that while he was in Auckland he was coming over to Patrick's for the day, on the Saturday, to do some work around our place, whatever we needed. He reinforced that with Patrick having treatment in just a week, and with it all coming about so quickly, he must have so much to deal with and do, so he was sure there would be some things he could help with.

He wasn't asking, he insisted and I can't tell you how much that meant to both of us. He was right. The coming weekend we were going to be away with the children and the weekend before Patrick had been doing what he could around the house knowing that coming up in the future he may not be able to. He had water blasted the decks, cleaned the windows and did most of the weeding. However there was still a huge garden area that had grown way out of hand at the back of the house, and clearing out of cupboards and the garage etc. That was one of Patrick's worries that he may actually not make it through all of this, and he didn't want to leave me with a mess to deal with, bless him.

So Mark's offer was a godsend. Patrick didn't say no, not that Mark left an opportunity to, and we were very grateful. Mark came that weekend with his brother's truck with a tow bar. We hired a trailer and he, and occasionally Patrick, cleared that overgrown garden out, it was a huge job and took all day, with a large trailer overloaded with weeds being taken to the tip at the end of the day.

I wouldn't let Patrick do much. I was in a real worried stage about him being in his first week of chemotherapy, needing to be conscious he didn't overdo it and have a heart attack. I knew from previous experience that this is a thing; a real thing and yes, I worried a lot about it. Patrick was pretty tired from his first week of chemotherapy, but he had mustered up with Mark coming and managed to do his bit. What a blessing Mark was in more ways than one, it was just so nice to feel that level of support coming from friends. I can't say enough how much that meant. Let alone how nice the garden now looked!

Back to people though, then there are the good friends and family who are shocked, feel bad for you, offer their support, and then you pretty much don't hear anything from them. The odd text or call but it's not going to interrupt their lives, or the ones who seem to care but make sure that you know you already have lots of support around you and don't need them. Seriously?

Then there are the ones who go on and tell you about so and so they know who got cancer and died recently or quickly. The insensitivity of that staggers me to be honest. The next person that does that is going to be sorry and we might not remain friends! Or the ones who really only care about themselves and even in the midst of cancer say, oh sorry to hear that, that's terrible but I've been having a hard time too lately, blah blah blah. (Basically those who don't really give a shit.)

That's just a few of the key responses. As a therapist I know this depends a lot on personality type. We have friends of all sorts of personalities, from all sorts of walks of life, living all sorts of different lives and I love that. We have friends we just go out and have fun with, friends for deep and meaningful conversations, friends for sport, friends for our spirituality, family we hang out with, family we don't. It's been perfect. Different friends, different personalities, all are part of the balance and I love it.

I myself am typically the one who wants to offer help, to be there for friends in need and give my time, energy, love and support… often at a cost to myself. It's my key personality type. Right or wrong it's who I am. As much as I don't want to judge others for being different personalities, they are values I hold dear.

Certainly when you are on the other end of the foot, as I have been with chronic fatigue and now Patrick with cancer, you can't help but feel sadness that the same support is not offered from a number of friends and family. On the other hand, expectation is one of our biggest evils, one of our sure fast ways to unhappiness. It's a dilemma and nearly two years later I'm still trying to work that out. How much does it matter? I can tell you now, it mattered a lot at the time. Going through cancer, it mattered a lot. I felt sad, and yes admittedly resentful, to those that I felt could have and didn't offer any support… but is that just my personality getting in the way? Is it fair I have those expectations? Should I just enjoy people for who they are and not judge or have expectations of them? To be honest this latter option is what got me through, it helped me to let go at the times I did feel lonely, let down, disappointed, even aggrieved.

Without being able to let go I would have found the journey so much more bitter and harder.

As we go on through this story you will hear of that struggle. Little bits here and there. To be honest, when I look back it was a constant struggle in me finding acceptance around this. Although I also have to look to myself. I should have asked. I should have asked for help, for support. Coming from nearly two years later, right here, it's fitting to say this at this point right now. We were in our first month of a 14 month journey of treatment, we should have got a support team together, we should have asked for help. I can't say it enough, don't do this alone, it's too hard!

The previous month, since finding out Patrick had cancer, everything seemed such a blur. Really not much got done. We were so busy, but really it was just spent coping with work, telling our relatives and friends the news, a few jobs were completed around the house, and our holiday with the children was thrown in at the end of it all. But then, getting things done just didn't seem to matter at the time, however now, three weeks later, we have relatively adjusted, and all of a sudden those things have started to build up, so an added stress has started to set in. At the beginning of the third week of chemotherapy I became very stressed with how behind I was with everything outside of Patrick and treatments. My work was suffering and I knew I had to rally up, pull myself together more and get focused. The head space seemed to be there more for other thoughts now, other than life threatening cancer, which is probably why the brain kicked in with this message, 'There is more to life and it's sorta falling apart around you right now!'

It's really quite fascinating watching the mind through this whole process. What it can and can't absorb. How overloaded it can get with shock and shut down. How foggy it can get when afraid, and how it slows down or speeds up to help you cope with situations around you. Now also seeing how it can protect you from worry when you can't cope with it, but then bring it back as soon as you can! Life had changed drastically and the mind was now catching up, we were learning to fit into our new week of two days of chemotherapy, and it was now becoming just a way of life, as many of the other small changes were too now. I thought we were settled, until this particular morning, week three of chemotherapy, the day after Patrick's last treatment for the cycle.

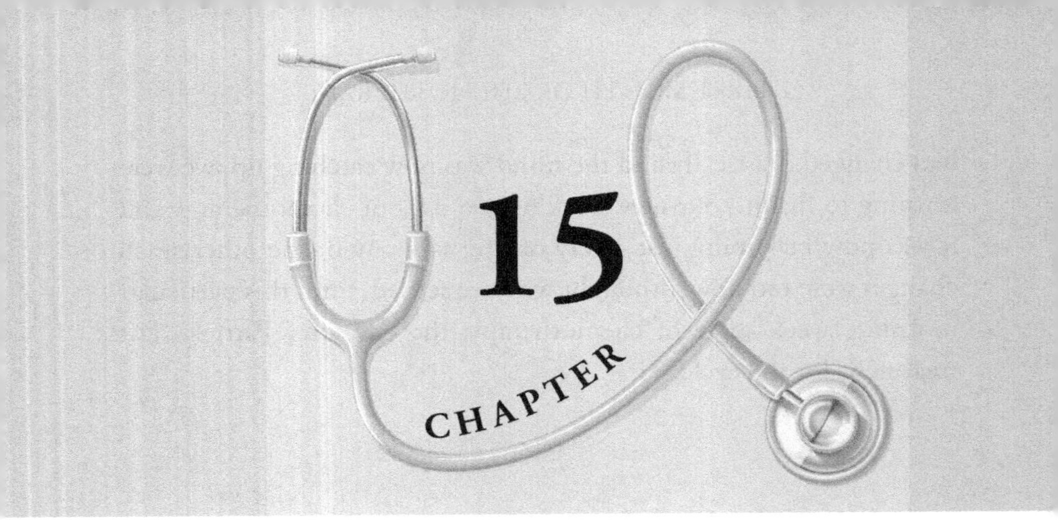

Chromosome 1p32 Deletion

"You may forget with whom you laughed
but you will never forget with whom you wept."
- Kahlil Gibran -

Poor Patrick had hardly slept and was already up when I woke at my usual 5.30am.

By now I wasn't really concerned when I would wake and find he wasn't there. I was used to his medication causing him to sleep so little over the first few days of treatment each week. I messaged him that I was up, the signal for my morning cup of tea, bless him. He came in not long after, just as I was sitting up about to grab my iPad and write for the day. He took one look at me and burst into tears, his face was wracked and he looked just awful. I put my iPad down immediately. "Oh darling" I said, "what's wrong? Come here." patting the bed next to me. Already my heart was aching for him. "Whatever it is," I said, "remember the chemotherapy makes you highly emotional you poor thing. It's probably not as bad as you think." Trying of course to be reassuring.

This was something we were learning to deal with. Each week, by day three after chemotherapy Patrick was highly emotional for one or two days. He climbed on the bed next to me still sobbing. "No it's not that, it's bad." he said. "It's really bad. I don't want to tell you but I have to!" "Oh God darling what is it?" I replied, already starting to hold my breath and feeling time stand still, waiting to hear what else had now been thrown at us. "I have been up all night researching the chromosome 1p32 deletion to find out what it means and it's not good. It's really bad news." he sobbed.

My stomach plummeted. Oh the poor boy. The chromosome 1p32 deletion was of course what had been discovered in the FISH test. We knew that as a chromosome deletion it was an extra complication, but of course I also knew I'd put my head in the sand as I'd not been ready to deal with it. With Patrick starting chemotherapy, it had swept us away over these last few weeks, I'd very successfully parked researching this, and thought Patrick had done the same.

I was so surprised at the state he seemed to be in. At the back of my mind I was still putting his emotion down to the drugs he was taking, they could easily cause him to be highly emotional around matters that perhaps didn't warrant it. Although I felt for him, I did wonder if he was overreacting. Little did I realise that I actually didn't fully know what a 1p32 chromosome deletion truly meant myself. I had read the article Patrick had found - 27 months overall survival with treatment... and of course we hadn't bought into that. On the rare occasions we had talked about it, we'd be dismissive, considering Patrick was now receiving the very latest treatments and we fully expected he would exceed any of these reported statistics.

This morning however this assumption was squashed as he sobbed "I have now got the full report on that study we read. Darling it's a condition that's so rare, this 1p32 deletion. It's actually a chromosome I have missing from every cell in my body." (Actually even now Patrick still didn't have that quite right but that's pretty irrelevant right now). He gasped for breath then continued, "With having multiple myeloma and this chromosome deletion, it means I definitely don't have the same chance as everyone else, I can't fight it the same way even at my age. This study was actually done on young people! People my age! It seems **the prognosis of 27 months is quite real.**" he managed to say through the sobbing.

I almost froze. "What?!" was all I could blurt out. I tried to say more but couldn't, shock started to set in. What was he saying? No way - 27 months - no way. I wanted to speak but I couldn't get the words out. I started stuttering trying to ask again "wh, wh, what?" My mind was trapped in what Patrick had said. Overloaded and stuck in these words of doom, I could not move forward. "Wh, who, what do…" The tears were pouring down my face by now. I felt so helpless and weak. "Pat…, what….?". I couldn't finish a sentence, I was so choked up in fear.

Patrick sat there just sobbing and sobbing. The silence hung between us. What dreadful news was he telling me? Poor Patrick couldn't speak, he seemed caught in such a huge wave of despair.

I sat there so still. I had never experienced this before other than in dreams, that type of dream where the fear is so strong that you can't move or scream as there is so much terror. This truly felt the same and I literally could not form words. Every part of me knew, for him to be this upset, this was a tragedy unfolding! I moved to Patrick and held him as he sobbed away, my own tears silently merging with his. Eventually I finally got out the simplest most obvious question I had been trying to ask. Stiltedly I cried "what… do…you mean?"

Patrick shoved some papers at me, he had been holding them all this time. I found myself staring at the full article of the survey done on 1p32 and multiple myeloma. It was clear now the page we had read a few weeks ago was just the top paragraph of a five page report. Having something tangible was a good thing, it moved me into action and gave me something to do, to melt me down a little into movement, and to help my brain start moving. I grabbed my reading glasses and started to pour over the article. I hadn't gotten far before needing to grab my iPad to start to google and decipher all the words in this article, I needed to understand exactly what on earth it was saying. This helped Patrick too. He rearranged himself and slowly stepped out of his very sad heart into his head, bit by bit, as we started to read the report.

Patrick was leaning tight into me as I had started reading. Quietly spoken he said "You have to read through everything in this article. We can't ignore it, it's all there in black and white." So once again, I started to learn a whole new language as I googled words along the way.

Cytogenetic abnormalities - a broken, missing, rearranged or extra chromosome. In this case for Patrick it is a missing chromosome.

Chromosome deletion - This is where a small piece of chromosome is deleted in each cell. Chromosome deletions are now often tested before treatment at the same time as your FISH test as they have a significant relevance to the complications for your body in fighting for overall survival, and the type of treatment you should undergo can change because of this.

1p32 - is a specific chromosome. Every chromosome type has its own number. With multiple myeloma common chromosome deletions that can be detected are del(17p), del(17/17p), del(1p22), del(1p32), del(13q), del(6q). Additionally in MM there are also translocations where one chromosome swaps with another such as t(4;14), t(14;16), t(14;20). The ones I have named here are ones that can lead to a poorer survival rate.

Progression Free survival (PFS). This term is commonly used. It means the length of time during and after treatment of a disease, such as cancer, that a patient lives with the disease but it does not get worse.

Overall Survival - (OS). The length of time from either the date of diagnosis or the start of the treatment for a disease, such as cancer, that patients diagnosed with the disease are still alive.

Pejorative - this seems to have different meanings depending on the context it is used in. In this case I'd sum it up as meaning 'terrible'.

High Risk Factor (HR) - Higher risk of shorter life span.

Prognostic factor - can be defined as a variable that can be used to estimate the chance of recovery from a disease or the chance of disease relapse.

Univariate analysis - when only one variable is involved. Can yield misleading results in cases in which multivariate analysis is more appropriate.

Multivariate analysis - data collected on more than one independent variable

I went through the report with Patrick at my side, going through it word for word, line by line, trying desperately to get my brain to grips with the content. Googling every word I didn't know as we went so I could fully understand what was being said. Just one word being unclear can change the whole meaning in a medical report.

Straight away the heading is significant.

'Deletion of the 1p32 region is a major independent prognostic factor in young patients with myeloma: the IFM experience on 1195 patients'

Chromosome 1p deletions were present : 7.3pc for 1p32 regions.

It went on to say that in **univariate analysis, 1p32 appeared as a negative prognostic factor for progression free survival (PFS). 1p32 showed : 14.4 months as opposed to without a deletion 33.6 months.**

It also had analysed in **multivariate analysis overall survival (OS) 1p32 showed : 26.7 months as opposed to 96.8 months without a deletion.**

And the result we had read also those few weeks ago:

In multivariate analysis 1p32 deletions appear as an independent negative prognostic fact for PFS and OS for patients with Multiple Myeloma.

Reading this now was so different to when I had first done so a few weeks ago. Patrick's distress left me no option but to take this seriously and acknowledge fully what it was telling us. They are saying life span just over two years. It was sinking in. I looked at Patrick, the tears streaming down my face. I didn't know what to say, and in fact I couldn't speak even if I did. I felt like I was holding my breath waiting to read the full report before I could breathe again. Poor Patrick must have been up for hours reading all this and getting his head around it all on his own, while waiting for me to wake. Bless him.

As we read on, we came to the chart shown here. Little did I realise, this chart would stay fixed in my mind throughout the coming months as a constant reminder of what we were up against.

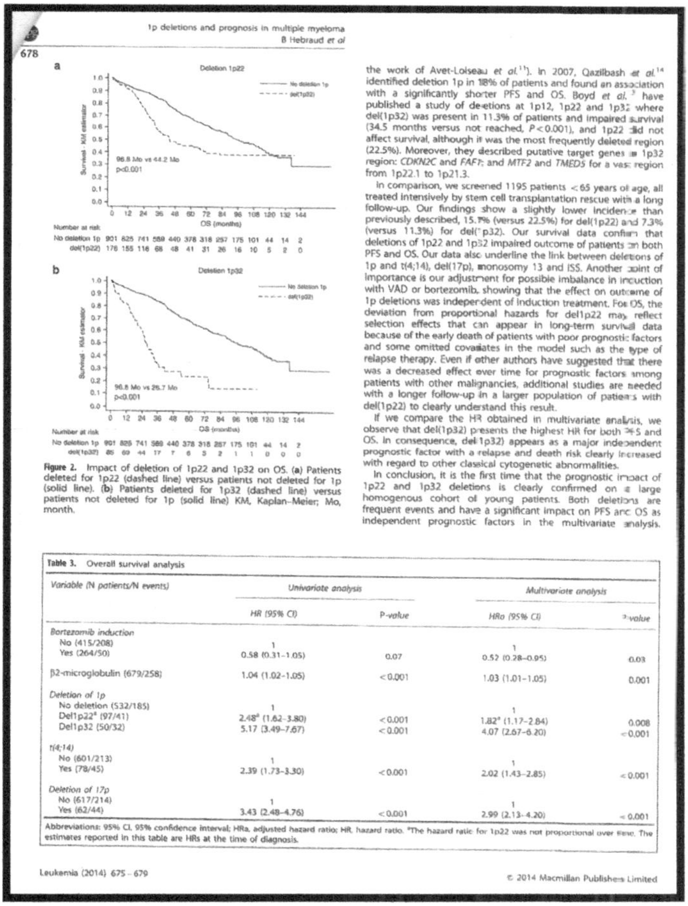

Figure 2. Impact of deletion of 1p22 and 1p32 on OS. (**a**) Patients deleted for 1p22 (dashed line) versus patients not deleted for 1p (solid line). (**b**) Patients deleted for 1p32 (dashed line) versus patients not deleted for 1p (solid line) KM, Kaplan–Meier; Mo, month.

the work of Avet-Loiseau *et al.*[11]). In 2007, Qazilbash *et al.*[14] identified deletion 1p in 18% of patients and found an association with a significantly shorter PFS and OS. Boyd *et al.*[3] have published a study of deletions at 1p12, 1p22 and 1p32 where del(1p32) was present in 11.3% of patients and impaired survival (34.5 months versus not reached, $P<0.001$), and 1p22 did not affect survival, although it was the most frequently deleted region (22.5%). Moreover, they described putative target genes [illegible] 1p32 region: *CDKN2C* and *FAF1*; and *MTF2* and *TMED5* for a vast region from 1p22.1 to 1p21.3.

In comparison, we screened 1195 patients <65 years of age, all treated intensively by stem cell transplantation rescue with a long follow-up. Our findings show a slightly lower incidence than previously described, 15.7% (versus 22.5%) for del(1p22) and 7.3% (versus 11.3%) for del(1p32). Our survival data confirm that deletions of 1p22 and 1p32 impaired outcome of patients [illegible] both PFS and OS. Our data also underline the link between deletions of 1p and t(4;14), del(17p), monosomy 13 and ISS. Another point of importance is our adjustment for possible imbalance in induction with VAD or bortezomib, showing that the effect on outcome of 1p deletions was independent of induction treatment. For OS, the deviation from proportional hazards for del1p22 may reflect selection effects that can appear in long-term survival data because of the early death of patients with poor prognostic factors and some omitted covariates in the model such as the type of relapse therapy. Even if other authors have suggested that there was a decreased effect over time for prognostic factors among patients with other malignancies, additional studies are needed with a longer follow-up in a larger population of patients with del(1p22) to clearly understand this result.

If we compare the HR obtained in multivariate analysis, we observe that del(1p32) presents the highest HR for both PFS and OS. In consequence, del(1p32) appears as a major independent prognostic factor with a relapse and death risk clearly increased with regard to other classical cytogenetic abnormalities.

In conclusion, it is the first time that the prognostic impact of 1p22 and 1p32 deletions is clearly confirmed on [illegible] large homogenous cohort of young patients. Both deletions are frequent events and have a significant impact on PFS and OS as independent prognostic factors in the multivariate analysis.

Table 3. Overall survival analysis

Variable (N patients/N events)	*Univariate analysis*		*Multivariate analysis*	
	HR (95% CI)	*P-value*	*HRa (95% CI)*	*P-value*
Bortezomib induction				
No (415/208)	1		1	
Yes (264/50)	0.58 (0.31–1.05)	0.07	0.52 (0.28–0.95)	0.03
β2-microglobulin (679/258)	1.04 (1.02–1.05)	<0.001	1.03 (1.01–1.05)	0.001
Deletion of 1p				
No deletion (532/185)	1		1	
Del1p22[a] (97/41)	2.48[a] (1.62–3.80)	<0.001	1.82[a] (1.17–2.84)	0.008
Del1p32 (50/32)	5.17 (3.49–7.67)	<0.001	4.07 (2.67–6.20)	<0.001
t(4;14)				
No (601/213)	1		1	
Yes (78/45)	2.39 (1.73–3.30)	<0.001	2.02 (1.43–2.85)	<0.001
Deletion of 17p				
No (617/214)	1		1	
Yes (62/44)	3.43 (2.48–4.76)	<0.001	2.99 (2.13–4.20)	<0.001

Abbreviations: 95% CI, 95% confidence interval; HRa, adjusted hazard ratio; HR, hazard ratio. [a]The hazard ratio for 1p22 was not proportional over time. The estimates reported in this table are HRs at the time of diagnosis.

Leukemia (2014) 675 – 679

© 2014 Macmillan Publishers Limited

The chart relates to overall survival (OS). The chart that is related to 1p32 is the bottom one. Patrick's line, with the deletion he has, is the broken line. It has a significant difference compared to without a deletion. Wow! Yesterday, we thought we were up against it, today it's a whole new ball game.

This chart was so mean. Staring back at us with such dreadful news, so blatantly, obviously and unashamedly pointing out to us that Patrick had high odds of only living a short life. Patrick put his arms around me and held me gently. "I'm sorry," he sobbed. "I'm so sorry, it's such terrible news." We started to rock and cry together, holding each other for such a long time. He sobbed "I don't want to die, I really don't want to die."

My man, my beautiful man. Only about 50% chance of overall survival over two years and about 30% chance of overall survival over three years. No, I didn't want to believe this. I too was sobbing now. Both of us just held each other crying. It was too much. Too much! I tried to speak but literally couldn't. I opened my mouth to speak but words wouldn't come. My brain was now literally frozen in shock and all that came out was a strangled sound. I gave up trying and we just held each other for a long time, holding each other tight, not wanting to ever let go. I don't know how long we stayed like this but finally the sobbing subsided, my brain started to thaw and all I could finally get out was "I'm so sorry, I'm so sorry." again and again and again.

Although I still really didn't understand it all, I knew that most likely Patrick did. He was obviously grappling with the evidence, right in front of his face that he didn't stand much of a chance of surpassing these statistics!

That's all there was for now. It was all I could say as I held him near to me stroking his face and his hair, feeling his lovely soft skin and looking at this gorgeous man. We were in a bubble just the two of us, a bubble we had created just for now, so nothing else could get in but us and our love for each other at this moment.

I have no idea how much time had passed. Slowly though, as we started to calm, the bubble started to dissolve. Outside noises started coming into our space and I began to notice how uncomfortable I was in the position I was in; Patrick started fidgeting. We were coming back to the present. Goodness knows where we had been but I was thankful for the safe place it had offered us, a place of security while we adjusted to the news.

I was the first to speak, blurting out, "How can this be real Patrick? I don't want this to be real," and there it was, my voice getting stronger, more tears, but more grounded ones now. I repeated again, "I don't want this to be real Patrick. How can this be real? Please let it not be real." The tears flowed as I repeated this again and again and again, these words spoken out loud bringing the stark reality into the room. The strength in my voice and my determination to want to fight this propelled me into picking up the report again continuing at where we left off. It wasn't long however before we came to the next bold black and white, in your face section of destruction.

26.7 months survival with 1p32 deletion vs 96.8 months survival without it!

Then to top it all off, at the end of this section:

'If we compare the HR (high risk) obtained in multivariate analysis, we observe that del(1p32) presents the highest HR for both PFS and OS. In consequence, del(1p32) appears as a major independent prognostic factor with a relapse and death risk clearly increased with regard to other classical cytogenetic abnormalities.'

In other words, del(1p32) is one of the worst chromosome deletions for multiple myeloma. So not only is it rare for him to get this, it's in the highest risk group of all cytogenetic abnormalities. What the!!

Having read this Patrick then directed me to another report showing a table of analysis on risk stratification for the key chromosome deletions. This table also was to forever remain embedded in my mind.

Table 3. Cytogenetic risk stratification of myeloma

Risk stratification	*Cytogenetic abnormalities*
Standard risk[a]	Trisomies
	t(11;14)
	t(6;14)
Intermediate risk[a]	t(4;14)
	Gain(1q21)
High risk	Del(17p)
	t(14;16)
	t(14;20)
	Del(1p)

Modified from Rajkumar.[1] [a]Presence of del 17p indicates high risk MM regardless of other abnormalities; gain(1q21) (without other high risk abnormalities) is considered intermediate-risk.

Here was a chart showing the degree of high risk for the chromosome deletions. Risk stratification basically means the level of risk you are at of dying earlier compared to other chromosome deletions. Each deletion has its own risk factor going from Standard to High Risk. Some deletions have a less serious effect than others. Any of these deletions were not good news and here was the graph on the severity of them all.

I started scanning down from Risk Stratification. It was clear that the top of the chart listed the best outcome of all the risk factors and it went down from there. As I went down the chart searching for 1p32 I felt like I got smaller and smaller until there was almost nothing left of me when I got to the bottom. The last line at the bottom of the chart, and in the highest group of all risk factors was the 1p deletion!!! By now I'd almost disappeared, the significance of this fully setting in, it was a death sentence handed out on this table. This simple black and white list staring me in the face, telling me the man of my life had the hardest chance of all to fight this terrible cancer. I felt so weak, so defenseless, so useless and so small. No wonder he was so distraught. No wonder the reality of this had hit him so hard. No wonder he wasn't coping with these findings!

I had to do something, and I found myself rising up with a fight of my own. "This is shocking Patrick. Why has the specialist not covered this with us at all? Why have we not been more informed? We need to call and talk to him today. We need to know if this is true, and what we can do, and find out more about what this means, and, and…." I felt myself growing bigger and bigger with each statement of blame. Throwing it back at someone seemed to help make me stronger. It was giving me strength that this was at least something I could do. My God. This changed everything and Patrick confirmed that as he quietened me down.

"We will darling, we will," he spoke softly, "but to be honest, I want to do more research on this first, find out as much as I can. We are seeing the specialist at the beginning of the second cycle so we can bring it up then." He continued quietly "I've got to think more now about what I really want to do with my life. What I want to do with what time I have."

Oh so sad. I realised he'd had time this morning to absorb this information and time to process it already. I had to put myself aside immediately, and try to catch up. Catch up to be present with him and where he was now. I was so very desperate to be able to support him, to be there for him. I knew I had to push through the fear and the shock even if just for this moment, so I could settle with him. In that, somehow, as we allowed ourselves to fall together into the acceptance of this new finding, we opened miraculously into a beautiful embrace and just like that, a new journey began. We lay there talking for quite some time and I couldn't stop holding him, stroking him, touching and feeling his soft skin, his silky hair, unshaven face, his manly body. I couldn't get enough of knowing he was right here with me now. The reality slowly was sinking in as Patrick went on to talk about what this meant to him.

"I've just got to think about what I really want to do with my time darling," he said countless times. I think saying it out loud was helping him to come to the realization that he really does need to do that. "I have to think seriously on what I want to do with my weeks off chemotherapy for starters." Then a big question "and I have to consider whether I want to do the stem cell transplant!"

I was shocked in one way to hear him say that, but in another way not surprised. I had already done a little googling on stem cell transplants, though Patrick had asked me not to, plus a friend of mine had been through it for leukemia a few years ago.I knew it was a gruelling experience that took a real toll on you, not just physically but emotionally too.

"Why are you questioning that?" I asked. He hadn't at all up until now, I had hoped it wasn't because he was giving up on treatment! He started to speak slowly, not a good sign with Patrick. This usually meant he was finding it difficult to say what needed to be said. "Well, it's just that in doing all this googling on this 1p32 deletion darling… It seems that with this chromosome missing… well, I'm worried I may not recover well from the stem cell treatment. Once they blast everything… I'm not sure it's a given that I will properly recover from it."

There it was, another indication of the possible enormity of the meaning of this 1p32 chromosome deletion. "I don't know." he continued, "I'll have to speak to the specialist… If that is the case I may choose not to have it, to enjoy what time I have left, rather than get trashed to prolong what may be a poor quality of life."

Oh God. I held him tight next to me. Are we really having this conversation?

"If I do decide to take it though… these next four months may be the best time left of my life… and so I really do need to consider what I want to do with that." I started stroking him again as I lay in his arms. His arm, his face, his chest; trying to soothe him, though I think in fact soothing myself too.

"Of course darling, you do. You so do! You really have to do that," The tears started to flow again and, in my pent up confusion, I burst out indignantly "but Patrick we need to see the specialist. This is huge. These are huge life decisions. This is huge for you to carry this burden and worry.

Honestly, NZ's health system can be so stretched. Our doctors and specialists work long hard hours. Their days are packed with an endless line of patients to see and then there are those who are waiting in an invisible line still to be seen at all; a continuous stream. When I thought about it more fully, getting an appointment would probably be virtually impossible before our scheduled one in two weeks anyhow… but maybe just a phone call? I didn't want to wait, but I didn't push any further so I let go, knowing this was Patrick's journey not mine. I had to leave it to him to make his own decisions.

It was Patrick's turn to now reach out and comfort me. He put his big strong arms around me and held me tight in a firm embrace. We lay talking for I don't know, another hour. Tears were shared as we became closer and closer talking about possibly a new future now. One that was not five to possibly ten years of being together, to possibly only two or three years together if we were lucky. With this new realisation, we both knew it could even mean less and life had become even more precious!

Finally Patrick and I got up to get on with the day. I hopped in the shower and the warm water was soothing, calming, a welcome relief. After drying, I wrapped the towel around me and walked back into the bedroom. There was the report still sitting on the bed. I decided to go through it again and this time I wanted to pick holes in it, this time to find a way it could be wrong.

I did come up with a glimmer of hope, it was under the title 'Patients and Methods'.

'We studied 1195 patients with newly diagnosed MM, younger than 66 years of age. They were all treated by induction therapy VAD (Vincristine-Adriamycin-Dexamethasone) or bortezomib-based induction followed by high dose melphalan autologous stem cell transplantation in IFM centres.'

Well right there thank you very much!

Firstly they are classing young as under 66. Patrick was only 53 so surely that would still give him an advantage.

Secondly the treatment drugs that Patrick was taking included Carfilzomib, the latest in chemotherapy drugs that was already getting better results.

And third but not least the trial did not include consolidation therapy of which Patrick was having four months (as part of the Kiwi Trial), nor did it include maintenance therapy which he was almost certainly going to have when he finished the Kiwi Trial.

So yep, a glimmer of hope. Patrick's treatment plan was going to be superior to the treatments in this study. Who knows what influence this might have. I rushed off to tell him my findings. "That's great that you've picked that up," he said "but it's still not good, you need to prepare yourself. This chromosome deletion is not good." It seemed to do nothing to alleviate how he felt. Damn! Hot damn! What were we to do?

At the end of this chapter I have included a photo of Patrick's FISH test. You really need to ask to see this report if you have a FISH test done. Don't just rely on being told the results! In fact if you're not scheduled to have a FISH test done, insist that you do. You need to know if you have any chromosome abnormalities!

The next two days were pretty rough and emotionally, very draining as the shock of this discovery slowly subsided. We seemed to be constantly adjusting and I'd like to think we were getting better at this. Life goes on. By Saturday I'd woken at my usual 5.30am feeling quite fresh and alive as we'd had a good early night and a good night's sleep after the exhaustion from the week's events.

It was a beautiful morning. Patrick and I both had good energy so we decided to go for a long early walk as the tide was fully out at 7.30am. We live in an amazing area in Auckland called the North Shore. The land is lined with sandy beaches, each one denoting a suburb of residential homes. There is a cliff walk that runs along through the beaches from where Patrick lives in Browns Bay, that goes for miles and miles, so you can literally walk from one beach to another. Even when the tide is in you can walk mainly on the beaches or on the cliff path, only occasionally needing to walk through the residential streets. It really is beautiful and I never take it for granted how lucky we are to be able to walk amongst the rustic stunning nature of NZ. We always take Indi on these walks of course. She walks off lead the whole way or should I say runs, sniffs, forages and swims. It's doggy heaven and she gets to catch up with lots of doggy friends along the way.

We drove to a nearby suburb, Mairangi Bay, and began the walk back to Browns Bay, a walk of around 45 minutes taken at a leisurely pace. It is not yet summer so the temperature at this time was about 14ºC/57ºF. It was a cloudy day but it was calm and still and peaceful. Not many people were up and about so we had plenty of opportunity to talk freely as we went on our way. It was Patrick's week off chemotherapy and he seemed to have enough energy today, thankfully, to go for this nice walk.

It wasn't long before the conversation turned to Patrick's latest findings about 1p32. He asked me what I wanted. He was coming to the conclusion that these next four months before stem cell transplant may end up being literally the best months of his life. I couldn't argue with him as it all felt so unknown. There were tough questions we still needed to ask the specialist however that appointment wasn't for another eleven days!

"What do you mean, what do I want?" I questioned. "Patrick, what do you want to do, is more the question? You have to really do some soul searching and feel into what you really want to do with this time. The last thing you, or I for that matter, want is for you to be looking back in six months time saying if only…."

So typical of him, thinking of others before himself. Honestly, that is Patrick to a 'T'. But that wasn't going to work today! "Seriously Patrick, you don't know how long you have of feeling good. Maybe we will get a clearer picture when we see the specialist, maybe we won't, but what we do know is you need to make the most of every moment that you do feel good. You don't want to be on your deathbed wishing you had done so much more when you could have. Seriously!"

Did I cross the line, was I too direct? Oh this is so hard, but who else is going to say it so frankly. The words hung in the air, not even the slight sea breeze taking them away. Even though I'd said it, a part of me was still not believing it. It was like I was split in two, the part of me who knew this possibility and the other part of me who felt it was a dream to be woken from.

I picked up again, going forward to encourage him to get positive and think for himself and his own needs. "There are so many things to consider Patrick, like for example where you want to live? Are you happy where you are?"

"Yes, yes," he jumped in. "I'm quite happy where I am living for now." Good I was getting him engaged.

"I guess I need some time to really think about what I'd like to do. If these are my best months, do I want to keep working for example?" Definitely on track now! "I wonder whether I want to go traveling, and where? On the weeks I don't have chemotherapy, what could I be doing with the children and things like that." he continued. "I think it's good that you're going away this week darling, it will give me some good space to really consider all of this."

I was going to Dunedin on the coming Monday. My son Taylor had finished university so it was time for him to pack up and come home. He was going to drive back, taking his time traveling up the country with most of his gear, including three surfboards, however he needed his cat, also called Indi, brought home by plane. We also had a couple of fun things we wanted to do in Dunedin together before he left. I had booked this months ago and fortunately the time away fell in the week Patrick was off treatment so I'd continued with the plan.

As we walked on, heading up the only slight hill we had to climb on this part of the cliff walk, the conversation turned to what we were going to do today. It was Katelyn's birthday, so we discussed the plans for the day and formed a list of things to do, all the way enjoying our beautiful surroundings. We have done this walk many times. It was always about exercise and enjoying the fresh air and beauty, we didn't normally stop along the way, but today was different. Half way along there is a lovely bench seat that Patrick suggested we sit on and take a moment. I gladly obliged and I sidled up right next to him. With his arm around me we sat there in silence and it was very romantic. We looked out over the lovely green park, looking out across the ocean and the islands in the distance, Indi was having a ball racing around. The sun was shining and right here right now all was good.

igenz

PO Box 106-542
Auckland 1143, New Zealand
Tel +64-9-307 3981
Fax +64-9-307 3983
www.igenz.co.nz

Patient Name: **HENSHALL, Patrick**	Lab Number: 17N1938	Date collected: 09/10/2017	Referring Doctor: Dr R Henderson Ross.Henderson@waitematadhb.govt.nz
DOB: 08/07/1964 Age: 53 Sex: Male		Received: 09/10/2017	Copies to:
Specimen Type: Bone Marrow Aspirate Tissue Origin:	Ref Number: 17B239933	Reported: 11/10/2017	

FISH Report

INDICATION:
New diagnosed multiple myeloma
Kiwi Study

RESULTS:

Probe	ISCN	Comment
Zytovision Zytolight Spec TP53/CEN 17 Dual Colour Probe	nuc ish(TP53,D17Z1)x2[200]	
Vysis LSI IGH Dual Color Breakapart	nuc ish(IGHx1)[174/200]	Loss of one copy
C[illegible]cell Aquarius CKS1B/CDKN2C (P18) Amplification/Deletion Probe	nuc ish(CDKN2Cx1,CKS1Bx2)[171/200]	Loss of CDKN2C

IMAGES:

Zytovision Zytolight Spec TP53/CEN 17 Dual Colour Probe

Vysis LSI IGH Dual Color Breakapart

Cytocell Aquarius CKS1B/CDKN2C (P18) Amplification/Deletion Probe

COMMENT:
Interphase *in situ* hybridisation analysis showed loss of one copy of CDKN2C (1p32) and IGH (14q32) in 171 and 174 cells out of the 200 cells examined.

There was no evidence of an IGH (14q32) gene rearrangement and the normal diploid complement of CKS1B (1q21), TP53 (17p13) a[illegible] D17Z1 (chromosome 17 centromere) was observed in all 200 cells examined.

SUMMARY / INTERPRETATION:
CDKN2C (1p32) - Loss of one copy
IGH (14q32) - Not Rearranged, loss of one copy
CKS1B (1q21), TP53 (17p13), D17Z1 (17cen) - Normal diploid complement

Loss of 1p is a recognised finding in myeloma and is associated with a less favourable prognosis.
(Walker et al. Blood (2010) 116:56-65; Qazilbash MH et al. Biol Blood Marrow Transplant (2007) 13:1066-1072)

Authorised by:

Senior Scientist

18/10/17

IANZ

In situ hybridisation analysis using DNA probes targets specific loci only and will not detect other genetic anomalies. Uncertainty of measurement applies to interphase analysis at a 95% confidence interval These results adhere to NPAAC guidelines at the time of reporting.
*Probe names used are those described by the manufacturer, which may not reflect current HUGO nomenclature.

CONFIDENTIAL REPORT
Laboratory Enquiries Tel: (09)3073981

Page 1 of 1

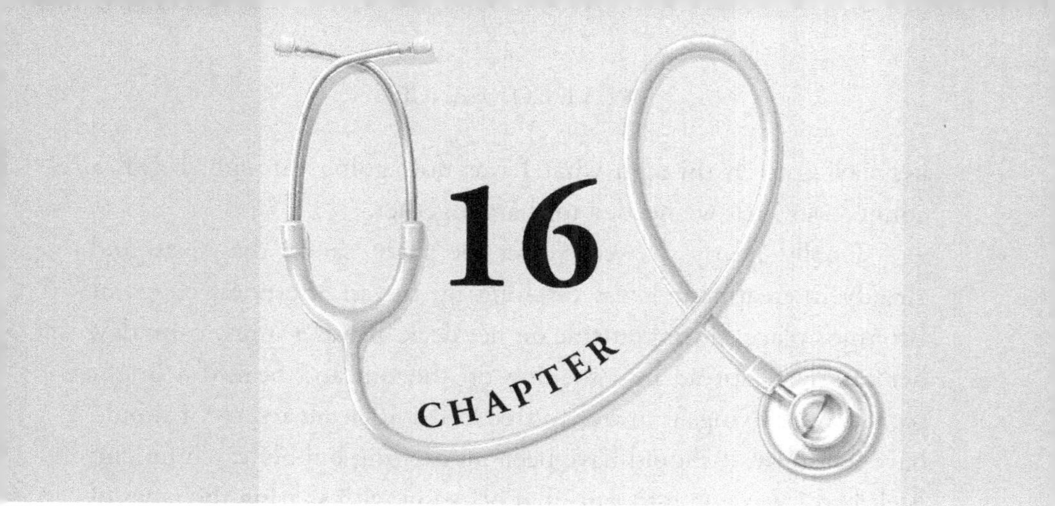

Faith

"Faith doesn't always mean that God
changes your situation, sometimes
it means he changes you."
- Steven Furtick -

I had been so caught up in Patrick's first weeks of treatment and coping with it all in so many ways that I still hadn't reached out to many friends to tell them of his diagnosis and it was starting to stress me out. One person high on my list was Bronnie.

Bronnie was a friend who I'd trained with, in one of the key therapies I use in my counselling work. She was top of the list for two reasons. We missed her 50th birthday party, if you recall, on the night Patrick's eardrum had worsened, (pre-cancer diagnosis) and I wanted to catch up and give her the gift I had bought. Everything had been such a whirlwind since and I hadn't been to see her yet. The other reason was that Bronnie lost her husband about 10 years earlier, after a long fight with cancer. I had been really wanting to share Patrick's diagnosis with her as kindred spirits. I also wanted to ensure she didn't find out about it from someone else first. With her having been through what I was now going through, it was a connection I felt we needed to share together.

Finally, nearly six weeks after the party, cancer diagnosis, and already in treatment I was catching up for an afternoon cuppa at Bronnie's place, sitting outside on her deck. It was a sunny calm day, her cats were spread out, soaking up the sun and beautiful bright parrots were flying from tree to tree in the adjacent reserve. I should have felt great, it should have been an exciting bubbly catch up and I felt bad I was going to ruin that occasion with sharing the news of Patrick's condition.

I'd become increasingly aware of how destructive this announcement can be with the handful of friends I'd told already. They may have called me to say hi, or when I had caught up with them in person, I'd have to give them this depressing news. We cry and it's devastatingly horrible. They don't know what to say, there is nothing to say really. Nothing can make it right, no one can make it right. Then we are left with this abyss of darkness and emptiness between us that can't be taken away.

So now, visiting Bronnie, I was very conscious about how this news was going to affect our afternoon. Of course she was shocked. Everyone is shocked… but like Nikki, Bronnie lost her husband to cancer too. Bronnie and Jock, her husband, had three children and were such a beautiful family. Dear Jock fought very hard and Bronnie was such a pillar of strength and determination for him. She is an inspiration to me in looking into my time ahead with Patrick.

So we sat over cups of tea and talked and talked about her experiences with Jock, what was happening so far with Patrick, how we were coping, how they coped, how the family coped with Jock's passing, and how they have been since. Bronnie has since gone into a new relationship, but Jock's memory sits right there on the mantelpiece in the lounge, still very much a part of their lives and of course, always in their hearts. Bronnie and her three children were going on holiday to Hawaii in just two weeks; being the anniversary of ten years since Jock's passing, she thought it would be a lovely thing to do with the children.

To be honest, I came away quite rocked. The reality of cancer and the long term effects hit me today more than ever as I saw in front of me a picture of the carnage it causes, the grief, and how that never goes away. Ten years later the family is still mourning and is still deeply affected by the loss of this great man they all loved.

I wondered what it would be like for me. Would Patrick's girls still be a part of my family then? Would my boys be so affected like Bronnie's children were, considering Patrick is not their actual father, even though I know they love and respect him very much and dearly value and love him as their stepdad. I suddenly felt very alone. I cried a little while Bronnie was sharing the beauty of the love they all still shared together, ten years later. But in the background I felt the reality that I would be alone as the years went on, carrying my own form of grief, different to Patrick's girls, different to my boys. We were not a whole family in the same way as Bronnie and Jock and their children were.

And what am I doing talking about all this death anyhow! That night I woke suddenly in the early hours with such a feeling of guilt, it was 4.30am. My heart was so heavy as I recalled leaving Bronnie's. I had made a light hearted comment that I had joined the club as I hugged her goodbye. Bronnie was friends with Nikki and she knew immediately I was referring to the club of friends who's partners not only had cancer but passed away from it. The conversation had just turned that way so easily, given Bronnie's experience, and the reality of cancer was so apparent, that we went there… but in these early hours of the morning I felt sick to my stomach that I had spoken this way before its time. Who knows, I may even die before Patrick. I felt like in some weird way that conversation about Jock's death and their experiences and impact, and our focus on that, had me giving up on Patrick before we had even started!

So it was interesting to observe. Right there and then in the wee hours I decided that in future I would fight for Patrick when talking to others. I will be true and honest with the situation but I don't want to discuss his passing away in any way with them. I decided not to invoke those words, entertain that conversation, or put it out there in any way that this was going to happen. It wasn't denial; we all die one day and none of us ever know when that will be. That is the reality for all of us, it could be tomorrow or even today. Sure Patrick's odds have increased and it looms as a threat now more so than a month ago. Sure we know he won't live to be an old man, but do any of us really know that we will ourselves?

Some people, when I tell them, say "It's not fair." That doesn't resonate for me at all. I guess the philosophical side of me is very strong. Years of studying at the school of philosophy plus my spiritual understanding holds me in good stead for acceptance of what comes. I'll never forget reading a comment from the Dalai Lama that the sooner people realise life deals you shit and accept that, the happier we will be. It perhaps wasn't said as forthright as that, but that's my version of interpretation. Expecting life to be perfect, to go your way, and to be disappointed or offended or hard done by when it doesn't, seems stupid and ignorant. OK so we can feel sad, distraught, shocked, traumatized, but 'that it's not fair?!' That only creates resentment and helplessness and we create that ourselves so unnecessarily. So thankfully that's one thing less on the load I'm carrying now.

I lay awake for the rest of the night. I had opened my curtains as soon as night started turning to day and I felt a shift in myself as I watched the sun start to rise and the sky start turning blue. The song comes to mind "It's a new day, a new way, a beginning." The focus of my conversations from here on are to be around treatments, remissions, mrd-, new discoveries in medicines and living life to the full while it's here, right here, right now, in this moment. It's all we have, all we really know, it's all we have truly got. Right now is what we have and this we will make the most of, whatever that will be. It may be a day of rest, it may be a day of chemotherapy, a day in the office, or it may be a day feeling good catching up on things, a walk on the beach, a movie or a picnic in the park. It may be watching the clouds go by, or feeling the sun on our skin, or laughing with family, or watching our dog sleep. Seeing the beauty in nature, or reading a good book. Right here, right now. That's what we have, and that's what we will focus on.

My spirit lifted and the room became even lighter… brighter. **You've gotta have faith right!** The dictionary meaning of faith - **'complete trust or confidence in someone or something'.** I invoked this in this moment, together with the 'law of attraction'! Believe, visualize, know, and you shall receive. MRD- here we come. I invoked my faith in Patrick, and I invoked my faith in his treatment plan… and then in this moment I let go.

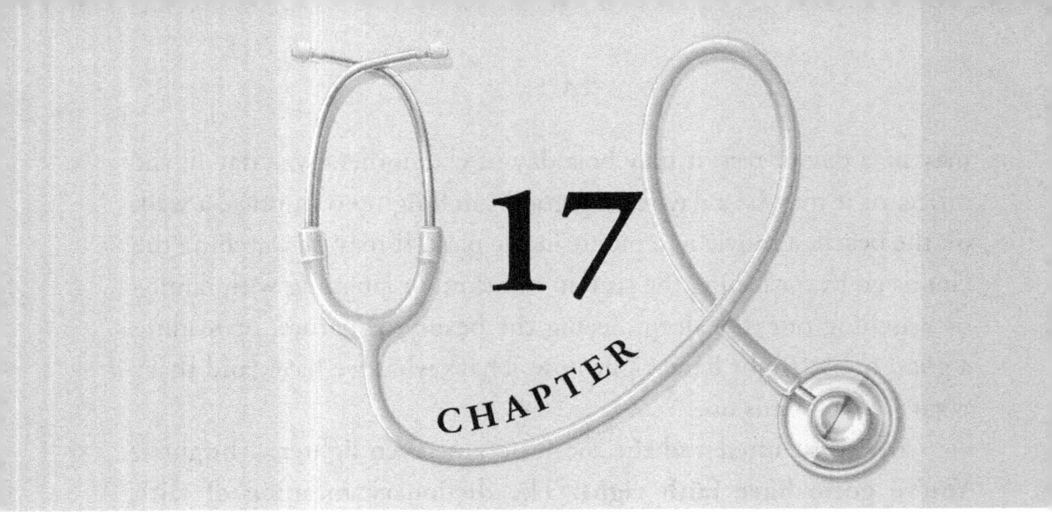

CHAPTER 17

Grief

"We choose our joys and sorrows
long before we experience them"
- Kahlil Gibran -

I was really looking forward to my trip to Dunedin. Taylor and I had so many lovely things planned and the weather forecast was looking great. In the same breath, however, I was uneasy about leaving Patrick. Thank goodness chemotherapy had coincidentally finished its first cycle, with this being his break week, or I really don't think I could have forced myself to go. I realised I was still very protective of him.

Patrick decided to take me out to the airport. Katelyn was off school and he offered to make it a driving lesson for her so she could get some good driving experience before sitting her license soon. On the way out to the airport, a 50 minute drive, I started to feel anxious and empty leaving him. I didn't say anything, I knew this would only upset him, and Katelyn was in the car. The excitement of going away fell away completely and I really just wanted to stay at home with him. I knew this couldn't or wouldn't happen, but I was surprised at how strongly I felt. By the time we got to the airport I was flat and quite low in myself. Patrick came into the airport with me while Katelyn waited in the car. Once I'd checked in I quickly said goodbye to him so he wouldn't notice how I was feeling and then worry.

As I walked through the gate to the departure lounge I shed a few tears. What was going on? Oh God, it was too hard saying goodbye, I didn't want to say goodbye, I never wanted to say goodbye. I didn't want to say goodbye now or ever, and the enormity that now one day, in possibly the near future I may have to say goodbye forever, really hit me. I fell into a deep sense of grief and sadness. So much for keeping positive about Patrick's future, or maybe it was because of this vow that I couldn't help what was rising. Sick to my stomach I went through the actions of getting on the plane. When I was finally seated with my seat belt on I quietly let the tears flow. I didn't care about the man next to me, I had said my hellos and blocked him from there, this was not a time for anyone else. This was my time to open into what was really here, it had come out to bite me and I needed to face the grief that was overwhelming me now.

I think in my new conviction it was bringing up what I had been storing, the depth of grief at the thought of losing my lovely man, the love of my life. My partner, who knew me more than anyone and loved me, warts and all. The man who shared so much of my life with me, my companion, my mate. Traveling alone I thought of how much we had traveled together, how great we were together enjoying seeing new sights and traveling the world. We had so much more we were going to do. Who would travel with me once he was gone? Who would be my companion? I quickly dropped into the loneliness that would be waiting for me when Patrick was gone, and there I met fear. It tried to swallow me up there and then. I couldn't let it right here on the plane so I pulled away from it. It tried to take me back, pull me back. I struggled saying in my head, NO! I can't see you right now, I can't deal with you right now, I have to move away. Get away from you until I have the right space and time to face you fully!!

Thank you again mind for rescuing me that day. With great strength I used it to pull myself away from these feelings and the emotion that was drawing me deeper into such a dark, scary and hopeless place. I'd had no idea until now that I had been holding on to such a deep sense of grief. Of course it makes sense. I had just thought I was handling it all so well, yet here it was, fear, right here in the core of grief. I knew to move on, free with positivity for Patrick. I would need to process the grief, but here on the plane just wasn't that time!

I drew my attention to the people on the plane. The emergency drill had begun and I focused on the inflight video. It was Air NZ and they have a different video every month, so my mind grabbed that as an excuse to focus on who was in this new video and I was saved. I was still left feeling extremely flat but now I could cope; I pulled out my iPad once we took off and the trip began.

My dear son Taylor picked me up from the airport and after a 'tiki tour' of some of Dunedin's amazing surf beaches he took me to my girlfriend Leigh's, where I was staying. I tried my best to be cheery for Taylor as he too had been looking forward to these couple of days together. By the time we got to Leigh's, however, I couldn't pretend anymore. Taylor had left and Leigh made the first of our many cups of tea; we sat on the couch and I poured my heart out. Like a true friend she was amazing, listening and crying with me until I was spent. I felt like a train wreck, exhausted and just a shell of myself. We mustered up and managed to pop out for a meal and by 9pm I was going to bed. Leigh came and sat with me and was sharing a story about herself that I duly fell asleep listening to. This pent up emotion had been too much and I drifted off and hoped tomorrow would be a new day. When I woke, the sun was shining and it was a beautiful day. I'd had a good eight hour sleep and I felt so much better. I let my mind only fall on what was ahead for the day. After my dumping the night before I felt ready to enjoy my trip to Dunedin, so I was very thankful.

Taylor and I had booked e-bikes to bike around the harbour inlet. It's an amazing paved road that runs flat right along one side of the harbour, suitable for both walking and cycling. The winding road takes you through a series of little beach inlets and suburbs, each with their own character and charm and biking along I felt I could be anywhere in the world, it was spectacular. The tide was in, the sun was shining and it was a beautiful, calm day. It couldn't have been more perfect. "Yeehaa!" I yelled as we moved the bikes into top speed and raced along... past watersheds, quaint homes and idyllic wee beaches that, on such a still day, seemed like pieces of art. Being a week day, almost no one was about. A smattering of cars would pass at times but it felt we had the place to ourselves.

After about five or six kilometers the path disappeared and we had to ride on the road. This was a little scary as the road was built into the cliff edge and quite narrow and winding with no room for a car to overtake us, especially if another car was coming the other way. Taylor and I decided if cars were coming behind us we would pull over so they could pass and, as there were not many, this didn't seem too big a problem for us to do.

I decided to tell Taylor to ride in front. "You ride in front Tooty," I said. Tooty being the affectionate childhood name that evolved for Taylor from when he was very young. "Oh, why?" he asked. "That way if a car comes up behind us and hasn't seen us, he'll get me first." I replied. "It's better that way, I've had a life, you haven't!" Taylor got this immediately and accepted it without question. Of course that made sense and was right. "Oh, OK." he simply said and rode on in front of me.

What Taylor didn't realise was the internal dialogue that was going on, for the first time in my life I really didn't care if I died. It was so clear and staring me in the face as I was biking and I couldn't believe the thoughts that were coming. Well then you won't have to suffer the grief and loneliness. Who knows there may be life after death and you will be with Patrick longer then. It all felt perfectly aligned and OK if I died today. I was loving what I was doing right now with Taylor and that would also be a great way to go. I wasn't feeling suicidal, or wanting an accident to happen, I just felt so at peace with it.

I felt at the time quite comfortable with this mindset, although of course later I realised this was not good at all. This trip and the space I was getting from Patrick was slowly evolving to show me how much I needed help myself! It didn't stop me having fun this day with Taylor though and we stopped en route to a cute little cafe in one of the seaside inlets for a cuppa on the way back. We biked for a good few hours before we handed in the bikes and finished with lunch at the gorgeous homestead there which had award winning historical gardens. We sat outside on the balcony and ate away all the good we had done with our bike ride, and then carried on seeing the sights of Dunedin.

We went to find some old army bunkers built into the hills. Thanks to a friend of Taylor's texting directions and Google we found them… a needle in a haystack really, but well done Taylor in finding them. It was a trek through gorse and a bit of bush to get there and on the way we passed a fairy flower… well at least that's what I call them. A Dandelion. I always pick one if I see them and make a wish. I picked it and out of habit, went to make a wish, but stopped short. It was like a brick wall had arisen and the flower couldn't reach me. Taylor had stopped behind me and was watching me. I immediately gave it to him. "Here, Taylor, make a wish," I said. "No you Mum." he replied, not taking the flower. I thrust it out at him and said "No please, I want you to." and I put it up to his mouth to blow. He graciously accepted, my sensitive boy knew something emotional was going on so he took the flower from me and made his wish, and then blew the fairy away to carry it out for him.

We carried on the path but my mind was racing as strong emotions arose. What was that all about? Why couldn't you make a wish? What's going on Kushla? I was scrambling in my mind when it came to me. What's the point? The one wish I want I can't have, there was no point in making a wish… then the tears started to prick my eyes. Oh God, what now! In my mind's eye I saw myself on my birthday blowing out the candles. That's what I wished for every birthday… without fail, for years and years, my birthday wish was always for everyone I loved to be healthy and well. I can't say my wish now. Because it didn't work, it's not worth saying it now, the spell has been broken. The wish didn't work! My wish wasn't granted. Damn wishes for me. Damn them! I was ignored, so they are not for me anymore. I was choked up, fighting the tears. I walked on ahead trying to pull myself together so as not to ruin this expedition for Taylor.

I felt my whole being shift. My heart, my soul, my mind, my emotions, my maturity, my outlook, everything shifted. I looked out over the pristine glowing blue waters below me and out to the land across the inlet which was surrounded by beautiful white sand. At that moment I felt I moved into another lifetime. Just like that I left the innocence of my old life of fairy stories and wishes and into a lifetime of a stronger maturity. I passed away the delight in magic and transcended into a life of harsh reality; I was reborn with a thud. I didn't like what I had landed into but as I looked out at the beauty around me acceptance was there. It is what it is and this new lifetime now goes on.

I thank God I was where I was at this moment. As I looked down the inlet now with all of nature's beauty opening before me, it helped me to realise I will be OK. I didn't feel so alone knowing nature is always an amazing comforter for me.

I turned around and there was my dear son quietly following. I had my beautiful children to follow me into this lifetime too, I would find my way. I was stripped of this childhood innocence and joy but I would find a new way to exist in this new lifetime. The universe was leading me and I would follow.

My urge to keep connected to nature grew and on the way home I suggested to Taylor we do the night trip to see the penguins come in. It's a sight I had always wanted to see but had never given myself the opportunity to do. Well this was interesting, this new lifetime was opening me; encouraging me to do what really feels good and comforting, and for me that often centers around nature.

What a treat that night was, it is one of the most amazing and cute nature experiences I've ever seen. The penguins come in stages. They form bunches out at sea and swim in en mass to protect themselves from predators. Watching on, all you see is a large dark mass in the water coming closer, then, as they get to shore their little heads pop up and they become individual penguins. Their white bodies then show as their feet hit the ground and they waddle together up the sand and over the rocks to rest in the dunes for the night. What a delight, as then another dark mass forms in the water and comes closer and closer to shore. Again on reaching the safety of land, their heads pop up, their little white tummy's stand out in the darkness as their feet plonk on the sand and another dozen or so penguins start waddling up the sand.

It filled my heart with joy, I was so delighted and happy. By the end of the night I truly knew I really was going to be OK. This new life, though beginning steeped with sadness, grief, and the fear in loss, I was going to be OK.

The following day was my last day in Dunedin. Taylor and I had our last mission to achieve, visiting the archaic churches built in the late 1800's… well archaic for NZ. These buildings of stature and magnificence are made of brick and stone and I had been wanting to visit them for years, so how appropriate, in this new lifetime I was now achieving this.

The Church that struck me the most turned out not to be the largest or grandest of them all; it was St Joseph's Church which on entering, had a lovely softness to it. Attention to detail was evident in the surrounds and arches where lovely flowers and birds were etched into wood or stone. Oh I've just realised as I write this, nature was present. No wonder I felt so struck by it.

However, the most moving experience was one of the statues at the front of the church. It's unusual to have statues of such magnificence in a NZ church, as well as the intricate detailed carvings as I described. The statue was at the left of the church and as I stood in front of it I was struck. That's the only way I can describe the feeling. There was Jesus with His robe open and His heart carved out and exposed, and He was looking down at me. His bare feet showed below his robe and He was standing simply, totally exposing himself, with His heart wide open. I felt compelled to reach up high, almost on tippy toes, and placed my hand over His heart. In my mind's eye I spoke to Him. "Oh Jesus you stand here with your heart so exposed but it is so painful to do this. How do you do it? You're so exposed to all the world's pain!"

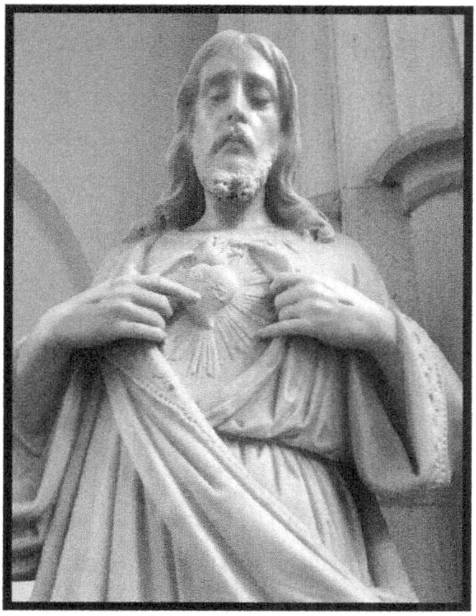

As I looked up I could see His eyes lovingly looking down on me and I asked, "Please, show me a way that I can stay with my heart open and not feel the pain?" At first there was nothing, I could just feel His softness as he kept looking down on me. I continued holding His heart, reaching up, holding on, waiting, waiting for the answer. Then it came. "Let go of your attachment." As I heard this I immediately let go of His heart and my feet returned firmly to the ground; I stayed staring up at Him as I got it. It's so simple yet so profound. Attachment is not necessary and only gets in the way of true love and happiness. Attachment is our cause of grief. With attachment we feel aggrieved, loss, and pain.

It took me back to my earlier days at the school of philosophy. Again and again it would come up that we should not be attached to those we love, that this is not true love. True love is the all encompassing, unconditional love. Let people be who they are, accept what comes and goes, and love that. Love everything for what it is. In learning this I learnt that true love does not come from our physical hearts, that kind of love is attached love. Detached love comes from everything, it runs through everything; good and bad, right and wrong, life and death. Detached love is so much stronger, so much more pure and so much more freeing, it is the place of joy, acceptance and presence. In fact when we know detached love we know it is really the only sure thing that exists and that is constant. In that, with death there is only love. We know that love is always here for us, it is not reliant on one person or thing, it is constantly here through everything.

Jesus stood there and in those few words reminded me of this knowing. How helpful it was at that moment to come back to this place, although I knew I would get caught up as the months went on, as we do, in the play of life, but I felt safer now. I remembered the truth and felt OK to open, as Jesus did standing in front of me, with my heart open and raw to feel, give and receive no matter what came my way. I was strong in the truth that nothing can take away this love and that life won't destroy me and will only make me stronger. What a healing experience, I no longer felt so helpless, so sad, so lonely and scared. I knew from here on in, no matter what, I could feel, and acknowledge what I felt in the knowing I was going to be OK.

I hopped on the plane leaving Dunedin that night so thankful for the trip. Thank you Dunedin for being there when I needed you. Xx

CHAPTER 18

Desperate for Answers

"Blessed is he that expects nothing,
for he shall never be disappointed."
- Benjamin Franklin -

So Tuesday finally came around, the day of our appointment at the hospital with the specialist at 11.00am. After the appointment, Patrick was to take his full monthly blood test to see what effects the past month of chemotherapy had achieved, and then the next round was to start. These tests are more comprehensive than his usual weekly ones. I had mentioned to him a couple of times in the week leading up to the appointment that I couldn't understand why he wasn't taking the blood tests a few days earlier before his appointment. Each time he dismissed me and the question fell into thin air.

Patrick was really off this morning. His face looked different, he was obviously stressed and he was very low. I asked a number of times what was wrong, each time he replied he was OK. I put it down to his being as anxious, as I was, about today's outcome. We were so keen to get answers on del 1p32! We arrived at the hospital and waited for the specialist to arrive. Patrick walked into the office first, then I came around the corner, following him in, just as the specialist was about to shut the door. “Hi there Ross.” I said, surprising him. He greeted me as I continued “Oh yes, there are always two of us.” The head nurse of the Kiwi Trial program came into the office with us also. I was really pleased she was there as I felt it was important she knew our questions and concerns, and could hear the answers from Dr Henderson.

Dr Henderson started searching the computer for the blood results so he could assess how Patrick had fared with his first chemotherapy round and seemed surprised that there were no recent results showing up. He looked to the nurse and asked “Have the tests not been taken yet for Patrick?” to which she replied “No, we take them on day one of the second cycle.”

Of course this had been worrying me leading up to the appointment so I jumped in suggesting that maybe next time we do the blood tests a few days before the appointment, quickly glancing at the nurse to see if this suggestion was OK. She and Dr Henderson both agreed this was a good idea, and we made a note to ensure we get the lab form from the Kiwi Trial team on our last chemotherapy appointment of this round, so we can take the tests a week after Patrick’s break. This way the results will be at the hospital in time for our next month’s follow-up appointment.

“Well then” said Dr Henderson, “let’s take a look at what is here.” and he looked at the few past blood results Patrick had taken at the beginning of each week of chemotherapy. He seemed pleased with those and he then proceeded to give Patrick the physical check required before the next round of chemotherapy. After the examination Dr Henderson wrote a few notes and then went to end the appointment. “OK, well when the results come through they will be sent to you, so you can view them too.”

I had tried to nudge Patrick a little earlier to get on with his questions, but he hadn’t picked up the cue. He is so polite, he didn’t want to interrupt Dr Henderson. As Dr Henderson thought he was finishing the appointment Patrick finally spoke up and told him he had a couple of questions he needed to ask.

"I guess" said Patrick, "the biggest question I have is about the 1p32 deletion that showed up a few weeks ago with the FISH test. I noticed the diagnoses in the letter that was sent to the insurance company, and followed it up by obtaining the FISH result. I have done a lot of research on it and it doesn't appear to have a good prognosis, I would like to know what your thoughts are on that."

Dr Henderson turned his chair back to his desk and started tapping on his computer to find the results of the FISH test. He eventually found it and turned to Patrick, acknowledging that the FISH test did indicate this. He went on to say that Patrick's results show deletion of **only** 1p32, and that this is worse when it's combined with deletion 17P or translocation 4:14. He said these combinations have a very poor prognosis when combined.

Hanging on for a glimmer of good news, this was a little of what we wanted to hear... so it isn't a worst case scenario however Patrick was not content with the answer. "It seems some research has been done in recent years around del 1p32," Patrick replied, "and it still seems to show poor prognosis on its own, I just want to know straight up if this is the case. I can handle the news, but I just want to know."

Dr Henderson started to explain what a chromosome deletion was which was helpful. Every time we hear or read an explanation it seems to help us to understand it a little more. At the end of the explanation Patrick bless him, persisted, saying "In all the research that we have looked at, it all leads to poor survival with del 1p32 though. I just want to know if that is the case for me."

Dr Henderson responded saying he'd have to go through all of Patrick's results to have a proper look which would take some time. He had patients waiting so he could not do that right now. He continued saying that of course he can't tell Patrick exactly how long he is going to live as everyone is individual and responds differently to treatment.

He explained that there is never an exact science behind this and we can never be definitive in an answer to 'how long you will live.'

I stepped in "I don't think Patrick is asking you to be definitive." I said quietly. "It's just that we have read of studies done, like the one in France recently where 1195 myeloma patients were studied, young patients in treatment. Under 10% had del 1p32. The study was done to assess the prognosis of this diagnosis and it was assessed at overall survival two years. It's pretty alarming to see this and we need clarity on this. If this is the case, Patrick will change his life quite significantly, so it's something we need more clarification on. Obviously we can't be exact but is this still a problem with this deletion, or does this new treatment help, or is there something more we can do to assist?"

Dr Henderson didn't know of the survey I had mentioned so I pulled it out of my bag and passed it to him. The first thing he did was point out that the study was completed in 2013. He said he would need time to review the paper, which he didn't have right now, but he'd do that as soon as he could and get back to us.

I knew we were now overtime in our appointment but I couldn't help myself. I pulled out the other chart Patrick had shown me showing a huge decline in survival rate with del 1p32 compared to standard multiple myeloma, and handed this to Dr Henderson also saying "This chart is also very alarming to us." Dr Henderson thankfully took this too and said he would look at this later also and get back to us. He kindly went on to say that he did expect with the treatment plan Patrick is on, even with this deletion, that he should achieve remission. This was promising to hear! He turned and started writing a few notes.

As we rose to leave Patrick, goodness he's a trier, dared to ask one more question, "What about replacing this deleted chromosome? I read how in China they are trialling this at the moment. Is there anything we can do like that?" I was surprised at the question as I had not heard about this treatment. Here is this poor guy trying to find a way to save his life, desperate to live long enough to see his daughters marry, be around for his grandchildren.

Dr Henderson sat up and back in his chair and thankfully took the time to explain to Patrick that he was afraid the answer at the moment was no, as those trials he said are in their early stages and there have been fatalities so we are a long way off having those types of solutions. He said he was sorry but he really had to finish up now as he had patients waiting and they agreed that Patrick could email him with any further questions he might have. When we walked out of the office I felt such a sense of guilt. The waiting room was full, and when I looked at the time I saw we had been there for 25 minutes. Well over the 10 minute appointment time. Dr Henderson would have a lot of strain on his morning now catching up!

The head nurse took us to the chemotherapy ward. To be honest we both were still very caught up in our questions. We had got to know the head nurse as she had been on duty for Patrick's first round of treatment. Usually we were very chatty but today we walked to the ward in silence. It was clear Patrick's chromosome deletion was weighing on us. The nurse was silent also. No one seemed to know what to say; it felt like a very long walk to the ward.

When we were seated in the ward another nurse joined us to take Patrick's bloods and the chatter between her and the head nurse helped to fill the space, but it didn't distract us from the disappointment we both felt in that we hadn't managed to get answers to all our questions. It wasn't until the nurses finally left us for a time on our own that we spoke to each other. "Wow!" I puffed out, finally able to breathe. "That didn't go so well did it?" Patrick responded quickly, "I should have sent the reports through to Dr Henderson earlier so he'd had a chance to read them before we saw him." His head was low and he seemed resigned. "I agree," I said. "Well at least he has the articles now and you can discuss it with him through email later." The unknown hung in the air. We'd been so desperate to gain clarity on the reports, and now we had to wait even longer.

We stayed silent as the usual processes eventually took place of inserting the line into his arm for the blood tests to be taken, the saline flush to go through and for the chemotherapy to be dripped through. Usually we are very chatty, so our silence would be getting picked up by the nurse. I didn't want an unpleasant environment for them, however there was nothing I could do, I could only be real with what I was feeling. Patrick was in the same space.

Eventually, once the nurse left, I turned my attention to the head nurse who had again joined us. "Do you think David would mind if we asked him a few of the questions we have around the del1p32?" David was the specialist in charge of the Kiwi Trial program. "It's just he travels around the world to all the seminars, hearing all the latest, I wonder if his knowledge might be of help?"

Thankfully she replied "No, I don't think he would mind at all. The best way is to email him your questions, as he's very busy and it's hard to get to talk to him. He is going back overseas for a few weeks before Christmas, so emailing him is best." She was looking at me sympathetically. "I'm sure he will get back to you, just give him a bit of time, email him soon though before he goes away."

"OK, thanks so much," I responded, "we will do that." Nothing else. I didn't say another word about the matter, Patrick didn't chip in and silence fell again. The head nurse left while Patrick's chemotherapy was running through. I suppose this wasn't unusual, there was no need for her to be there and she didn't usually stay on. But today, it felt like she couldn't get away fast enough and I didn't blame her one little bit.

After some time another nurse we had come to know on the Kiwi Trial team appeared. She often would pop in and visit us each week to see how both Patrick and I were getting on. She always arrived with such a beautiful smile and cheery manner with words of encouragement adding a breath of fresh air to the ward. Today however she didn't show up to us in this way. Instead her face was full of compassion as she stood in front of us and it was obvious to me she had tagged the head nurse on her way out and got the 'heads-up' on our concerns.

This was more evident as she spoke. "I hear you didn't get quite the answers you were looking for about the studies today." This was more a statement than a question. The previous week Patrick had emailed her the studies and voiced his concerns in regards to the del 1p32. (This is the correct way to write it by the way. Del 1p32). She was our main point of contact in regards to queries, processes etc and she had been the one who initially suggested he bring up his queries in the specialist appointment today that she herself had booked for him. "That must be disappointing for you," she continued "it's important you get your questions answered. I hear you are going to write to David as well so that's great." It felt so good to have her understand, also to care and validate to us that we weren't out of order for wanting more clarification.

She continued, obviously seeing the concern on our faces and wanting to help, "I did speak briefly to David about it last week," she said "and he said at the time he did still fully expect you to achieve remission, to not worry about it too much." "Well that's good to hear." I replied. "Thank you for talking to him, we really appreciate it." I turned to Patrick saying "That's good to hear isn't it Patrick?" Patrick was still very quiet, he hadn't spoken at all since she had arrived. "That's David and Ross both saying they still expect remission for you. That's one positive thing." I continued.

Patrick just grunted in return, he was making no effort, he just didn't have it in him and he felt so despondent. He had so many questions around 'remission' I knew. All well and good to get remission, but for how long is it expected with this deletion? That was the first big question of course. The nurse, bless her, made no attempt to try and lift the mood. She was sympathetic, and that was enough. She didn't stay long, like everyone else. We were pretty hard to be around today, however we were very appreciative of her efforts and concern.

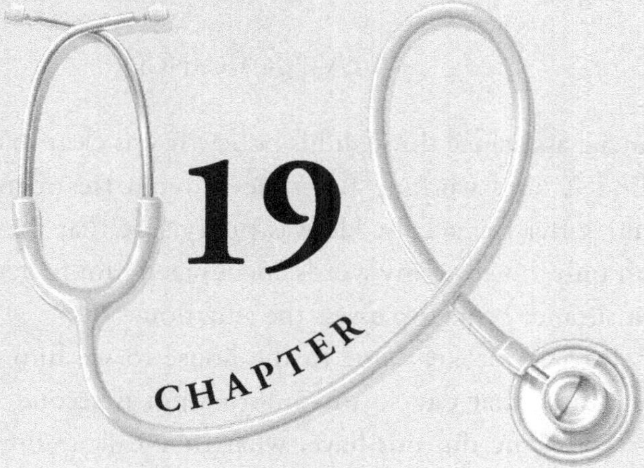

Life Insurance

"The world of will is not at
the discretion of randomness."
- Georg Hegel -

We finally left the hospital, still very quiet. Our spirits hadn't really lifted and on the way home in the car I reached over and held Patrick's hand. He turned to me and said "You know, I had the insurance form with me to give to the specialist for him to fill out but I forgot to bring it up."

The life insurance saga has been another huge stress on Patrick that he could have done without. Patrick had decided we both should take out life insurance policies some four years ago; we had bought a house together at that time, so he'd considered this the best option for financial protection if anything happened to either of us. Wow I had only been thinking of something sudden like a car accident, honestly, it never occurred to me that it would be useful for something like cancer.

When Patrick was diagnosed I was actually the one who suggested he enquire as to whether there was any way he could get financial assistance through his policy. It was clear that he was going to find it hard working full time through treatment and that we would suffer financially. He was pretty sure that the policy was for death only, however my words encouraged him to get in touch with his insurance broker to assess the situation.

Patrick's broker came to the house to see him immediately. I wasn't there that day so this information is second hand. He told Patrick that he did not have, what they call, trauma insurance or critical illness insurance, just as he had thought. He did however say that if his expected **life span *without treatment* was 12 months or less, it is possible to get an early payout of the whole policy!**

Patrick had phoned me that afternoon feeling a little relieved and hopeful as he expected that his life expectancy **without treatment** may fit in that criteria. It seems a little crazy being excited that your condition without treatment is that you may not live that long right! Patrick obviously thought the life insurance policy coming through early would be a godsend for him in a lot of ways. Though we believed that **with treatment** his life expectancy would be much longer than that.

This was sometime ago now and I hadn't heard anything since from Patrick. I had presumed it had been dropped due to him being on the Kiwi Trial and the hope that these treatments would serve him well. I hadn't taken into account the later diagnosis of Patrick's chromosome deletion, which I presumed now must have prompted him to follow this up. I questioned him asking "I didn't realise you were going ahead with this, or that you needed forms filled in. Even though you are having treatment and will more than likely live longer than 12 months, can you still apply?"

"Yes," he replied, "apparently that doesn't matter, it can go on what the expectancy is without treatment. I suppose it's because no one really ever knows if the treatment will work, so they can take it on the worst possible scenario." Patrick let that sink in with a pause before continuing "When I heard about the chromosome deletion one good thing was that I saw it as good news to help towards my case with the insurance company to get an early payout to help out financially. I decided to follow up again with the broker, and since then we have been getting all the information together that they need."

I could see how Patrick, not managing to get the life insurance form filled in today, hadn't helped with how he felt, combined with the events of the day. Patrick didn't lift in spirits at all through the afternoon and neither did I. It was such a depressing day and we both stayed very morose for the rest of the day and night. It was not just the insurance company details of course, but also having so little information still on the consequences of the 1p32 deletion.

I guess we both knew in our hearts the outcome wasn't great but we really needed to know more. What does this mean? Will Patrick get a long remission considering his condition and the treatment plan he is on? Is he even on the right treatment plan considering this condition? What should we be doing with our lives now?

Patrick had taught me the saying over the years 'tomorrow's another day', being that it will be a new day, a better day, and I bought into the hope of that as I went to bed that night… however, by morning we both woke feeling the exact same way.

It was a slow morning for us both and we really only got ready just in time to go to the hospital. Walking into the hospital for day two of chemotherapy for the week I tried to lift things a little and talked with him about a couple of positive things. I really didn't want to go back to the ward feeling as low as we did the day before and I didn't want the nurses to see us that way again.

Patrick had been given his own room today, the one and only room in the ward where he previously had the bone marrow test taken. I wondered if it was because they felt sorry for how he was feeling yesterday, though nothing was said. The nurses were super nice but that was usual. We were quickly coming to realise how amazing the nurses were and we were very grateful that, although we came feeling so vulnerable each day, we always felt welcome, and that we were in a friendly, caring environment.

Patrick was incredibly tired. He hadn't got to sleep until 4.30am again. The Dexamethasone seemed to be keeping him awake more and more and it made it so difficult for him to function on a day to day basis around chemotherapy time. He welcomed the private room and a bed to lie on for his session today. The usual procedures had taken place and now the Carfilzomib was set up and flowing into Patrick's body yet again. The lovely nurse from the Kiwi Trial program who had checked in on us yesterday dropped in to see us again. Cautiously it seemed, she came into the room, to see how we were.

I greeted her with a smile, Patrick's was less forthcoming. It was still hard for him to make the effort, however it was soon apparent she was bringing us good news. "I spoke to David about you yesterday." she said to Patrick after the usual pleasantries were made. Both of our ears pricked up as we waited to hear what she had to say. "He said he is very happy to have a chat with you. You just need to send him an email with your questions and he will give you a call before he goes overseas next week."

I surprised her by leaping off my chair and giving her a big hug. "Oh thank you, thank you so much," I exclaimed, "that means so much to us that you did that." I felt a weight lifting immediately. Patrick piped up "That's great to hear. There are just some critical points unanswered, so it will be really great to hear from him." She continued, "Well he is happy to have a chat, he just wants an email first, so I'll give you his email address. OK?" she asked, standing there, giving us both such a caring smile. "That's awesome," I replied "it's just what we needed, thank you so, so much."

From that moment both of our spirits lifted. Maybe now we will get some answers. Patrick emailed David before we had even left the hospital and I got home from work the next day with the good news that he'd had a twenty minute phone conversation from him!

Patrick seemed almost high from it. He was so happy that his concerns had been heard and that David had taken the time to call him. He didn't seem to know where to start in filling me in. "Start at the beginning." I said, trying to get him focused. We were by now sitting down on our outdoor couch with a nice cold drink on this beautiful sunny day. I was excited to hear what had taken place.

Patrick had so much to say. David had been so good to him hearing out all his questions and answering where he could, however it soon became apparent that this del 1p32 was so rare that he didn't really have key answers. He actually told Patrick that he had not yet had a patient in New Zealand with this deletion, or if he had, he didn't know it. Apparently the FISH test hasn't always been available so it may have been in some patients in earlier years and they wouldn't have known.

It came back once again to the fact that David really considered the most important thing was that we had to fight the cancer the best way we knew how for multiple myeloma and that is what we were doing. He said that Patrick's best opportunity was to get into as good a remission as possible and for as long as possible, which would also be the best outcome for fighting this deletion. With this deletion, how long would Patrick's remission be? Well no one knows, but the best thing and the only thing for us to do right now is to rid his body of the cancer to give him that fighting chance. This we were doing, so we were on track. No other answers were available.

So really, so much to say but still unanswered questions. Patrick accepted this for now, however it didn't stop him in the future from continuing to research the shit out of this question and it wasn't good what he eventually uncovered!

I now wanted to know more on how Patrick was getting on with his claim so I grabbed this opportunity while we were sitting down and he was in a good mood and asked him. He was happy to fill me in with what was sadly turning out to be a fight with the insurance company.

Patrick had apparently passed the specialist's letter with his **untreated prognosis of 6-10 months**, to his broker some time back when he had first received it. At the time the broker had been shocked and sympathetic. He said he would put this letter forward also and try his best to get a good outcome, being an early release of the money. Patrick had then put this matter to one side as the Kiwi Trial program had started, and he was caught up adjusting to its effects on him, and also adjusting to less time in our week to achieve things with the frequent trips to hospital. Two weeks on and Patrick was getting concerned he had not heard anything. He said he had 'mustered' himself up to contact his agent. When he said 'muster' I could imagine that as I knew how very tired he was physically and emotionally from the chemotherapy. He had enough to cope with trying to work part time around the treatments also, so I could imagine how difficult it was to take on chasing this up.

When he contacted his agent he was told they had needed more information from the specialist. Apparently they had requested it but the specialist had not gotten back to them yet.

By the time the first round of chemotherapy had finished and he started recovering on his week off, he started getting really annoyed with the insurance company as he had still not heard anything. Yet again he was sitting in the dark wondering what was going on. He became determined to get to the bottom of it all and started pushing them along, as he was beginning to feel he was getting mucked around. Patrick felt that surely a prognosis of 6-10 months without treatment would fall into their category of an early settlement, that's what the agent had basically said. If your prognosis is under a year to live without treatment, they will often pay up early… however this is at 'their discretion'.

Apparently it was the day I flew to Dunedin that Patrick phoned and asked the broker to come to our home. In his defense he was always available immediately for him to talk to. By now Patrick had decided to look further into his results of the 1p32 deletion.

He had found the study on the French trial and to be honest he was still getting over the shock of the realization of this result. Actually I don't know if he'll ever get over the shock of this trial, however he felt the report was something compelling to pass on to the insurance company also.

So unbeknown to me, Patrick had passed this report to his broker that day. With the broker being a friend, he too was shocked, and was genuinely sorry for him. They apparently had a cup of coffee together and sat and chatted about the implications of this result. Patrick then asked how his case was progressing. Apparently they had received some answers from his specialist now but had gone back with further questions and were again waiting for the specialist to respond.

Patrick knew Dr Henderson was a busy man so it was at this point he offered to help his broker. He asked him if there was anything he could do to speed up the process or assist in any way and the broker had responded that yes, it would be great if he could help get the forms they needed filled in by Dr Henderson since he was seeing him in a week's time. Patrick agreed, feeling good that he could at least be a part of trying to pull all of this together. The forms were emailed to him and these are the forms he had with him two days ago to take to his specialist appointment.

I had been unaware of these latest developments and that Patrick was endeavouring to have these filled in at our last appointment. Looking back, it helped explain why he was quiet on the way to the appointment, however I totally get why he forgot to ask once we were there. He had been too absorbed with his life and death questions!

It was clear the delays with the insurance company seemed insurmountable to Patrick and it was all getting too much for him to deal with. As Patrick finished filling me in, my heart went out to him big time.

Unfortunately this conversation had dampened his good mood. Dejectedly he sighed "I feel I just have to give up on this insurance thing darlin', it's just not going to happen." I didn't know what to say. Honestly that's unusual for me, but I know I've been put in this position so much lately. We had stepped into a world of so much unknown. I just held his hand and we both actually had a wee cry. I felt Patrick's helplessness. These struggles were leaving him feeling useless and yes, worthless actually, and that feeling was rising for both of us right now. But right here, thankfully, as we sat together for some time, I managed to reach for gratitude. A saviour thank you. I squeezed his hand and said "Darling, at least we still know you are on the best treatment plan. You know the specialists have given you that and you are on the best possible path for recovery, and that is the main thing!" However, to complete the life insurance saga, I'll go ahead in time and tell you how it went, with the full story abbreviated.

A couple more weeks went by and still Patrick had not heard anything from the insurance company. He was very agitated at the lack of response and with always having to follow up. When he followed up with his broker yet again he was told that the specialist had in fact now communicated with them supplying them with the latest information required and all their questions had been answered. Patrick now had to wait for their decision. Apparently it was very complicated.

Patrick first contacted the insurance company on 17 November 2017. On 8 December he received a copy of the letter from his broker's boss that had been submitted to the insurance company. The content of the letter really upset Patrick as it was clear the line his broker's boss was moving towards in his submission was not in his favour:

1. The chromosome deletion 1p32 had not been considered or addressed in the lifespan prognosis that was provided to the insurance company, stating median survival would be 83 months and 5 year overall survival of 62%.

2. It also appeared that the broker's boss was presenting to the insurance company to look at his 'possibility of overall survival **with** treatment' as opposed to 'overall survival **without** treatment'. The reason he had gone through this process at all was because he had been told this was possible to get an early payout if your prognosis was under 12 months without treatment!

Patrick felt the data given to the insurance company was not current and he was concerned that current data had purposely not been supplied. He was also concerned that they were only addressing the best possible scenario as opposed to the worst.

Patrick's broker advised him that he could, personally, take this further with Sovereign, the Life Insurance Company, directly if he wished… and Patrick wished. He made an appointment through the correct avenue and, together with his broker, he went to see the Chief Medical Officer of Sovereign. It took 6 weeks to get this appointment, taking it to mid January 2019 with a lot of stress and concern to carry in the meantime for Patrick!

When they arrived for the appointment, it appeared they were not seeing the Chief Medical Officer after all, they had been fobbed off onto a Claims Manager… and unfortunately it went nowhere. They had received the information on the chromosome deletion 1p32 now from Patrick weeks earlier, and the studies done around it. They sat in front of Patrick and told him that even in consideration of this they declined the application. They said that because he was having treatment, they expected him to live longer. It was at 'their discretion' as to releasing a policy under the 'terminal within 12 months without treatment' policy! They felt it was not warranted in this case as Patrick was having treatment and was expected to live longer.

6-10 months life expectancy without treatment was clear in black and white as Patrick's diagnosis. His chromosome deletion showed poor prognosis. His policy allowed him to be paid out early under the clause if terminal prognosis without treatment is under 12 months - **BUT 'at their discretion.'** There was nothing more he could do. **Read the fine print in your policies** is all I can say. If anything is up to discretion, pretty much you're probably not going to get it. Insurance companies will not pay out unless they have to… at least that's what I've heard time and time again telling this story to people over the last few months. It's a business, so go figure.

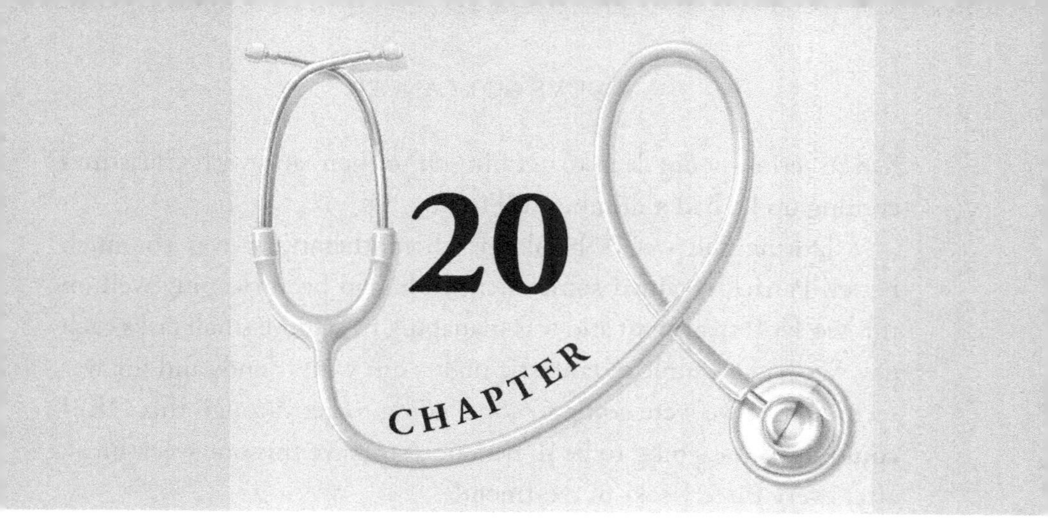

Tiredness and Chemo Fog

"The way I see it,
if you want the rainbow,
you gotta put up with
the rain."
- Dolly Parton -

Patrick was finding it so hard to cope with the tiredness he was experiencing from chemotherapy. In the first round we put it aside, we were just so grateful that he wasn't throwing up, that his hair wasn't falling out, and just that he could still function at all. I think too, we were so concerned about the cancer invading his body that we were just pleased he was getting treatment. The letter from the specialist with the words in black and white still flashed in front of me constantly - 6-10 months without treatment.

However, by the second round of chemotherapy this acceptance of tiredness started to change, it was really starting to take its toll. Patrick was finding it increasingly hard to manage his business even part time and I noticed his focus was very limited. He also had a couple of magic shows to perform during the first round where he'd had to seriously dig deep to get himself to them and with Christmas coming up he had a number still to do.

During the week's break off chemotherapy it was so much better. Patrick regained some energy. He had been sleeping well on this week off treatment and was managing to achieve small tasks each day. We had a couple of fantastic nights out with friends and life was seeming like we were going to cope, going to get through this OK. I could see it was going to be so beneficial to have this one week break after every three weeks of treatment!

Just on that, I have to say how important a role your good friends make in such a journey as this. As said earlier, the responses have varied depending on the type of person, or the closeness of friendships. As much as it has been interesting to observe, it has been heartwarming to experience the thoughtfulness, care and kindness shown by some. A few of my girlfriends have been amazing, always texting, not just to say hi, how are you coping, but let's catch up. Do you feel like coffee, lunch? That kind of thing. Really wanting to connect and show they care.

On Patrick's week off chemotherapy one friend invited us out to such a lovely dinner at our favorite restaurant, Gusto's. It was like the maitre'd knew we deserved a treat too, as when we arrived he offered us the chef's table for the evening. This is where you are practically sitting right in the middle of the kitchen and the chef decides the food for the evening for you. You get to experience the hustle and bustle of the kitchen, see all the food coming out, watch all the finishing touches as food is plated, all the while meal after meal of delicious Italian food is being served to us. It was so great to be out having such a treat of a night.

The following night another couple we are very close to invited us to a show - Pleasure Dome with music from the 80's starring Lucy Lawless. It was so much fun. They had booked a table and did the whole nine yards with drinks and food. The show was funny, and sad, and groovy, all in one. We were whisked away from the realities of cancer and laughed and sang the night away.

So after a twelve day break from chemotherapy, Patrick had begun the second cycle of chemotherapy and the tiredness kicked in again and with it the damaging effects on both of our quality of life. I woke up suddenly. "Oh my God!" I said to him the morning after his second day of treatment on this second month of chemotherapy. "I've just got it! You have to take sleeping tablets Patrick. I know you are worried about it interfering with your chemotherapy treatment, but I am sure it won't. In fact I definitely remember Liz saying if you need them, they will prescribe them. I seriously think this will help you a lot."

Patrick had just had two nights in a row again with just a few hours sleep. The first night he couldn't sleep until 4.30am and the second night 2.30am… but was awake again at 6.00am! His voice had faded so you could hardly hear him, he was so tired. He was constantly collapsing on the bed during the day to sleep, and it just felt we couldn't go on this way.

I'm not going to lie. A part of this was for me too. We had to find a solution as I was losing sleep these nights as well and I wasn't coping at all with that. I'm an eight hours a night kinda girl, so I don't do well at all with lack of sleep. Patrick was skeptical. "I don't know about getting caught up in sleeping tablets, I don't want to get addicted or disrupt anything," he quietly said. But I could feel his resolve had dropped. I grabbed the opportunity and pushed it exclaiming "We can't go on like this Patrick, it's too tough. At least try it! I think we have been blaming and accepting the cancer and the chemotherapy too much for your tiredness. I think if you get your sleep it will make a lot of difference, we have to give it a go!"

Patrick was silent so I took that as agreement and mentioned it to a couple of people over the week that this is what we were going to check out with the nurses next session. So we did, and they not only agreed it was the best avenue, they insisted! They stressed to him how important sleep was, not only for his quality of life but for his well being too. In fact the head nurse of the trial program stated it firmly to him. "Your body needs sleep to recover and regenerate," she told him. "It really is essential, and it will not have a negative impact on your treatment at all."

I could have jumped up and kissed her. Instead I gave her a sneaky thumbs up, but thank God she convinced Patrick and he duly got his subscription from the pharmacy on the way out. What a difference it made. Actually for the first night maybe too much of a difference, he snored so loudly all night it kept waking me up… but of course I let him sleep, so pleased he was getting some decent rest.

The following night was the same. For the first time since chemotherapy started Patrick was now only needing to rest in the afternoons during the day, and then again in the early evening or early to bed. He was functioning at a much better level without the sleep deprivation. Trust me, it was a huge improvement. At least he had a few hours of the day when he was reasonably functional. His voice still faded about two days after his second day of chemotherapy but it seemed to be now evident that this was a side effect of the chemotherapy.

Chemo fog was still a problem too. We hadn't been sure if this was from the lack of sleep or not, but it quickly became apparent it was the drugs Patrick was taking. His memory was shocking and organisation was difficult for him. When we spoke to the nurses about it that's what they called it. Chemo fog. Yep it's a thing.

In the second month of his chemotherapy cycle it was coming up to Christmas. Companies had started their Christmas functions and Patrick had accepted performing two, one hour shows right smack in the middle of this second month. The first one was a Saturday night. The second one was on the following day, Sunday, in the afternoon.

Patrick was beside himself. With the difficulty of focusing, the brain fog, and still so many errands to do, he wasn't coping. There had been so much to do following up on his health insurance, so much time spent having treatments, so much to do for work, so much to do clearing things out around the house, so much to do, so much to do, with so much limited time feeling OK to do it in. In reality not much was getting achieved at all.

By Saturday he really wasn't prepared for either of his shows. He wasn't too worried about the Saturday night show as it was close up magic for which it is relatively simple to prepare. Patrick knows his magic inside out, and his performances around it, so it was just a matter of deciding what to take.

My nephew was up for a tag rugby competition near the venue of the Magic Show and I was catching up with him for dinner. We all decided to go to the restaurant where Patrick was performing. Although Patrick was performing in a private room it would be nice to go together and he could have a bite to eat with us afterwards. Apparently the magic went really well and everyone enjoyed it, but I was shocked how much it took out of him when he later came to join us. He only had a bowl of soup to eat and you could barely get a word out of him. It had wiped him out.

When we woke the following Sunday morning we lay in bed planning the day ahead. Patrick still had to put together his show for the afternoon which it seemed was going to take him quite some time. This was a stage show which involved so much more preparation, yet he already felt very tired and wasn't sure how he was going to get through the day. I'll never forget him saying to me very emotionally as we lay there "I think this will be my last show darling." I turned to him startled. "What!?" I asked. He simply replied "I don't think I can do this anymore, truly, I think it will be my last show."

I couldn't even look at him. Another heartbreaking moment, another deep acknowledgement that my dear man had cancer and it was getting to him. Patrick loved his magic and loved performing. It was him in his element, him with his chance to express. He loved to be able to make people laugh and put on a show.

I tried to encourage him. "Darling it's just because you aren't organized. If you had planned the shows during the week, it wouldn't have felt so hard when you just had to perform on the day, instead of preparing as well. Once you've put together this show today, just use the same show for next time, and the same with the close up show you did yesterday. There is nothing wrong with doing the exact show again, all magicians do that, then you may be able to handle it better." "Even then," he went on "it's too hard for me to find the energy. No, I think this is going to be my last show." he repeated as he threw back the covers and got out of bed. I couldn't say any more, I had seen how exhausted he was after last night's show, I knew it was taking its toll on him. Bloody cancer. Bloody, bloody cancer.

The rest of the day felt like a funeral in its own right. I wanted to go to the show with him if only for moral support, but he insisted I head off to the beach. It was a beautiful sunny day and I had been hanging out for my first swim of the season. I hung around until he went to the show. I knew he just wanted to be on his own and he told me later he was very upset on the way and in tears at times. He was wondering how he was going to cope, how he could possibly do a show everyone can enjoy feeling the way he was, and so sad it would be his last show.

I made sure I was there when he got home. He came in exhausted but thankfully all smiles. "They really loved it," he beamed, "everyone had a lot of fun and the tricks went down great."...and he proceeded to fill me in on all the minute details of a show really well done!

I was so happy for him. So happy that, if indeed this did end up being his last show, that it was a great one... but also secretly hoping that he may find it in himself to not give up on his passion quite so soon.

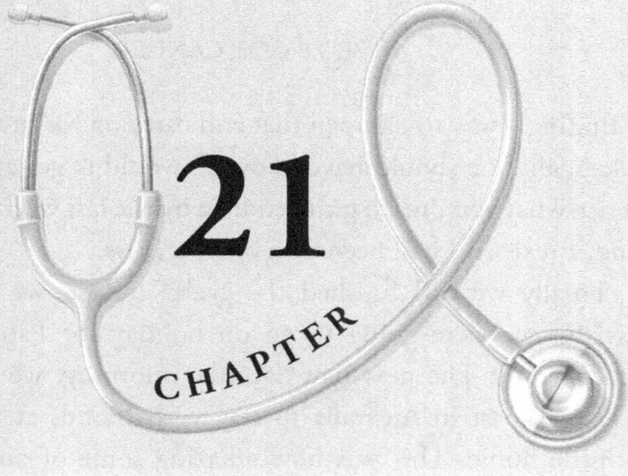

Take A Break!

"Women are meant to be loved,
not to be understood."
- Oscar Wilde -

So quickly it seemed, we rolled into the last week of the second cycle. So quickly because three weeks had gone by and it felt that so little had been achieved in that time. We were feeling stagnant.

I found my stress level very high. Taking two days out of your week to go to the hospital had proven very tough and now I had to take clients on these days too. The children had taken turns to be with Patrick on the first month's cycle so I'd not accompanied him for three of his sessions. However by this second month there had been no mention by any of them of going again. I didn't want to ask, I wanted to protect them. If it wasn't easy for them to offer then I didn't want to make it hard for them so I took the bullet and went every day myself.

With work, I would either book a session before chemotherapy began, or for later in the afternoon or evening. It was taking its toll; it was still such an emotional day going to the hospital. Somehow I was finding a way to dampen that and carry on for my clients, but at a price! Silly me should have known I wouldn't get away with that. Practice what you preach girlfriend! So by the last week of this second round, I realised I had become a bit of a mess.

Finally we had finished the cycle, and, as we had promised ourselves, we were going to go on holiday for Patrick's week off chemotherapy. The next day, Saturday morning, we were flying to the Gold Coast in Australia to stay with friends at their stunning beachside home. This was how amazing some of our friends have been. A number of offers had come forward from friends of staying at their holiday homes whenever we needed a break, so this was the first opportunity we were taking up and I couldn't wait.

We were booked to leave Saturday. Friday was my dearest 'antenatal group' girlfriends' and our yearly Christmas lunch, never to be missed! Each year, the four of us book a special lunch, which had started off initially as simply a celebration of us getting through another year with our babies. 25 years later, we are steadfast friends and now we meet because we can!

This year it was Ostro for lunch. Ostro is a stunning restaurant on Auckland City's waterfront. The food and service are fantastic and the whole experience was to be, as always, a real treat… however I woke in the morning highly emotional. I'd had a bad dream in the night, and actually woke sobbing my heart out. Patrick, bless him, as usual, had brought me in a cup of tea, unaware of the bombardment he was about to get.

I was surprised to notice, as I slowly poured out my soul to him, that everything was getting on top of me; the list of things undone! The fear and worry of cancer seemed to be wearing off, and in its place was awareness of the effect it was having on our lives.

Patrick, being a bit of a hoarder, had the garage packed with mostly unnecessary things. For the last two months he's gone into the garage many times, gone around in circles, moved things around and got nowhere. I hated seeing this every day when I would go to my car… the car that was parked outside the garage as there is too much gear inside it for any cars to reside. There was only room for his motorbike. On top of that, there was his magic apparatus. Preparing for his recent magic shows, he'd been bringing props upstairs to sort through. Usually I insist this is always put back but it had seemed so unimportant then and I'd let it go. Now it wasn't only the garage that was looking like a bomb site.

I knew there were elements of his business work that still hadn't been done and this also bothered me deeply. Two months on and he still hadn't completed certain things, like what I knew was a time consuming invoice, to his biggest client… as if he didn't need the money! What was going on that he couldn't apply himself to do this? It was getting embarrassing that he would finally send this so late, to his biggest client… and how was he going to cope financially through all of this? All of a sudden this was so important and needed to be resolved now! If he wasn't functioning fully with work, how was he going to survive?

Oh, and then the list went on of all the things I had got behind in over the last couple of months. Initially it hadn't seemed to matter, but I realised now it really did and it was all falling on top of me. I poured this all out to Patrick between tears and sobs; the poor guy had just thought he was bringing me a nice cup of tea!

Patrick didn't know what to say, he just sat on the edge of the bed holding me. I am so thankful he didn't even try to solve the problems right there and then. It probably would have just taken me deeper and deeper into distress as really, there were not a lot of appropriate answers. Then the guilt of pouring all this on him, as if he needed the worry of how I felt, had me sobbing more.

Finally I stopped emptying out, the sobbing calmed down and the tears dried up. Patrick just started talking about the day ahead. He is so good at that, diverting was his specialty. Maybe this was why he was such a good magician being good at misdirection! It worked however! I allowed it to happen as there was nowhere else to go.

People say it's really good to get things off your chest and to have a good cry, that it's healing. As much as I agree with this it is also really not enough. My emotions remained stuck with no resolution and the worry stayed bottled inside. I knew in myself I needed to really free myself of these worries and that the need to do this on an emotional level was evident to me. However I couldn't sort the physical aspects like Patrick getting well, or even cleaning up the bloody garage, so I didn't feel ready to release the concerned feelings I was holding on to!

It's crazy how we do this really. It's like we feel if we let go of the worry, or fear, or pain, it will mean we accept the situation. And the fear of accepting the situation is too great, so we think it's safer to stay holding on to the worry. It's a continuous, never ending roll of stress and helplessness.

I had my cup of tea, made a bit of a plan in my head for the day, and then felt I was ready to pull myself out of bed and carry on. Well I thought I was ready. In fact I was pretty much a cot case as I cried at everything that day.

The next lot of tears I had to fight back was when talking to a client on the phone about a child she knew who was being physically abused by her father. It would have been so unprofessional to have let her know the impact this was having on me. I'm supposed to be emotionally stable and strong as a therapist, ready to support my clients like a pillar of strength but I was feeling so vulnerable and open I nearly had a wee melt down on the phone while hearing the story.

When I arrived at the restaurant for lunch and saw my dearest friend Kay, finally home for good after years of living in Singapore, I held her tight for ages with tears flowing, telling her how happy I was she was home. "I'm so highly emotional." I apologised to her, realizing I really was in a heightened state of emotion all round today. Continuing on with tears, I couldn't stop them when one of my other dear girlfriends at lunch gave me A$100 she'd had at home to spend on a lovely brunch or something with Patrick while we were away. Acts of kindness too! Good God, I was ready to cry at anything and everything.

When I got home later, my youngest son and I were in the car driving to take Indi for her walk, and I cried simply telling him about how bloody highly emotional I was! It was quite unbelievable really, all this heightened emotion flowing. On our walk along the beach, with the cool sea breeze, the fresh air, and the lovely space that is often there between Taylor and I, I suddenly remembered that it was a similar experience after week three of the last month of chemotherapy. In a different way, but looking back, it had all got on top of me that week also.

It was one of those 'aha' moments. Anyone would think I was having the chemotherapy myself, I was getting affected so deeply at the end of each cycle. But there you go. As Patrick's partner, I was going through this so fully with him, it was deeply affecting me too, just in different ways.

I could see clearly how each three weeks of chemotherapy had taken its toll on me too. The strain of time out for hospital visits and treatments was one thing, the emotion of going through that another. Watching him struggle was hard enough, let alone that I was also picking up a lot of the slack on things he couldn't do anymore… actually I was getting physically shattered too. On top of this, last month Patrick had not felt up to doing anything during the chemotherapy weeks and life seemed to be becoming quite a drag.

At that moment on the beach, I was doubly pleased that tomorrow we would be going away on holiday, I clearly needed some serious destressing!! And fun! I also knew I needed to address my worries on all levels. I couldn't keep going on this way, so it would be great to have some space to do that.

Worth mentioning, we didn't ask the Kiwi Trial team if we could go overseas, we were too afraid they would say no. Patrick had checked out the medical side of things in Australia and had learnt that if he was to run into any trouble, he was entitled to free treatment as part of a reciprocal arrangement between the two countries. That was enough for us… so we sneaked away, totally undetected, under the radar, incognito. It was fun to be a little naughty actually.

Honestly, within 12 hours of being on the Gold Coast at our friend's beautiful relaxing home in the heat and sunshine, with nothing we needed to do, I felt myself finally start to unwind a little. I literally felt like a screw, so uptight, and even in just this short time I noticed I was unwinding just a slight notch. The analogy was giving me a good indication of where I was at on the stress level and how far I needed to go to release!

Sitting on our friend's glorious deck enjoying this beautiful warm and bright day I couldn't help but feel sadness that I was not getting the real sense of joy in being here. I just couldn't get that holiday feeling or relax into the comfy outdoor couch I was sitting on. I said to my host "Oh dear, I think it's going to take me a few days to unwind." I had such a sense of my body being this corkscrew, all twisted and tight.

We didn't do much the first couple of days. We would wake early because of the time difference and be walking by about 6.00 or 6.30am. We would take a half hour walk along the Gold Coast boardwalk to a local cafe, have a nice healthy breakfast and coffee, then walk home again where Patrick would rest for a lot of the day. I'd read and swim, or chat with our friends; it was very hot which is always great for relaxing the body.

By the third night though I felt I had come to a road block. The screw was no longer releasing and I felt stuck and anxious. We were lying in bed in the dark, trying to get to sleep, when the floodgates opened. Just out of the blue, I sat up and threw my hands on either side of my head and sobbed, "I can't do this anymore, I can't do this anymore." Patrick sat up leaning over, "Oh darling," he whispered. "what is it?"

"I just can't do this anymore," I sobbed. "I can't. I want it to stop. I don't want this anymore. I need it to stop. I just can't do this anymore!" Sobbing and sobbing, I just kept repeating these words again and again. I was really overwhelmed so suddenly with such a deep core feeling of helplessness.

I had been so strong over all this time, managing to continue on with normal life through it all, but it was time to realise that actually this has all been too hard. Too much. It was all too much pressure, too much to deal with. I was overloaded with stress and I just didn't want to cope anymore.

I don't know how many times I kept repeating these words as I held my head, rocking myself as I sat up on the bed. The impossibility of it all seemed just as endless as the darkness in the night. "I just can't do it anymore, I just can't Patrick." I had no idea what that meant really, neither did Patrick… just that it was all too much, and the realization of that was enough for now.

After some time I came to see that in just that awareness alone, this was allowing the screw to start to unravel a few notches. How I truly felt, how I was truly being affected, was being seen more fully now and I needed to accept and acknowledge just how tough this is. This alone seemed to be enough to help release some of the strain I was under. It is such a perfect example of how important it is to not push aside how we feel.

A lot of the therapy techniques I work with are about this. As humans, we tend to constantly hold on, block or push aside our feelings so we can carry on not affected by how we feel… supposedly. Of course that wee trick doesn't really work. The feelings are still there, and get more and more embedded as we ignore them! Then stress forms, anxiety, depression.

Patrick kept holding me until the rocking slowed down, the tears yet again dried on my face, and I became calm. Nothing else was said. It was what it was. We eventually lay back down, cuddled up, and both just drifted off to sleep.

As the days went on, notch by notch, my body slowly but surely unwound. I found myself laughing out loud and cracking a few jokes and I realised how foreign this sound had been to me lately. In fact when I first burst out laughing, I actually gave myself a wee fright!... I expected everyone else too as well and looked around for a reaction, but no one had noticed of course. Someone laughing was perfectly normal to them, it just hasn't been my norm lately!

Honestly, we so have to take care of our emotions and bodies when dealing with trauma. They are such a huge indicator of where we are at, how we are coping, or not, and can be an amazing tool for helping us to cope better if we just listen and give ourselves what we need. My body needed rest and a break. It needed to feel fun and laughter. This time away was turning into the best medicine ever and I found that after these few days of unwinding I no longer wanted to talk or write about chemotherapy or diagnosis or research or anything. It was lovely to allow it to not be at the forefront for a while and relax!

We were away for six days and I slowly relaxed more and more. Patrick continued to do a lot of sleeping and resting, and after a few days he started doing a little more swimming and socializing with our friends. The weather stayed warm and the sun seemed to just soak all our worries away. It was so lovely to have nothing we needed to do, nothing that should be done and wasn't getting done. None of it mattered over here, and for this brief time it felt like none of it really mattered at all. By the time the holiday was over we were ready to go home. As much as I didn't want to go back to the same old in one breath, I wanted to get Patrick back in treatment in the next breath. Time to kick that cancer's butt again!

The trip to Australia proved to be so healing. I can't recommend it highly enough to get yourself away from it all when you can. After this week away, and that significant emotional release, I went from crying several times a day, to now only once every few days. In fact even a week can go by now. What a difference it had made.

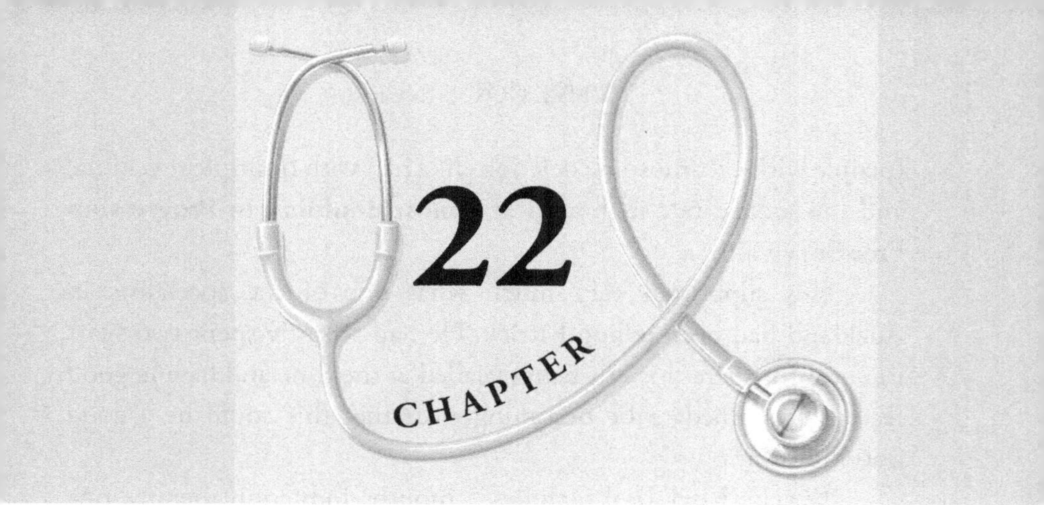

Double Stem Cell Transplants

"A man doesn't know what he knows
until he knows what he doesn't know."
- Laurence J. Peter -

Patrick had loved our Gold Coast holiday but it had highlighted how much the chemotherapy was affecting him and his need to rest. He did sleep a lot. He also couldn't get himself away from research while we were away and spent many hours on his laptop looking for more information on the 1p32 deletion. It seemed to have become quite an obsession which was worrying me.

By now Patrick had spoken to a number of key specialists in Auckland about their knowledge around the 1p32 deletion. Unfortunately it's so rare, many could not offer specifics, leaving him always coming back to the information in the French study.

He had learnt of a conference that was held in the USA just before Christmas on multiple myeloma and chromosome deletions. While we were away Patrick found papers online that had been presented at the conference. One paper was in regards to research around a **double stem cell transplant trial for high risk factors** (people with chromosome deletions like his) with multiple myeloma, and the success rate it showed of **almost doubling in Progression Free Survival!!**

This supported very much what one of the specialists in Auckland had been telling Patrick. He had recently spent two years in Toronto where this was being trialled at the time and having good results. It seemed to be becoming clear that this could be a good option for him.

Patrick's Kiwi Trial includes 5 months induction therapy, one stem cell transplant, and then 4 months of consolidation therapy. Double stem cell transplant is when you receive two stem cell transplants given within a short space of time of each other.

When Patrick told me about it, we were pretty excited. This could really help his outcome given his chromosome deletion! But the Kiwi Trial program didn't include double stem cell transplant. If this is what Patrick needs, how do we get it? Can we break the trial program if we need to? Will this affect him getting the bonus of the extra drug Carfilzomib, as this combo was deemed to be the best of therapies?

I asked Patrick to let it go for now - we'd ask these questions when we get back to the hospital. I also made it clear to him that it doesn't concern me that he is on the Kiwi Trial program. If you're not allowed to break it, we just will. What are they going to do, sue us? Fine, they can go for it. I told him nothing would stop us getting what is the best treatment for him. We knew we would take the steps one at a time starting with asking about this at the specialist appointment on day one of chemotherapy, cycle three, when we returned.

On our first day back for chemotherapy we were met by a new specialist. It was Christmas, so she was filling in at North Shore hospital. Gosh she was lovely. She greeted us with one of the nurses from the Kiwi Trial program, telling us how excited she was to see Patrick's blood results that had just come in.

Patrick's paraprotein levels had gone from 45 down to 3 already in just two months! This was apparently an excellent result. She explained that this meant the cancer was really not liking the chemotherapy and was dying off rapidly and he was responding brilliantly.

I was so delighted. I asked the specialist, if this was the case, would we need to do a whole five months of induction chemotherapy as per the Kiwi Trial, somewhat hopeful for a brief moment that this could be shortened.

The specialist kindly went on to explain how it works. She said that she likened it to a garden. Now we have rid most of the surface weeds however the next three months chemotherapy will give us a chance to weed the remainder, and get underneath to the roots and obliterate the cancer more fully. It made sense. It was also very familiar to hear a similar description that had been applied to our late friend Darryl for his chemotherapy treatment.

I knew this new result meant that already Patrick would be good to go for stem cell transplant. Some people don't respond well to chemotherapy and don't get as good a result even after five months, so this was all such positive news.

We then discussed our concerns about being committed to the Kiwi Trial program when it might be deemed Patrick would be better to have double stem cell transplants as per the studies presented at the conference. Both the specialist and the nurse, almost in unison, chimed in "Oh no you don't have to worry about that." The specialist then went first. She said that if Patrick's condition shows that he would fare better with double stem cell transplant then this will get presented to a board for assessment. If they approve, they can either break the Kiwi Trial program for him, or incorporate it. She enforced that it was their priority to give him the best treatment possible.

The nurse, bless her, the one that is always so cheery and positive, then said that it is our decision at all times whether we wish to stay on the Kiwi Trial program or not, we are not bound at all.

Their concern also, first and foremost, is that Patrick gets the best care possible, and it is important for him to know he is free to make these choices. Well what a relief all that was.

Patrick however remained subdued. Towards the end of the session he revealed the reason saying "It's all well and good getting these results and while this is a good indicator that I am heading towards remission, remission is not my biggest worry. In fact I already feel quite convinced I will achieve that, however, with this deletion I have, it's how long will I get remission for?"

The specialist did a big pause. I felt for her, I knew she didn't know the answers. I could feel her go from her mind to her heart as she talked to him. She was open and honest as she said she didn't know the answer to that. She went on encouragingly though. "What you do know is that you are young and your body is responding well. You are having the best of treatments and there is a lot available to assist you as time goes on. You can be confident with how your treatment is going now and we take it one step at a time." Patrick tried to smile back at her but it was a grimace really. All the right words but this boy had done way too much research to find any appeasement in them.

The following day, day two of the third cycle, we asked our Kiwi Trial nurse if it was possible we could talk to the cancer trial specialist again, Dr David Simpson, about the survey that had been presented at the latest conference in America, the one that spoke about double stem cell transplants for high risk factors. Patrick had found out that David had actually been at this conference, so we were curious as to what his thoughts were.

The next thing we knew he was at Patrick's side willing to talk to him. What a treat! His comments were interesting. He said that the trial Patrick was talking about, where the double stem cell transplant was implemented as part of the treatment plan with good results, had not included the use of the latest chemotherapy drugs that Patrick was now on pre-stem cell transplant. It was considered that with these latest chemotherapy drugs that he was taking and the excellent results they were having, it was not deemed necessary to have a double stem cell transplant.

Hmmm, interesting. David went on, reiterating what he had told Patrick on the phone some time ago when he was enquiring about what he knew about del 1p32. He said that even with the deletion Patrick has, we still need to take a step back and see it as multiple myeloma, and look at the treatment he was having and the effect it was having. This was the most important thing. He spoke about Patrick's results and said they were extremely good and it was unusual to have such a good result so soon. This was a good sign, and positive for his outlook for just the one stem cell transplant and achieving remission.

We fired so many questions at him… poor guy, but he kept his ground and gave us his time and solid answers. We felt clearer by the end of the discussion on a number of things and were very thankful to talk to David about all this latest research that had come out of the conference.

Week two of chemotherapy in this third month was the week of New Year's Eve. There is no rest for the wicked when it comes to chemotherapy. We were there the week of Christmas and due straight back after New Year's Eve, not interrupting the cycle at all. The nurses were working so hard up to Christmas coping with the extra workload of people coming in for treatment and less staff due to statutory holidays. Not once did they drop the ball in efficiency, capability or kindness even under this pressure. All of them were such angels!

At the beginning of week two of the third cycle, Patrick unfortunately had a scary incident. We had decided to attend a protest against rodeos on New Year's Day and so Patrick had stayed at my house in Warkworth for New Year's Eve. For many years, on New Year's Day, a rodeo has been held in Warkworth amidst protest from animal lovers. Over the last couple of years I canvassed against rodeos with SAFE, so I was keen to be at the protest on the day this rodeo was being held.

Patrick had insisted he wanted to come, as did my dear girlfriend Nikki who was staying with us. She is a huge animal lover and activist in her own way. So we showed up at 10.30 am New Year's Day with the 100 odd other supporters to protest. We stood outside the A&P showgrounds on the main road with our signs protesting at the atrocities going on inside the showgrounds. Cars honked in support as they passed and we smiled for the press as they took shots, hoping for a good article to be written to help raise awareness of this disgusting practice.

We had been standing roadside for about fifty minutes under shade. Patrick all of a sudden said he needed to sit down as he wasn't feeling too well. We were only going to be there another ten minutes or so, but when I looked back at him he looked really grey and not at all well. I turned to Nikki and told her we needed to go. I suggested she get Patrick's car keys and bring the car around as I wanted to stay and keep an eye on him. Patrick being Patrick refused to give them to her, he wanted us to stay until the end. There was nothing we could do, he was adamant. He got up after five minutes to join me, however he only lasted a minute before he went back to sit down. I was talking to Nikki debating what we should do in regards to insisting we leave or stay, when I heard a kerfuffle behind me and I turned to see Patrick on the ground with people all around trying to help him up. He had fainted!

Apparently, a minute after sitting down again, he just fainted and fell to the side! When he came to, he didn't know where he was at first and struggled to get up. He was so pale. I sat down next to him and started to pour water on him to cool him down while Nikki got the keys and ran for the car. I gave him the water bottle to drink and noticed how much his hand was shaking as he put it to his mouth, then he seemed to go off into a sort of unconsciousness nodding his head uncontrollably. Holy shit, this was serious! Someone suggested we call an ambulance and I agreed. I gave my phone to a lovely lady there to make the call so I could focus on Patrick. Twice he went off into this unconscious type state, then came back again and could speak, although he seemed far away.

It was so scary. I was so worried about him having a heart attack and you can imagine how Nikki felt. This is the same Nikki whose husband had died of a heart attack created from the effects the chemotherapy had taken on his body!

It seemed to take forever talking to the ambulance operator. In that time, Patrick started slowly coming round and he seemed to be out of the woods before the lady had finished talking to the operator. I took the phone off her then, preferring now to talk to the operator myself and asked if there was an ambulance in the show grounds. I said he was coming round and seemed better but it would be good to just check his blood pressure etc. She said that even if there was an ambulance just one minute down the road she was not authorized to ask it to come. She would need to place a call through the correct channels and an ambulance would be called, from probably the closest town, Warkworth. I told her to not worry as he was now feeling better. Patrick was insisting in the background he didn't need it now also. He did seem better and was able to get up so we got him into the car that was now waiting, and got him home to bed. He slept all afternoon and night, and actually in the end took him about a week to fully recover.

It was quite a scare and one we didn't take lightly. The next day I encouraged him to call the hospital and advise them of what had happened and he got the very helpful specialist Dr Henry Chan. He suggested Patrick have extra tests taken when he came in the next day for his chemotherapy session, including an ECG, so they could assess more fully how he was.

The tests all came out fine and Henry himself came to see Patrick to discuss where to go from here. His assessment was that it was probably the blood pressure medication he was on. It seemed that the chemotherapy was adjusting his blood pressure making it too low, so his usual medication needed to be dropped to compensate for that.

Patrick had suffered from high blood pressure for a few years before he was diagnosed and was on medication for this so it was the obvious place to start from. It was interesting that now he was on chemotherapy his blood pressure had changed from being high to now being too low. For another chemo friend of ours, going through the same treatment plan on the Kiwi Trial, her blood pressure had risen. Go figure, it affects everyone differently!

Of course while we had Dr Chan with us we decided to make the most of this time with him, as we do. Patrick broached the double stem cell option and also asked his thoughts on the recent study. This was the specialist who had worked in Toronto for a couple of years where they were doing a lot of double stem transplants for high risk patients.

He basically said that it is not something that NZ routinely does for patients with del (1p) as there hasn't been much published evidence to support that double or tandem transplant can improve the outcomes for patients with del (1p). There is some evidence, but not a lot compared with other deletions. Del(1p) is singled out in some studies as a high risk factor, but to what extent is difficult to tell due to other contributing and confounding factors, so there is still so much not really known specifically about it. It was very helpful to hear this, and we thanked him very much for his time.

Hmmm, I turned to Patrick after he left and said "It seems globally they still don't know a lot about the 1p32 deletion. Patrick, you need to do more research and find out what you need to do for this deletion!" Thinking at the time, he needs to find out more to support double stem cell transplants. Little did I know, actually, we could be barking up the wrong tree!

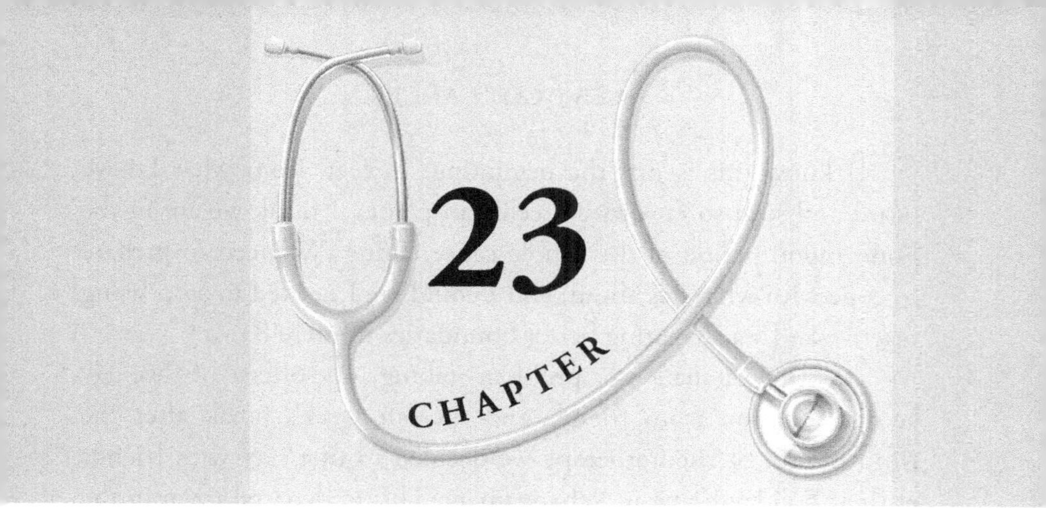

We've Got Cancer

"Muddy water is best cleared
by leaving it alone."
- Alan Watts -

We are now soon to begin the fourth cycle. It's 4am and I can't sleep. We had just got back yesterday from our week's holiday after the third cycle of chemotherapy.

Three months of chemotherapy, I have great sadness for myself. Great sadness for Patrick too. It was proving to be real shit, what we were going through; it really was. Having treatments through Christmas and New Year and the height of New Zealand's summer really had been awful, allowing very little opportunity for celebration or enjoyment as we were exhausted through it all. For the first time in my life I felt I was deserving to accept from others. For the first time in my life I can easily say no to helping others. For the first time in my life I feel OK not chasing friends to catch up. For the first time in my life I am OK with not pushing myself. For the first time in my life I feel it's OK to say no to some of the 'things to do'!

I know this is just the beginning. In fact, from what I have heard and seen so far of stem cell transplants, I think we are in the honeymoon period of this whole cancer thing. We need to prepare to cope with what lies ahead, and I could see I needed to stop being reactive and start creating better boundaries in myself!

In this, I had no problem taking up offers of holiday accommodation from friends and for our week's break after the third month of chemotherapy we decided to first stay with friends at their holiday home in Whangamata. This is a coastal town in the Coromandel on an eastern beach in the North Island and they have a stunning home right on the beach. It must be one of NZ's most beautiful spots! It looks out over the sand dunes to pristine beach, the sand running gently out into the pure clean green NZ ocean, as it should be! Then, in almost swimming distance, lies Donut Island, full of Pohutukawa which were still half in bloom. I could have sat on their deck all day never tiring of it!

Patrick loves it here. He is such a water baby. He loves the gentle surf as he's a keen body surfer. He also enjoys their land yacht and running around town on the mopeds when we stay here, it's just such a relaxing place. We didn't arrive until late on Saturday as there had been a bad storm but by the time we got there the weather was a lot better.

We had finished this round of chemotherapy on Thursday so he was still feeling the effects of it and was really tired. It was quite sad that over the two days we were there he didn't swim, he just wasn't up to it. That's unheard of for this water baby but there you go. He still managed to stay positive as usual and enjoyed some time on the beach land yachting, and joining in on small walks.

We then moved on to a friend's place in Tairua, another smaller seaside town in the Coromandel. This was her home but she was away, so we had the place to ourselves.

Once we got to Tairua and the days moved further away from Patrick's last treatment he started feeling better and his energy started building again. In fact by half way through the week he stopped taking naps during the day, which was really lovely, and started swimming which was fantastic to see. He bodysurfed for up to an hour on a couple of days, he was enjoying himself so much, and still managed to stay up for the day and night without a rest.

Tairua is one of those real kiwiana seaside towns... small, slow, and peaceful. The property we were staying in has a lovely fenced yard so we could have our dog Indi stay too. It also has a couple of cabins so we invited Patrick's daughter Katelyn and my girlfriend Nikki. Friends of Katelyn's came and went as it was school holidays so it became a really lovely time away.

Patrick was looking great again. This time away was helping to bring him back to life, as the effects of the drugs were leaving his body. Here we are, three months of chemotherapy down and still surviving... not only surviving but kicking that cancer to touch.

The weather was glorious! Every day was a stunning 27°C/80°F with no wind. We couldn't have hoped for better beach weather. We spent the first couple of days lazing on the local beaches and then ventured out further, to New Chums beach, about an hours drive away, and then a half hour walk to get there.

I had wanted to go to New Chums beach for a year or two as I had heard how stunningly beautiful it was and I really wanted to get there this trip. In the back of my mind I was worried it may be our only chance this summer as Patrick may not feel up to it as time goes on... and further back in my mind I worried it may be our last chance to ever go together. I kept tucking that thought away, not really wanting to acknowledge it, but that underlying threat was there, always there!

Patrick was feeling so good he didn't hesitate about going. We had taken two cars to accommodate us all and I went with my girlfriend Nikki, with Patrick taking Katelyn and her friends who had stayed the night. He didn't even get upset when I got us lost and ended up on some dirt track in the middle of God knows where.

Honestly, he has the patience of a saint so it was about an hour and a half just getting to the walk to the beach.

The photos following don't begin to give this idyllic piece of nature anywhere near its full justice, but they're the only shots we took. We had sneaked our dog over as there was no way we could have left her behind for so long. We kept her on lead, and proceeded to the end of the beach so she didn't bother anybody. No one was at this end, so it became our own little slice of paradise.

In looking back over the holiday I feel so blessed we had that opportunity… but we are back home now and I am awake, feeling anxious and worried and sad.

Reality has kicked back in and I am in wonder that the week ahead of us is real. Back to the hospital, back to chemotherapy, and the stem cell transplant process looming. Oh my God! It's not alright. Life is not good and it's not alright.

My mind was talking to me hard out "Your dearest partner lying next to you asleep right now is going to go through hell and back again in the coming weeks. He's going to start getting more tired and listless again. He's going to be wandering around in circles again. He's going to get highly emotional and he's going to need to go to hospital twice a week and get that toxic crap injected into his body… and soon, all too soon, he will be in hospital for weeks, losing his hair, throwing up, losing weight, and losing himself in this what seems to me to be, horrid process of zapping away his entire immune system and leaving him helpless through the stem cell transplant."

Lying here, I realised the negative place I was in. I was becoming so resentful for Patrick and what lies ahead for him. I have seen him get worse with each round of induction chemotherapy and the side effects seem to get tougher for him each month. I realise this five months of induction therapy really is probably the honeymoon period. I expect the shit is really going to hit the fan with the stem cell transplant process. We won't be able to pretend this doesn't exist for even a moment once that starts!

Since Patrick started treatment I have worried about him having a heart attack but as time has gone on and he has been OK I have relaxed about this now. An alertness without the stress. I knew now he was not going to throw up with his standard chemotherapy treatments, I knew what we were up for with the induction chemotherapy treatments and how he would be affected, but stem cell transplant, well that was a huge unknown. It was coming closer and closer and I could feel the fear closing in with it.

The holiday on this last week off was again, so worthwhile, it was so lovely to have that time together. It was fantastic to have fun and laugh, and get away from the harsh realities while we could however, as I lie here, it is coming to me how in the not too distant future we won't be able to 'get away' from it all with stem cell transplant looming… and I'm scared, really scared. As I open into it, it is so overwhelming. Like a dark black terror wanting to wash over me and engulf me, swallow me up. As it comes I distract, move away from it with my mind to another thought, another focus, but when I turn back it's there still, it never left. It's lurking there at my core, just waiting for the months to come and to have its way with me. Stem cell transplant!

When I look back I'd had three years of fighting in the high court with my ex, and again in court supporting a girlfriend with her case for a further couple of years. Then, when I'm finally free of all the court stuff and feeling a lot better with little stress in my life, now this with Patrick. Cancer! It felt like I was not meant to get a break!

The high court situation was awful. It disturbs me how the court system doesn't appreciate what people go through when fighting for their rights. It's all dragged out for years and years and it's horrific. So much negativity and a threat that takes away your fundamental core of a right to happiness.

But oh, oh, oh, it's nothing compared to this cancer trial. A pittance compared to what we are now faced to deal with. It doesn't even come close to this real life and death possibility. It doesn't even come close to having your whole body destroyed and your existence as you know it taken from you. Not money or things or rights… LIFE!

I started to feel myself drifting back off to sleep and I tell myself as I am sinking away, that it's not me, it's not me with cancer, but it may as well be. I'm so sensitive and caring I am going through this with Patrick like I am going through it myself. It's always WE. We've Got Cancer. Is that a good thing or not I wonder, as I drift off into momentary oblivion?

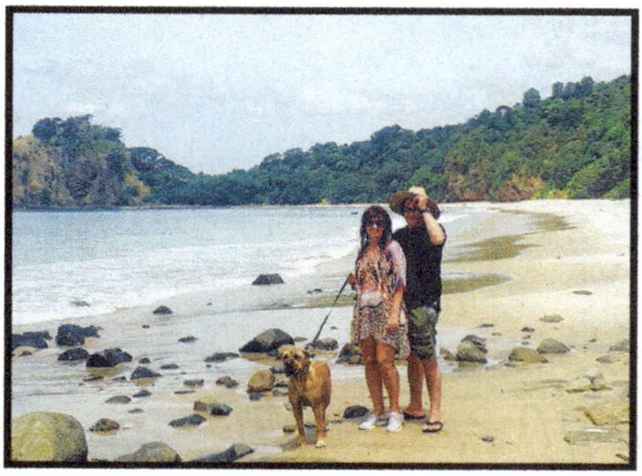

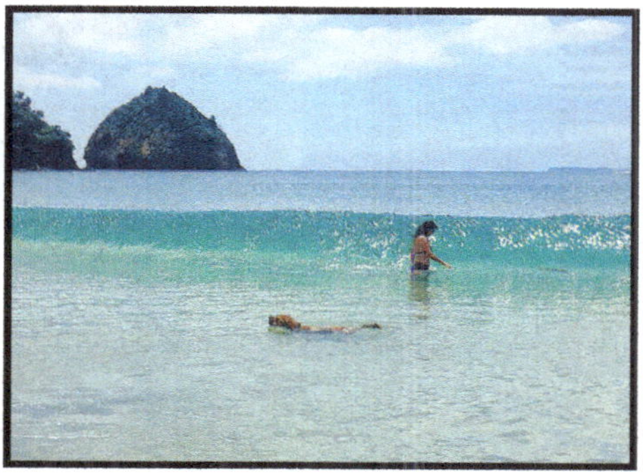

You have to swim in these beaches to know how lovely they really are. The water is clean, pure and silky. The white fine sand is so soft to walk on and the surroundings of NZ bush and Pohutukawa really make the backdrop spectacular. We all had such a special day together there.

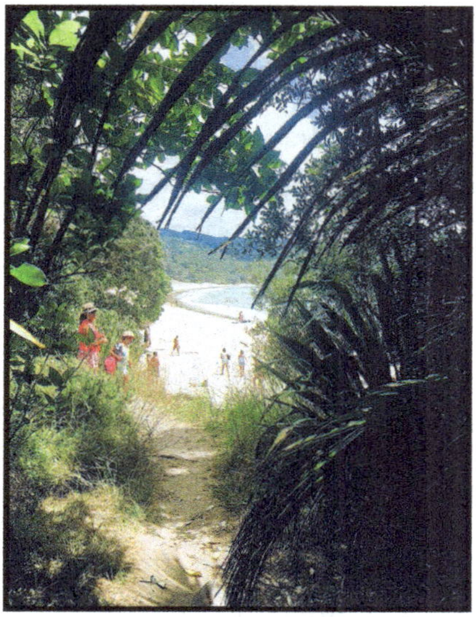

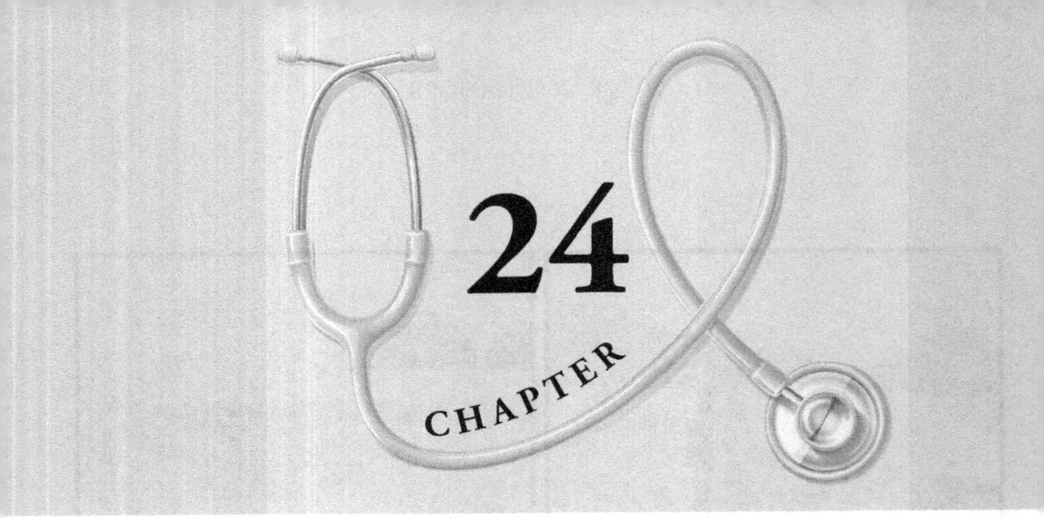

No To Stem Cell Transplant

"I refuse to answer that question
on the grounds that I don't know
the answer."
- Douglas Adams -

Today we were to meet the specialist to have the usual monthly check before chemotherapy begins for cycle four.

Unbeknown to me Patrick had, a couple of days earlier, through googling yet again, discovered another survey done on del1p32. Oh dear, in one way I wish he hadn't. It threw us into total turmoil yet again.

It was another early morning with Patrick bringing me a cup of tea in bed. As he sat down on the side of the bed he said "Hey darling, I think you should know before we see the specialist today that I found another paper of research done on del1p32."

Of course he had my immediate attention and I could see tucked under his arm, what I presumed was the paper he was talking about.

"I hadn't wanted to worry you before now," he continued, "but I have to bring it up at our appointment today, so you need to know about it." Patrick, it seemed, had been keeping this latest paper to himself, absorbing the enormity of it and finding a way to process the information before telling me.

He was speaking softly, with such kindness and care for me, I immediately stepped into 'I can cope' mode for him to try and alleviate his concern.

"No worries" I said, "maybe it's best you just give me the paper and I read it." which he did. It wasn't terribly long. It was a summary of a report done but it was very scientifically written and hard to get your head around.

The heading was:

"Mapping of chromosome 1p deletions in myeloma identifies FAM46C at 1p12 and CDKN2C at 1p32 as being genes in regions associated with adverse survival."

Immediately didn't like that heading at all. Another reinforcement of the consequences of Patrick's 1p32 deletion, 'associated with adverse survival'.

It basically went on to say that through their studies it was found that **1p32.3** was deleted in **11% of cases** and the deletion was **strongly associated with impaired overall survival in patients treated with autologous stem cell transplants (ASCT).**

In patients treated less intensively, del (1)(p32.3) was not associated with adverse progression-free survival (PFS) or OS (Overall survival).

There was a whole lot of scientific jargon after that and then the conclusion.

CONCLUSION: Deletion of 1p32.3 (which apparently is still part of 1p32) **and 1p12 was associated with impaired OS (overall survival) in myeloma patients receiving ASCT (autologous stem cell transplant).**

Oh God! How much more bad news were we expected to take? And how confusing when everyone at this point had said a stem cell transplant as part of treatment would provide the best result and increase remission time. This totally contradicted everything we'd been told. Let alone that **double** stem cell transplants for high risk patients were being recommended overseas.

Patrick lay down next to me. I looked over in disbelief. "Oh my God, what now?" was all I could say. "I don't know," he said "but I'm sure as hell not going to have a stem cell transplant now!"

My stomach sank. What does this mean when we are on the Kiwi Trial program. Will they stop our treatments now if we tell them this? Is this the right thing to do after all we have been told? What do we do?!!! My mind was racing! Support chief though that I am, I said firmly to him, "Absolutely. If that is what you think is best then we won't. They can't make you just because you are in the Kiwi Trial. Remember what they said, we can pull out of the trial any time we want to!"

We were so green, so new to the system, the hospital regulations etc, we had no idea what consequences this could bring or problems it could raise, but we were going to do what is right for him and that was that. However, we still worried… worried and worried about how to best deal with this situation now. Patrick had been surfing the internet to find more details on this study, yet could find nothing more. He had even tried to get the full study report but was not permitted access.

It was quite ironic really. Here we had been pushing for double stem cell transplant to the specialists thinking this was the best option, only to find now, in fact maybe we need to push for not having one at all. Will we start to look like idiots? Does this show we know nothing of what we are talking about and confirm their opinion that we should just leave it all up to them and stay out of it?

I brushed those thoughts aside. This is medicine, a constantly evolving industry where new things are discovered all the time. New illnesses, new drugs, new trials, new research. This study was the last thing Patrick had found on del 1p32, completed only five years ago, a few years after the French study, by some of the same people that did the initial French Study. So yes it should be listened to and heard. No, we shouldn't feel like idiots for chopping and changing direction, we are just trying to be informed and up to date on what is best for Patrick with his complication of this chromosome deletion.

So we were back to being concerned about the impact on the Kiwi Trial program if he was to pull out, and how the specialists would react to this new discovery of research.

We didn't have long to wait before we were in our appointment. By now Patrick was taking his bloods days before the appointment so we could then discuss the results when we went in. We were to see Patricks main specialist, Dr Henderson. This time we were prepared to ensure we used our appointment time wisely, and had agreed we would bring up our concerns sooner rather than later. Also, rather than surprise Dr Henderson with this report and expect immediate answers, we decided to just discuss that we had uncovered this research, ask if he was aware of it, and if not leave it with him to read for his comment later. I wasn't sure how he was going to take yet another study to be questioned over!

We were both really pleased when we sat down that Dr Henderson went straight into discussing the French Study we had left with him in our previous appointment with him, which by now was two months later. He said he had read it carefully and proceeded to give us his thoughts on it. It was encouraging to us to know he had taken our concerns seriously and read the report. He pointed out a couple of significant factors about how the report was combined with other major deletions. His consideration was that we can not take too definitively the graphs and life expectancy. He also pointed out how old the research was and said that the treatments had come a long way since then. He went on to explain how he felt that Patrick's treatment regime is still the best possible for his condition and his results to date suggested he was doing excellently and should expect remission, which was the best possible outcome at this stage.

So this was Patrick's opportunity to introduce the next report. The study had been done by a Specialist in the USA who was an internationally recognised clinician scientist, someone we knew Dr Henderson respected as a leader in the field of multiple myeloma. Patrick simply said to him as he handed over the new report "That's great in regards to my getting remission, but my concern, after reading this report is for how long and whether I should be doing the stem cell transplant at all."

I jumped in quickly. "We don't expect you to answer this right now, but if you can read it and get back to us that would be great." Dr Henderson had taken the report and was already reading it. He noticed immediately that it was just a summary of a more extensive report. Patrick told him how he was not able to get the full report as apparently you needed to be a medical body of some kind to obtain it. Blow me down, Dr Henderson offered to get it for him, and said he would email it to him, as well as read it himself. Patrick was very thankful. We then moved to the main purpose of these appointments which was to check Patrick's health before he began his next round of chemotherapy.

I'll just note here that we received the rollout letter about a week later, which is always sent out by the specialist following your appointment summarising the test results, recommendations and anything significant that occurred in the meeting. The letter commented on how well Patrick was doing, citing the paraprotein results. It also mentioned that we had passed on the survey to him and that he would review it and get back to us. When we went in for chemotherapy the following week, one of the nurses passed on the full report as provided by our specialist. It really helped to feel so supported by Dr Henderson. It meant a lot to be heard and to have him take the time to access and supply us with the full report. We felt honoured in our concerns.

A quick zoom forward… right up to the last week of our fifth cycle, almost two months later, we had not seen Dr Henderson again, so we did not get the opportunity to discuss the report. On day one of Patrick's fifth cycle a different specialist was on duty. At the point of almost finishing the full cycle of induction chemotherapy, and the stem cell transport looming, for us the question remained as to whether Patrick should indeed have a stem cell transplant at all. It was now pressing. Patrick decided to search further for answers. Thankfully, as you will read later, he spoke to many other specialists who gave their advice and with that knowledge he was able to make his decisions!

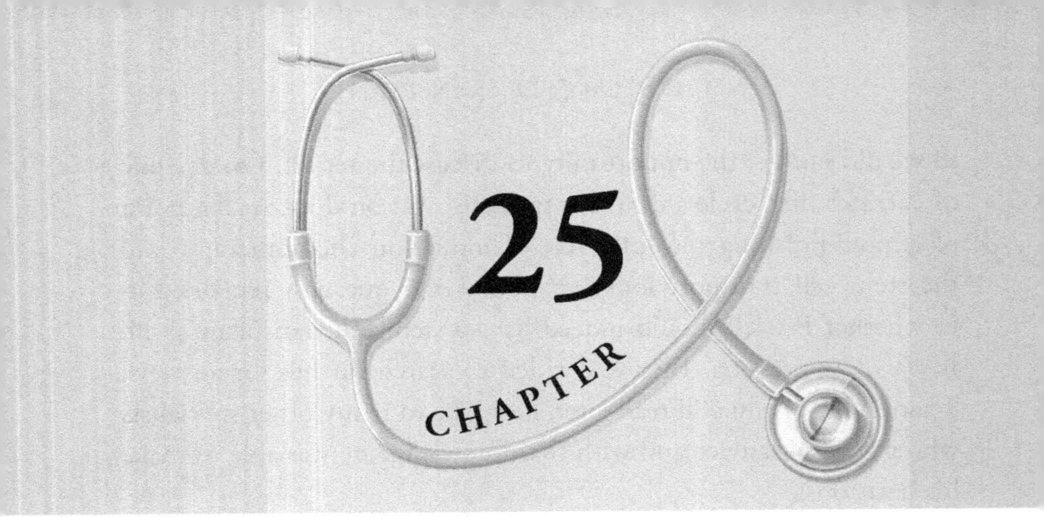

Peripheral Neuropathy

"I have woven a parachute
out of everything broken."
- William Stafford -

At the end of the second week of the fourth cycle it suddenly feels like there is a light at the end of the tunnel. It's Saturday and the beginning of a long weekend.

We have faced a lot of fear over the last four months and it's been physically exhausting. This last month I had ended up crashing with chronic fatigue despite doing my best keeping up with all my vitamins and creams. It's almost not worth mentioning as it still seems so inconsequential in the whole scheme of things, however it feels right to honor that this is a difficult road for the support partner of a cancer patient.

I had been finding it harder to take on so much as Patrick continues to take on less. As he steps down I have to step up. I had come to a point before diagnosis with chronic fatigue that if I was careful not to overdo things I could manage it pretty well. I couldn't do that now, it was virtually impossible. Things needed doing and someone had to do them. Hello! Thankfully it only took me about ten days to recover and here I am now ready to go again!

Patrick initially thought he was handling the chemotherapy better than usual at the beginning of this fourth cycle. He didn't seem to be wiped out as much the first week of treatment, and the tingling and numbness from the peripheral neuropathy that he had been experiencing as a side effect, was nowhere near as bad. He had started taking vitamin E so he was hoping it was getting a grip on the side effects, however by the Thursday and Friday of the week following treatment, the heaviness in his body and the numbness and heat in his feet had worsened. Over the last couple of months Patrick had been strapping ice packs on his feet some nights to calm the heat down, however, now the ice packs were also coming out during the day to give him some relief!

The peripheral neuropathy had definitely worsened with this month's treatment and he was not coping with it. At the monthly appointments the specialists regularly checked this, and along with the usual questions would ask 'can you do up your buttons?' If the answer was 'yes', he was considered good enough to continue. However during the second week of cycle four it got to where he felt he just didn't want to continue with the Cyclophosphamide anymore. He wasn't sure whether it was the Cyclophosphamide or the Carfilzomib that was causing the peripheral neuropathy. He didn't want to stop the Carfilzomib as he felt it was too important a drug, but he felt he needed to change something.

Patrick was terrified of ending up like his brother's friend in England. He had been under the same treatment plan as Patrick and went from being an athletic runner and cyclist to post treatment only managing a shuffle of a walk. Another of Patrick's biggest fears was not being able to perform magic ever again. Already it was starting to prove difficult for him for certain effects, in particular card tricks. The loss of feeling and tingling in his hands was affecting his movement.

On the last day of his treatment this week, Patrick raised it with the head nurse of the Kiwi Trial program. She in turn spoke to Dr David Simpson, the head specialist of the program. David happened to be at the hospital that day and he actually came and spoke to Patrick. I know I've said it before, but he is such a lovely man, always giving his time if he can.

He was very understanding of how Patrick was feeling and suggested that instead of cutting out a drug altogether that he was better to reduce the dosage of the Carfilzomib first to see if that helped. He said with the success Patrick had had to date with his response, it would not affect his treatment too much if he dropped the dose. This was apparently much more preferable than him stopping the Cyclophosphamide completely.

Patrick agreed to give that a try. He was relieved that something was getting done and it was something that everyone was comfortable with. Secretly so was I. Again, this was Patrick's journey and his decisions to make, but I had been worried about going cold turkey on a drug that obviously, combined with other treatments, was knocking the cancer out of the park!

As mentioned, it felt like the light was at the end of the tunnel, even amongst all this going on. Maybe it's that we know Patrick has responded so well to treatment that we can relax the dosage a fraction. Maybe it's that there is almost only one month left to go of the first stage of treatment. Or maybe it was because there was a possibility Patrick may not have the stem cell transplant. That was still a big question mark for him.

Right now, it feels incredible that we have just got through another month of treatment, with nearly four months of chemotherapy behind us. In one way it seems to have been a lifetime, in another it seems to have flown by. If I stop to analyze that, it makes sense, it has been a lifetime. I have a way of seeing my life when I look back, as different lifetimes. Life has had so many dramatic changes for me over the years, it's like one life has rolled into another.

My first lifetime was my childhood. My first real boyfriend, my first job, my first flat, my first marriage.

My second lifetime was separating from my first husband and traveling overseas as a free spirit with many adventures unfolding… then coming back to NZ and moving to Auckland to live with a man who was to be my future husband, working with him and growing a computer supplies company together. We lived and breathed our work; it was the 80's and party time too. This then flowed into starting our property development company, the beginning of the 90's with champagne flowing and more good times.

Lifetime number 3 was 6 October 1992. Becoming a mother when my dear son Chase arrived, then Taylor, three years later.

Then separating from my husband in 2003 after some 14 years of being together definitely became lifetime number 4. Coping with separation, bringing the children up on my own and helping them adjust too.

About five years later, lifetime number 5 began… the day I met Patrick. Our new love, eventually incorporating our two families together, and 10 years in on what I thought was to be a whole lifetime of growing old together.

Now it's Lifetime No 6. Living with a partner with cancer.

It really does shake, rock, and change your whole world. No longer does the future have the certainty you thought, as the underlying core of every day is threatened with the possibility of doom coming, difficult, hard times coming. Uncertainty, pain, sadness, loss and grief are all a real threat for the future. In fact, when you allow yourself to open, it's not in the future, but right here, right now. Our worry for what will happen in the future means you feel and experience it emotionally right now! It's not the sort of lifetime I like to be in for sure but we now seem to be finding a way through and thankfully being a therapist I had the opportunity to open and work through what I was feeling at times.

It feels like we are catching up on ourselves. The two holidays I know certainly helped, and I had given myself some good emotional therapy that had probably been very overdue. And then there was, just simply, time. I really should have taken more time off work over these past months. It was too hard working even part time, and going through this upheaval. On the other hand it did help keep me grounded, so who knows. I'm shrugging right now, it doesn't matter. It was what it was and what's important is going forward from here.

I've feared chemotherapy for years. Ever since my dear girlfriend Shane went through it some years ago. Yet here we are, doing it. We are coping. Does this seem strange that I say 'we' and talk as if I have been through it? I can't help it. It feels WE have, given I have been so on board with Patrick.

It emerges to me how important it is to see this and I am beginning to see that is what a lot of this writing is about. Everyone cares about the person who has cancer, but what about their closest loved one going through it with them too. Not just for their pain, but they are literally going through the whole process too.

Oh yes, it's all about me! Goodness no, that's not what I mean. I am not the one whose life is threatened, who only has possibly such a short time on this planet where all lifetimes will be terminated. I will probably form many other lifetimes and my dearest Patrick may not.

I am not the one who is having this toxic product injected throughout my body twice a week, taking sometimes 25 pills in a day, and who has the effects of this in their body! I am not the one who has to worry about whether he will be there for his child's 21st or graduation, or who knows he will have to leave his loved ones so much sooner than he had thought.

I'm just saying. It's really tough for us partners too. We go through it in more ways than I ever realised. Everything is 'we' in our partnership, and 'we' are going through this.

As the light starts coming through though I am enjoying feeling some relief. I can physically feel a weight lifting from me. Intuitively it seemed, without my doing or thinking anything, the light was bringing some space, some life, some joy. I welcomed it into my whole being.

We have got through more than three quarters of this sometimes gruelling process of chemotherapy and the awful impact it has had on Patrick. It has been healing writing as we have gone through this. It helps so much to take time to be present with my thoughts and feelings, consider them and get them out of my head and into black and white. I highly recommend this process! It helped even today as I am writing, to take the time to stop and acknowledge what is here and what has brought a ray of sunshine.

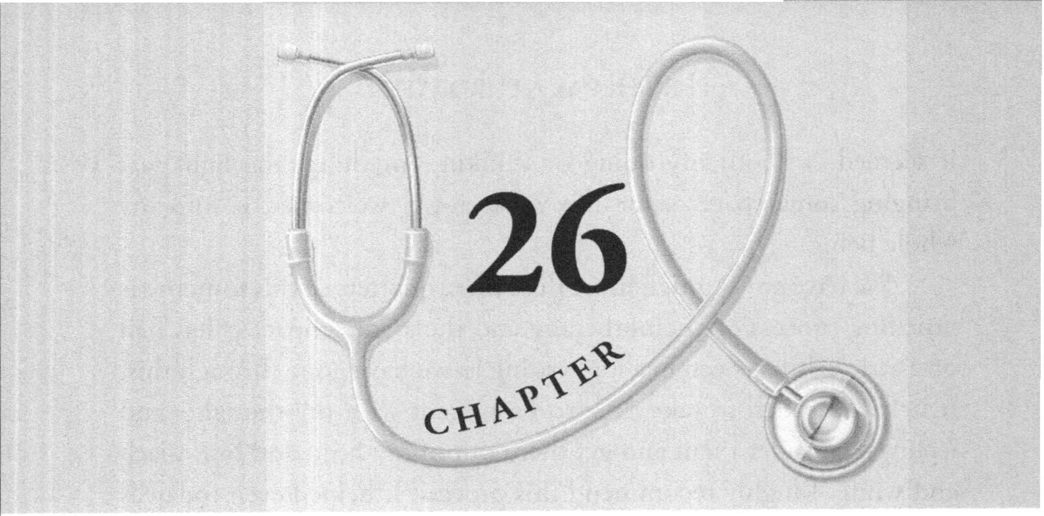

American Specialist

"In the middle of difficulty
lies opportunity"
- Albert Einstein -

It has turned out for Patrick that the last week of the fourth month was harder than we thought it was going to be. He seems to be struggling more and more. Can you believe the lightness I'd raved about last week has all but faded away. I felt quite sad and rocked at the shift he was experiencing now.

The drop in Carfilzomib seemed to have helped a little with the peripheral neuropathy. Although it still was a problem, it had eased a little and at least wasn't getting worse.

They say chemotherapy is out of the system in a week... well maybe that's true. As the week goes on Patrick eventually feels better. Chemotherapy Tuesday and Wednesday makes him so tired and he needs an afternoon and evening rest after treatment.

Thursday, Friday and Saturday mornings are the worst. He loses his voice quite a bit so it is hard for him to express. He is very tired, spending a lot of the afternoon resting in bed and goes to bed early also.

The numbness in his fingertips, the metallic taste in his mouth, and the heat under his feet is still a bother, even with the drop in dosage of Carfilzomib. This week he also now has been getting a sore gut and a discomfort in his throat he describes as a dragging ball type feeling. By today, Saturday morning, the tears are flowing and he is sobbing his heart out. He has started to worry that maybe the cancer has worsened and that is why he is experiencing these feelings in his stomach and throat. Oh poor baby it's so heartbreaking to see him like this.

He was lying on the bed and I sat next to him stroking his hair trying to reassure him that this isn't the case. We do bloods every Tuesday and nothing has escalated, it can't possibly be the case. I try to reassure him this is just the drugs upsetting him, taking him there, bringing him down, and that this will pass. For the first time I said to him "Patrick if this chemotherapy is too much for you, and you want to stop now, just say the word. I will support you in whatever decision you make!"

And I meant it. Every word of it. I don't know how he has got through so far. I really don't know if I could have done it. All the pills alone to take each week would have done me in. I'm so proud of him and what he has gone through. He has still managed to work a little through it all and managed a modicum of normal life, but if it's getting too hard he just needs to say the word! The treatments were taking more and more of a toll on his body.

Patrick's results have been consistently coming through as showing that he is now <3 for his paraprotein level… remember that's from where he began at 43! This has been consistent again with this month's results. He is already doing so well fighting this cancer and the specialist has indicated this is a sign he could already be in remission. Do we really even need to continue anyhow? Surely we've got down to the roots of the weeds by now.

So that leads me into the following week. We have been called in to Auckland Hospital to discuss stem cell transplant. Auckland Hospital holds the specialised stem cell transplant ward where everyone goes to have this done. I was at first a little disappointed, our specialist assigned was not our Kiwi Trial specialist's wife. She is a specialist at the stem cell transplant division at Auckland Hospital, I had thought it would be great if it were all closely linked.

However it was such a treat to meet the specialist assigned, Dr Richard Doocey. What a lovely man, who was happy to sit and listen to all our concerns and be open to all options that may be appropriate for Patrick.

Ultimately the conversation was around the upcoming stem cell transplant that had been booked for Patrick, which was why we were seeing him. However Patrick found the opportunity to give him a copy of the report from the **conference in December 2017, saying double stem cell transplant was having better success for multiple myeloma for those patients with HR (High Risk).**

Richard read the basis of the report right there and then. It was wonderful to hear Richard say after reading it, that should it be deemed Patrick would benefit from double stem cell transplant he would have no problem in allowing this to proceed. Wow, that was awesome to hear!

Patrick then went on with the dilemma of the more recent findings of the report done in December 2015, the one that the Specialist who was an internationally recognised clinician scientist was a part of, pointing out that the report was saying that **with 1p32 deletions it was better NOT to have a transplant at all!** Patrick gave him a copy of this report also.

Patrick had by now googled more on this Specialist and had discovered he was practicing in private practice in the USA. It turns out he was a Director of the Myeloma Institute at the University of Arkansas for Medical Sciences (UANS). Sounds pretty qualified, right?

Richard was very interested and could immediately see the dilemma but unfortunately didn't have the answers for us there and then. However, he advised that he had met this particular Specialist and he was a very approachable man, and suggested Patrick get in touch with him directly to discuss his queries. He thought that considering he was particularly interested in chromosome deletions and also considering Patrick's del 1p32, he may well get a response from him. Well we hadn't thought of that. I guess with all of his credentials, we had thought of him as unreachable. Richard went on to say that if we did have difficulty he would be happy to call him himself and get his thoughts on Patrick's case.

By the time we left the room I was in love with Dr Richard Doocey! He's a top Auckland bone marrow transplant specialist who is prepared to go the extra mile for us!

So Patrick did just that. He first emailed the Specialist's secretary advising of his chromosome deletion and dilemma in regards to stem cell transplants. He asked if he could have a Skype or phone appointment. We weren't sure if this was a thing, but it was our preferred option. Patrick stated that he was a US citizen as well as a NZ citizen, to see if that added any weight as we thought there may be regulations on who he could take on as patients. Unfortunately the response from the secretary was that he did not do Skype or phone calls, however, she said she had spoken to him and he'd be happy to view Patrick's case. We were ecstatic. So Patrick wrote immediately outlining his dilemma in regards to the conflicting reports he had read and whether to have double stem cell transplant or in fact not have one at all considering his del 1p32.

We were delighted to get a response from the Specialist's secretary the very next day asking us for ALL Patrick's records since the date of diagnosis up to now. Wow! That's impressive right?, we were extremely grateful. Patrick sent them immediately.

26 January 2018, the secretary replied… only six days after we had sent the information! She said that the Specialist had viewed Patrick's records and he has stated that transplant with maintenance is a good option. She said he would be delighted to have Patrick come to Arkansas and meet with him and added that if Patrick decided to travel to Arkansas she would be happy to set that up.

To be honest we did consider it. We actually considered flying over there just for that one appointment. The question was so important and pressing, a life threatening question really. What would the consequences be for Patrick either way? To have the opportunity to sit with him and discuss this in depth would have been wonderful but Patrick, in the end, decided this wasn't necessary enough to incur this sort of cost. What mattered most at the end of the day was the Specialist's opinion, and he had given that.

As soon as we came to that conclusion Patrick emailed back stating that he was under the Kiwi Trial in New Zealand which incorporated stem cell transplant and maintenance therapy. Patrick said again that he would still love a chance to discuss with the Specialist, or even through paid correspondence, the paper he was involved in with del 1p32 and stem cell transplants in relation to his specific case.

The response came the following day. The recommendation was **that transplant or 2 with maintenance was a good option.**

Her response was very clear. The area above in bold was written in bold by her also. Well there it was, from what we felt was one of the heads of all heads of expertise in del1p32. Go ahead with stem cell transplant and maintenance. It was very brief, no explanation, but that was his expert opinion… not just one stem cell transplant, but possibly two.

It was also very clear that he did not consider Patrick should not have a transplant at all. This is the same man who was part of the study six years earlier that had recommended not to have a stem cell transplant with del 1p32.

It was enough. We knew that drugs and treatment plans for multiple myeloma were progressing rapidly and changing constantly, therefore of course, opinions would change. It was all we needed to hear going forward. Every top specialist in New Zealand and it seems now also, one of the leaders in the field of multiple myeloma, were all saying stem cell transplant was the best option for Patrick, and as Dr Richard Doocey had said, possibly two if it was deemed necessary come the time.

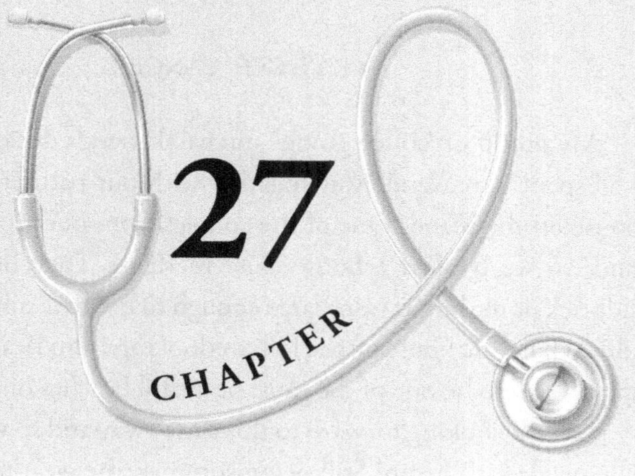

CHAPTER 27

Waiheke Island's Spiritual Message

"I have realised that the past and future are real illusions, that they exist in the present, which is what there is and all there is."
- Alan Watts -

It was the end of the fourth cycle and it was Patrick's week off. He'd had such a tough month so I was really thankful that we had booked a long weekend away to Waiheke Island with friends; Waiheke Island had most recently been voted one of the most beautiful islands in the world.

I love it there! I nearly bought a house there. It has traditionally been seen as a hippy lifestyle to live on 'The Island', despite it only being a half hour ferry ride from central Auckland City! It has developed considerably since then and the community now comprises a wonderful mix of people.

My group of 'coffee group' antenatal friends decided it was time we all spent a weekend away together with our partners, so we rented a house on the island. One of the couples from our group lives on the island, so we booked a house close to them. They have a gorgeous mudbrick home but it wasn't large enough to house us all so we managed to find a fantastic house on the hill overlooking Palm Beach. Palm Beach happens to also be one of the most beautiful beaches on Waiheke.

I was so looking forward to this time away and so was Patrick. We really needed it!! Again! Still being summer, the weather was fantastic and the long weekend was spent swimming, eating, laughing and relaxing... a perfect combination. Patrick was still pretty tired from his treatments however he managed to rally himself to have a good time.

Something a bit freaky happened that weekend on Waiheke Island. We were shopping in the small town of Oneroa on our first day there. I had forgotten my sunglasses and couldn't go without in this gorgeous weather.

Waiheke is well known for its natural, organic, environmentally friendly consciousness. There was a set of sunglasses in a gift store that were made of bamboo; they were just cheapies but looked alright on me so I bought them. It wasn't until later that day when I was wearing them that Patrick said to me "What's that on the side of your sunglasses?" I had no idea what he was on about, so I took them off to have a look. Blow me down, there were letters embossed on the outside of the glasses. MRD- !!!!!! I kid you not!

Wow. We had no idea why that was written on the sunglasses. In fact we didn't want to know. We just took this as a sign. MRD- Patrick - right there!

Minimum Residual Disease was the only MRD we knew of. This of course is exactly what Patrick was going for as his best possible result from his treatments. Such a simple thing somehow that gave us a real lift in positivity. We felt like it was a sign giving us confidence that yes, we were on track. Yes it's tough, but keep it up, you're on track!

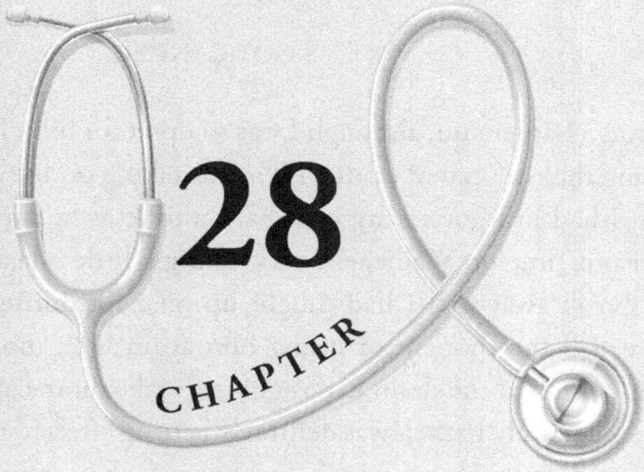

CHAPTER 28

Fifth Month Induction Therapy - Depression

"The more a thing tends to be permanent,
the more it tends to be lifeless."
- Alan Watts -

It's the end of the fifth month now and four days after Patrick's last day of chemotherapy (for the first stage of the Kiwi Trial), five months of induction therapy done and dusted!

Even now I still can't celebrate it. I feel so jarred and down from the last month and it hasn't lifted yet. The light at the end of the tunnel had dwindled completely through the fifth month to almost darkness. Patrick had found the last month of treatment very difficult and is still recovering.

When I woke on the first day of cycle five, knowing we were going back into the hospital for more, again I felt incredibly sad and low and I had a feeling of dread wash over me. He was finding it all so much harder and, although I was so upset for him, I was also really feeling the true extent of the toll it was taking on me as well.

I had just gotten my man back a little as he was feeling better after our time on Waiheke. I was feeling a little relaxed myself after our break away and I had caught up on a lot during his week off. I dreaded the thought of losing him again into another month of treatment, and the drain it was going to take on me also.

Physically Patrick was definitely getting affected more and more after each month's treatment, but not just that, he was also getting more and more frustrated and irritated. Honestly, as the months have gone on I now hardly recognize him for about four days out of seven each week. They say it's the steroids. He has been rising easily to frustration which is so not like him and he also voices his irritation at others which is definitely not like him. Even his face and appearance changes and to be honest it's becoming harder and harder to bear. On top of this, with his tiredness, concentration and memory recall suffering, his lack of energy, lack of enthusiasm and ability to get out and enjoy life, not to mention the peripheral neuropathy, it was all leaving life very flat and increasingly difficult to live with.

Patrick existed for treatment and recovery, I existed to do everything else. Through treatment we really have been doing just that, existing. I'm sorry, I would love to sugar coat it, but it's the truth. It's good to know right, so you can prepare yourself.

Months earlier I was just so pleased he was on chemotherapy and that it was fighting and killing the cancer. I was just so grateful he was alive, that he had been diagnosed in time and was being treated. The first few months we had taken the ride OK; we were more relieved than anything else and all that relief really did override the consequences of the treatments. Over time, as the side effects have worsened, I have got more and more exhausted, and the knowing is there - that this gratitude is coupled with one big chunk of a pretty shit time.

Gosh, I almost don't want to write this negativity. How do I say this without knocking Patrick or the treatments? It's not Patrick of course, it's the drugs, and the effect they are having on him. He really has been doing so amazingly. Still five months later, he hasn't felt sorry for himself at all. Ever! There has been no 'poor me', no 'why me', no 'it's not fair' and no resentment or judgement... just plain acceptance of his situation and what he has to do to get well again.

I'm so proud of him in this regard. This is why up until now, as Patrick has struggled with the treatments and its side effects, I've bitten my tongue... sometimes almost literally.

Honestly, thank God we have just finished the last month of induction therapy, I don't know how we would have done another month. Where I had bitten my tongue in these last months, knowing it was the treatment and not him, I was now, just in this last week or so, protesting. I couldn't help myself, it was getting too much.

Patrick too felt he only just managed to complete the fifth month and could never have done another round. But he did it right! We did it although now a new problem was presenting itself. It was to be our week's holiday after treatment and I had taken the week off work to go away... however Patrick was now not interested in going!

Forward planning has become almost non-existent for Patrick so I had understood why we hadn't booked anything for our time away this coming week, however I hadn't banked on him wanting to bail out completely. It's hard to describe what was going on. It was like he had lost the comprehension of the enormity of what we have just been through, how hard it was, and how we needed this time out. He seemed to have lost concern of how much both of us really needed and deserved the break to help to regenerate, remember to laugh, and help to create distance from it all for a time, which I knew would help us through the next stage - Stem Cell Transplant!

Whereas in earlier months Patrick had been considerate of the toll this was all taking on himself and me, he now seemed to have stopped acknowledging this. He seemed to be too accepting that he should just feel the way he did and now had no desire to shift it. I was actually devastated. I was so desperate for the break and I had been so looking forward to it; I had blocked the time off work and the thought of it had been getting me through this last month.

Is he depressed? I'd considered this after the fourth month and the Kiwi Trial specialist suspected it too. He had come to see him in the ward about his problems with peripheral neuropathy and suggested putting him on a drug called Gabapentin or Neurontin. This is a drug that treats partial seizures, but is also used for neuropathic pain, hot flashes and restless legs syndrome; it is also used off-label to treat anxiety. It was interesting as the specialist commented that its antidepressant qualities might be helpful for Patrick too. The attending nurse who had gotten to know him over the last few months, chimed in with an agreeable 'hmmm.'

At the time I was a little shocked but it made sense. Yes he was suffering in that way. I had previously put his moods down to the impact of the drugs and felt there was nothing much we could do about it, but yes, maybe this was creating a form of mild depression, and if that could be helped, I'd be keen for sure!

I couldn't help myself at the time, and had piped in quietly saying that yes, maybe Patrick was suffering from some form of depression. How do I say this? Looks were exchanged. An agreement formed amongst everyone without words. Nothing more was said as the specialist ordered the script to be written for him, nothing else really needed to be said as Patrick had agreed to take the drug for peripheral neuropathy, so it was deemed this would help him now.

We picked up the script from the hospital pharmacy after his treatment and I was feeling a lightness in myself that we may now get on top of how Patrick was feeling however, when we got home Patrick googled Gabapentin and checked out its side effects - dizziness, drowsiness, unsteadiness, memory loss, lack of coordination, difficulty speaking, viral infections, tremors, double vision, jerky movements and decided right there and then he wasn't going to take it. I tried to encourage him to. I brought up its benefits for depression and felt that alone could be a good reason to give it a try, let alone to help the peripheral neuropathy.

I reminded him of our old neighbour who was also having chemotherapy at North Shore Hospital; we ran into them in the ward occasionally. He started suffering from depression during his treatments which was considered a side effect from the combination of drugs he was taking and I suggested to Patrick that maybe he was being affected also by the drugs he was on. Patrick didn't say much around that, he just insisted he was taking enough drugs with enough side effects and felt he couldn't tolerate any extra problems to deal with. How could I argue that? It was dropped and never discussed again.

I had tried to persevere through his 'moods' during treatment as kindly as I could but now, over this past week I seemed to have had enough of it and I found myself fighting back. I was all of a sudden sick of it being always about him… so there you are. Do I feel guilty? Yes. Do I wish I didn't feel this way? Yes. Do I feel selfish? Yes. But I also feel very unheard and hurt and so exhausted from this ride, I really just want to get off!

Yep something switched at this period. It was a significant shift from deep within. I realised in the future I had to somehow take better care of myself as Patrick was mainly concerned about himself, and really quite rightly so! I was the only one who was going to take care of me and I was doing a really bad job of it.

I saw right here and now that I couldn't continue this way or I would end up really sick myself, even just from the emotional drain this was having on me. The stress of watching him in this state, the time spent going to hospital and caring for him, that and taking care of everything else… not to mention the huge financial burden this was now having on us both now. We were going backwards every day.

It was all too much. Something had to give and I realised it was me. I had to give… to myself!

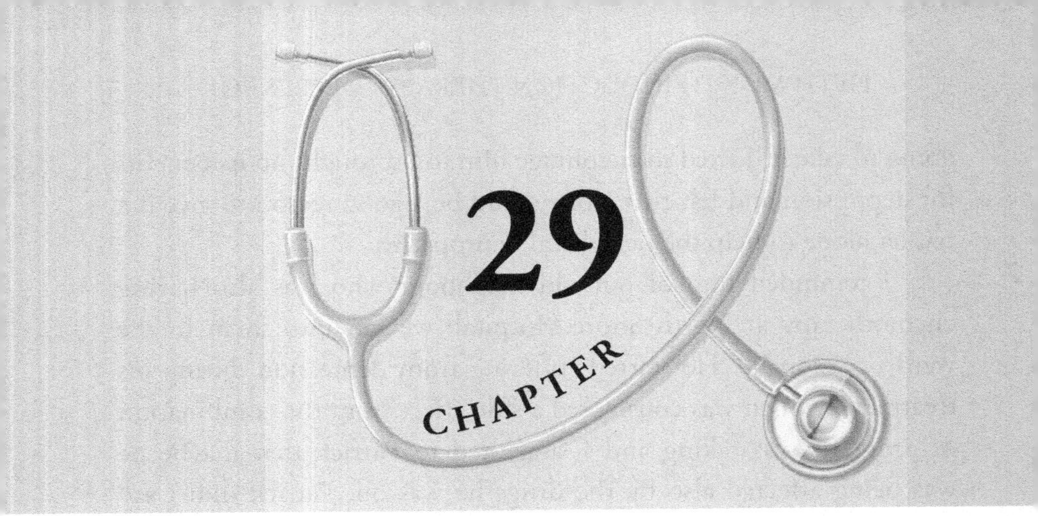

CHAPTER 29

Autologous Stem Cell Harvesting

"An investment in knowledge
pays the best interest."
- Benjamin Franklin -

As much as I had created a healthy resolve to take care of myself more, it wasn't long before we were about to start the stem cell transplant process and of course I needed to be there for Patrick through this. It was such a huge unknown, scary prospect, that he shouldn't go through alone.

Embarking on this journey we really had no idea what we were doing or what we were in for. We would have loved to have known, and for that reason I decided to document the whole process in detail, thinking at the time it might be useful for someone one day. So here we go…

Stem Cell Transplant.

A stem cell transplant is when the patient receives an infusion of healthy stem cells into their body.

You either have to harvest your own stem cells or obtain stem cells from someone else.

The stem cells used are blood stem cells and these are found in the peripheral blood… that is the blood circulating around your body.

The blood is first obtained in a process called **Peripheral Blood Stem Cell Process.**

Blood stem cells are collected from a person's bloodstream by removing blood through an IV line with two tubes attached. The blood runs through a machine that separates out the stem cells, then returns the blood back through the second tube in the IV line. This procedure is called **'apheresis'**.

There are two ways of obtaining the stem cells.

Autologous:

The stem cells come from the same person who will get the transplant. This type of transplant is mainly used for leukemias, lymphomas, and multiple myeloma. It is sometimes used for other cancers like testicular and neuroblastoma.

Allogeneic:

The stem cells come from a matched related or unrelated donor. This type of transplant is also mainly used for certain types of leukemia, lymphomas, multiple myeloma, and melody's plastic syndrome and other bone marrow disorders such as aplastic anemia.

Possible disadvantages of autologous stem cell transplant is that cancer cells may be collected along with the stem cells and then later put back into the body, also your immune system is the same as it was before your transplant. This means that your cancer cells were able to escape attack from your immune system before, so may be able to do it again.

Patrick is to have the Autologous stem cell transplant and here is a brief summary of the process and what he first needs to do, what they call **Mobilise and Harvest stem cells**.

Mobilizing is when you are given a drug, **Filgrastim**, to increase the number of stem cells in your bone marrow and move them from the bone marrow to the blood.

Before you begin mobilization, you receive **induction therapy,** of which Patrick had just received five months. This is to ensure as many cancer cells are killed off as possible before harvesting your stem cells.

The week before mobilization you also receive a single **high dose of chemotherapy, Cyclophosphamide**, to kill off as much of any possible remaining cancerous cells in your body.

The mobilizing process then begins to generate as many new, and now healthy, stem cells as possible for harvesting - peripheral blood stem cell process.

Harvesting happens next. This is the **process of stem cell collection** - the peripheral blood stem cell process. An IV line is first put into the vein in your arm or other part of your body, and blood is slowly taken out and put through a machine which separates the actual stem cells from the rest of your blood. These by now are, hopefully, new healthy stem cells. The blood is then returned to you through either a line in your other arm for example, or back into a second tube that is attached to your initial IV line. The stem cells are then frozen until you are ready to have them returned through the actual stem cell transplant.

Following that is the **Conditioning Treatment.** Once you are admitted into hospital for your stem cell transplant you are given a further very high dose of chemotherapy that kills any further possible remaining cancer cells, in preparation for your return of healthy stem cells. This is called Conditioning Treatment. Twenty four hours after this high dose chemotherapy treatment your frozen stem cells are defrosted and returned to you through a drip line in your arm.

Bone Marrow Recovery comes next. These stem cells will start to travel to the bone marrow and develop into new blood cells, allowing the bone marrow to recover, proliferate and continue producing healthy blood cells. This is called **engraftment.**

So we have quite the process ahead of us!

Patrick was scheduled to begin this process with his first appointment of receiving the Cyclophosphamide two weeks after his last day of induction treatment. The Conditioning Treatment and Bone Marrow recovery itself is booked for the month after the stem cells are harvested and frozen. That's the usual procedure. So we had a two week break, of which for one week we were supposed to be going away for a break on 8 March, the day after my birthday, before this main part of this process was to begin on 14 March 2018.

Before you start the process you have to have a dental check and a vein check to make sure everything is OK and in place for the procedure. These were booked for just before we were to go away. You will see a picture following, of the full schedule.

With a week break scheduled between the first and second appointments, Patrick had finally come round to my thinking and agreed to go away. We were going to stay with my girlfriend in Tairua from Thursday 8 March to Monday 12th March, after my birthday on Wednesday 7 March. I was really looking forward to it all.

On 5 March, the dental check had gone fine, but the vein check showed that Patrick's veins in his arms weren't good enough any more. We had pretty much picked that would be the case as he now had to soak his arms in a basin of hot water to get the veins up just for chemotherapy treatment.

In this situation, when the veins are not good enough you need to have a small hospital procedure where a line is inserted in your neck, which stays in for the whole harvesting procedure until it is complete… which can be for a few days or more. The line has two tubes attached to allow the blood to be taken from one tube and returned to the body through the other.

Peripheral Blood Stem Cell Collection Schedule 2018

Name : **Patrick Henshall**

GCSF dose: 5mcg/Kg/day
Patient weight: Actual GCSF dose:

Aiming for transplant week of : April 30th 2018

DATE	TIME	PLACE	PROCEDURE	LENGTH OF STAY
Monday March 5th	Anytime	Any community Lab	Virology blood tests – take envelope **1**	
	1pm	NZ Blood Service: 71 Great South Rd, Epsom Auckland	Vein assessment and signing of consent	30 minutes
Wednesday March 14th	Anytime	Any community Lab	pre chemo blood test - take envelope **2**	
Thursday March 15th	2.30pm	Haematology Day Stay	Appointment with registrar in haematology daystay to get go ahead for chemo on Friday	30 mins
Friday March 16th	8.30am	Haematology Day Stay	Cyclophosphamide chemo and GCSF education STOP COTRIMOXAZOLE	8 hours
Wednesday March 21st	8.00am	Home	Begin GCSF injections - continue until advised to stop	
Monday March 26th	8.30am	Haematology Day Stay	Blood test and waiting for results. Possible cell collection at NZ Blood service	1-3 hours All day if collection takes place
Tuesday March 27th	8.30am	Haematology Day Stay	Blood test and waiting for results. Possible cell collection at NZ Blood service	1-3 hours All day if collection takes place
Wednesday March 28th	8.30am	Haematology Day Stay	Blood test and waiting for results. Possible cell collection at NZ Blood service RE-START COTRIMOXAZOLE WHEN COLLECTED	1-3 hrs All day if collection takes place

BMBx : 15.3.18 *Echo* *Dental*

Transplant education booked:

Final appt booked with consultant :

Patrick was very disappointed to hear he would have to do this. Two of his friends who had this line put in told him it is very unpleasant to live with. C'est la vie. He just had to accept it.

When Patrick went in to have his vein check, we'd discovered he was only booked in for collection of two million cells. This actually set us off in a bit of a panic, the harvesting was supposed to be for five million cells. It had been agreed between Patrick and his specialist that, because of his chromosome deletion 1p32, he would try for more stem cells so he could hopefully store enough for two stem cell transplants, this way if he needed an extra transplant in the future, healthy stem cells would be readily available. This request, it seemed, had not been passed through! I must say, this was the first time we had encountered something not properly followed through since his initial diagnosis.

Susan[3], a nurse specialist for myeloma at Auckland Hospital, had to see how she could arrange this, as the existing booking could not accommodate the additional time needed to collect five million cells. It was expected that it could take days to accumulate that many. She told us she'd be in touch.

The morning of Wednesday 7 March arrived, my birthday, one I don't think I'll ever forget. I woke up in the morning just so happy, it was a day for me. So happy I had such a great excuse to not think, worry, or care about anything but me for the day. It was so liberating, such a sense of freedom and joy. As I write this tears come to my eyes of how sad that is. I knew at the time it was showing me how tough life is at the moment and how sad it really was that I was getting just this one day of freedom. I ignored the sadness in it, blocked it off and went for it. Honestly I felt like I was on a huge holiday. That feeling when you've already been away for a couple of weeks and still have a couple more weeks to go. That's how liberating it felt to be free for just one day. As I write this now I allow myself to feel the extent of negativity and drudgery we had been mostly living in!

I know it is starting to sound like I am a negative person but nothing could be further from the truth. In amongst all of this troubled

---

3 Name has been changed to protect the identity of the individual.

time I was proud of how we had still managed to find many times of happiness with friends, family, or just together. OK, so it was usually on Patrick's week off chemotherapy that we managed this, but still, we took the opportunity when it was there… and it had got us through. The rest of the time we had just been staying as present as we could as we moved through whatever each day brought us. We never lost acceptance of his diagnosis, we never lost being grateful for the treatment he was on, and we never lost sight of where we were heading, to MRD-, but the reality is, that this is a really difficult time.

Anyhow, so I had my day. That one, glorious, fun filled, joyful day, and woke Thursday morning feeling so happy we could continue on now, as we were going away today… only for Patrick to get a call from Susan first thing in the morning, delighted to tell him she had rejuggled the dates and had moved everything forward so he could get the five million stem cells!

Yep, you guessed it. So now tomorrow, on Friday, 9 March 2018, we were to go to the hospital. A bone marrow test apparently had to be done before the stem cell collection process could begin, and Susan had incredibly managed to get Patrick an urgent appointment. She carried on telling Patrick that she had rearranged everything, telling him that this Monday, 12 March 2018, he was now booked for his high dose of chemotherapy! Honestly what an achievement that she managed to do this. We were so grateful and appreciative that she had gone to so much trouble to arrange this, and that it had all come together.

But yep, there went our four days away! Right down the drain, along with the timing of everything we had organised our lives around for the next couple of months as per the provided schedule. It was now completely thrown. Holidays, work, etc, now all needed to be reshuffled. I felt in turmoil, but hey it was worth it, right? Obtaining five million stem cells to enable two stem cell transplants was more important than anything else right now, right?! It really was fantastic that Susan had gone to so much trouble and had managed to arrange this for Patrick.

We were very keen to do the bone marrow test, of course. This would help us to see more clearly how well Patrick had done through his induction therapy. I was, however, begrudging, as it was really just such rotten timing. I was torn between being so thankful that we have all this free fabulous treatment and tests available to us, to being resentful it had destroyed my break away… only because I really so desperately needed it!

The high dose of chemotherapy had to take place on Monday 12 March. That was needed before mobilization could start for the stem cell collection process. Sorry, but holiday plans ruined right there; if we went, we were only going to get two days away!

I plummeted and sank into a very low place. I felt very sorry for myself and actually I didn't really know how I was going to cope. I knew I needed this break just to go on; I had taken a week off work for goodness sake. For me that means I'd had a huge week before I took the time off, seeing clients and getting other things complete before going away. I also knew I would have another huge week when I started back in a week's time, catching up on everything. It's worth it for a break away though right!?

Now I was to have all of this new pressure without a break in between… well two days, basically a weekend. Barely enough to recover, let alone rejuvenate and now, in amongst that on my week off, we would now be thrown straight into the stem cell collection process.

Oh, it wasn't a good day that day. When Susan had called with the 'good news', I'd become overwhelmed at the prospect of all this treatment coming up so soon. I wasn't prepared for it. Not physically, or emotionally and I sank lower and lower as the day wore on.

We decided in the end we would still go to Tairua on Friday afternoon, after the bone marrow test, and come back Sunday late afternoon. It was a short time away but we were grabbing it! Even though Patrick was not likely to feel great after his bone marrow test, and we were really only going to get one full day to relax. Pretty ridiculous really but I was clutching at straws.

Something else I realised was really troubling me. Patrick was going to lose his hair. I have always loved his hair which is quite long (for a guy). I loved that look on him and have loved stroking his hair. Monday's chemotherapy was the type that causes complete hair loss and I wasn't prepared for this to have come up so quickly now.

This first stage of stem cell harvesting that uses this very heavy dose of chemotherapy, Cyclophosphamide, invokes the vomiting process as well as the hair loss. It was going to be a tough week ahead. I wasn't prepared emotionally and it was all happening way too fast. This built up and built up within me as the day went on. That night I phoned my eldest son Chase to give him the update and before I realised it I was crying my eyes out when I started telling him Patrick would be losing his hair. Something I rarely do with my children!

My poor son was so patient, so kind, as he listened and talked me through it. I ended up having such a good empty out as he let me cry and voice how I was feeling. I blabbed it all... about Patrick losing his gorgeous hair, the holidays now ruined, my fears of him being sick and how he would cope, how I would cope, juggling work now, and how exhausted I was.

Boy I needed that. I hadn't wanted to disturb Patrick with how I felt, he had enough to deal with right now, so Chase just happened to be the one at the end of the phone at the right time and he was amazing. I will always be grateful for his ear and kindness that day.

After that I was OK. Honestly I can't stress enough how important it is to always stop and address how you feel. Stop and allow yourself to feel the tension, what's troubling you, and the emotion that is caught up in it. Feel, allow, and release! Carrying it around is such a recipe for disaster. Even knowing this as a therapist it is still so easy to get caught up in your feelings and forget to do that. Sometimes I think I stay in it for a time to punish myself, or punish the situation, or punish Patrick, or punish, just punish! It seems the right thing to do at the time to feel how awful it is, but really it's not worth it. Process it through as soon as you can.

After my big empty out, somehow I now felt ready for Patrick to lose his hair. So much so that while away over the weekend we decided to deal with it early. We have heard so often how horrible it is the day your hair starts falling out. Apparently, emotionally it is hard to handle as all of a sudden as you pass your hand through your hair and a clump of it comes out. It seems to be one of the most emotionally difficult parts of the whole process.

Patrick decided that he would just shave it off early to avoid that trauma altogether and do it in his time, his way… it felt good for him to have some control over the situation. Patrick arranged with Chase that he would come over and give him a hand to shave it when we got back from Tairua on Sunday night. We knew that was early as it can take a week or two to fall out after the chemotherapy, however we also knew that over the next two weeks we would have enough to deal with so we wanted to get it out of the way now.

Over the coming couple of weeks after receiving Cyclophosphamide Patrick will first expect to be nauseous and have episodes of vomiting. Then he would be caught up in the process of injecting himself with Filgrastim. This is the product that is used to stimulate the generation of new healthy white blood cells, by helping to strengthen the immune system. The process is called a G-CSF (granulocyte-colony stimulating factor) and it can bring on a lot of pain for a few days. Next we would be retrieving the stem cells… all going to plan. Yes, we would have enough going on so we chose to get the hair shaving stage out of the way early!

We went in for the bone marrow test on Friday morning and this was now the second bone marrow test Patrick was to have done. The first one that he had before treatment even started, at North Shore Hospital, had gone so well and so quickly that we did not anticipate this one was to take too long or to be too painful afterwards. We had the car packed and were ready to drive straight to Tairua as soon as it was done.

We were unfortunately somewhat mistaken. Firstly Patrick's veins were playing hide and seek and it took four goes and two people to get a vein to lightly anaesthetise him. Each week that had gone by having chemotherapy it got harder and harder to find the veins. After this was finally accomplished the doctor on duty then found it very hard to get access into his bone marrow. Poor Patrick had to endure three attempts screwing into different areas and it wasn't until a second doctor was called in that they finally got through to the marrow. He ended up with three holes in his back instead of the one, which made it all the more uncomfortable for him later on.

But nothing was stopping us from getting away. The car was packed and we were off. Check out the following picture of the bone marrow removed from Patrick! Yes it's the red piece in the container!

My dearest girlfriend was so welcoming when we arrived at her home in Tairua. We had such a lovely time with her but I did feel a bit bad as we were still pretty uptight; a little niggly at each other and stressed with all that was going on but, as a good friend does, she was just kind and caring to us and we had a lovely time with her.

It ended all too soon and we were home in no time getting ready for the head shaving performance… and what a performance it was. Patrick decided to do it around a magic trick. He didn't disclose to us what he was going to do, but he decided it was too good an opportunity to pass up to not do some magic around the event.

Chase also being a magician was totally up for the challenge of being filmed through the trick. Patrick thought it might be fun for the family to watch later, as his hair was shaved off bit by bit every time he got a part of the trick wrong, which of course was deliberate. Each time he got it wrong Chase shaved more and more hair off until eventually all his hair was gone. I was filming it. It was all a bit of a laugh and I must say it really helped the process being light with it and something useful coming from it having it on film. There was a great twist at the end where Patrick finally got the trick right, which neither Chase nor I knew was coming, and we actually ended up really enjoying the whole experience.

So now I had a bald fiancé and he actually looked pretty hot! What a nice surprise. It was like having a new man and I was so pleased we were over this hurdle and now ready for what was to be a pretty heavy week ahead of us.

Patrick by now was feeling a lot better as it was now almost two weeks since his last chemotherapy. He had good energy and was positive and back to being more like his old self. He said he felt better than he has felt in years.

That made sense really as his bloods showed he was in fact better than he had been in years. For years he would have been getting tireder and tireder with this myeloma growing, without even realising it. The chemotherapy had 'hopefully' killed off all of the myeloma cells, his iron etc was on track, and with being off chemotherapy for nearly two weeks, he was back and stronger. I was pleasantly surprised at how well he was and it was a welcome relief in more ways than one!

It was so lovely to have him back. His temperament was so much better and he was great to be around again but it was sad to know that tomorrow the poor bugger was about to get blasted more than he had ever done before and would be sicker than ever before. Honestly, it takes courage for everyone to go through these treatments, it really does… and when I say everyone, I mean not just everyone with cancer, but everyone supporting them too!

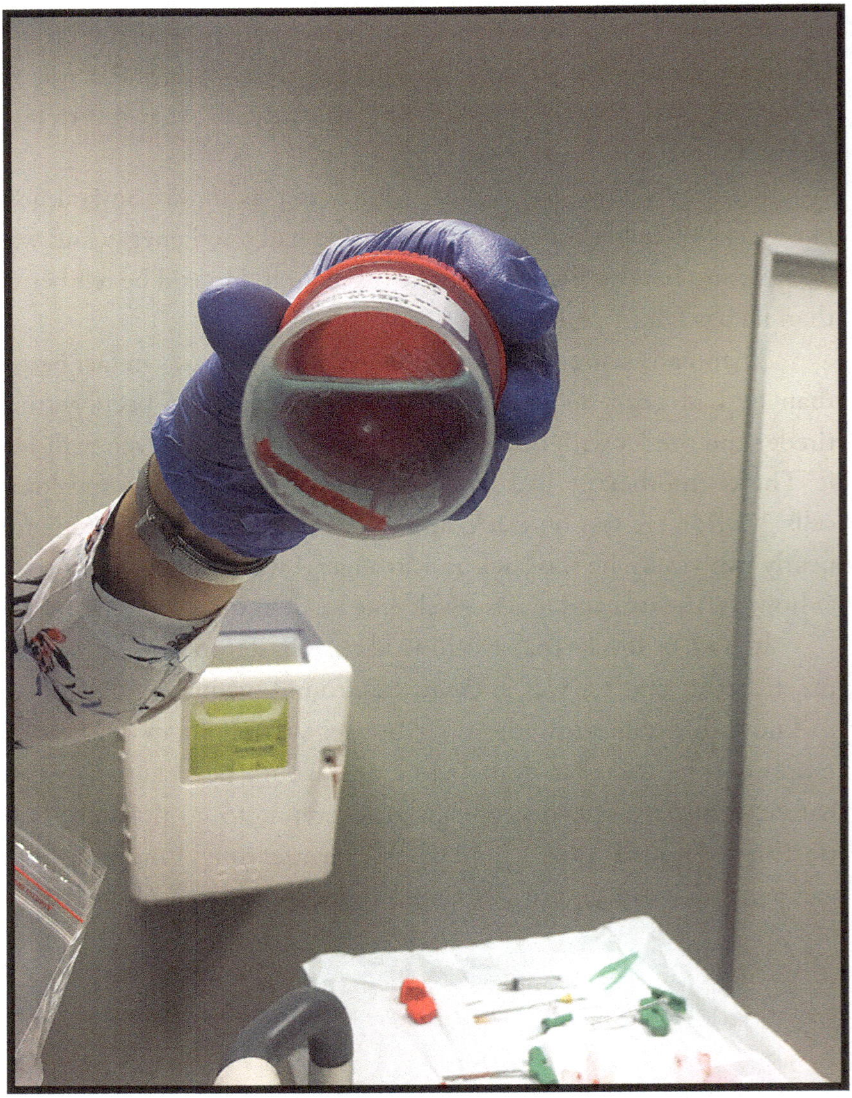

Bone Marrow Sample

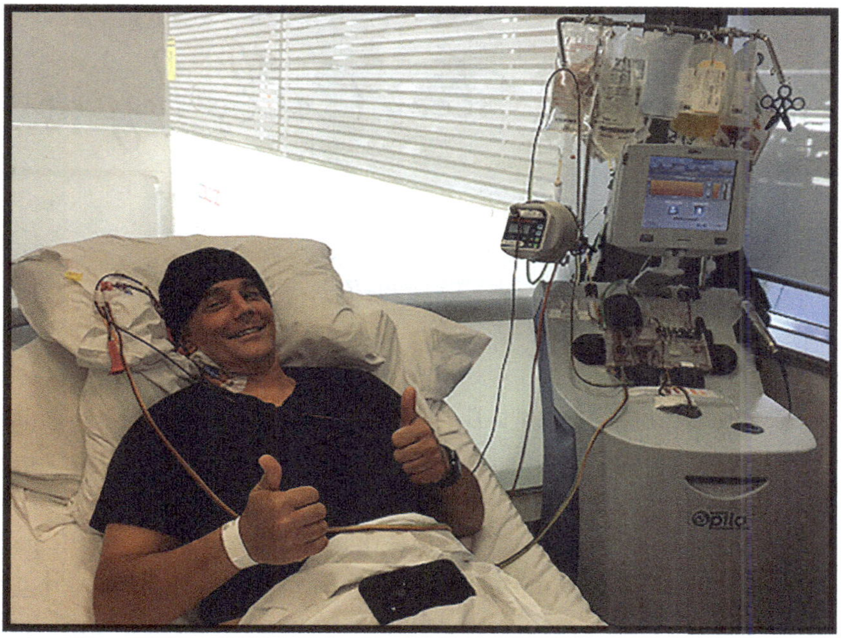

Harvesting Stem Cells

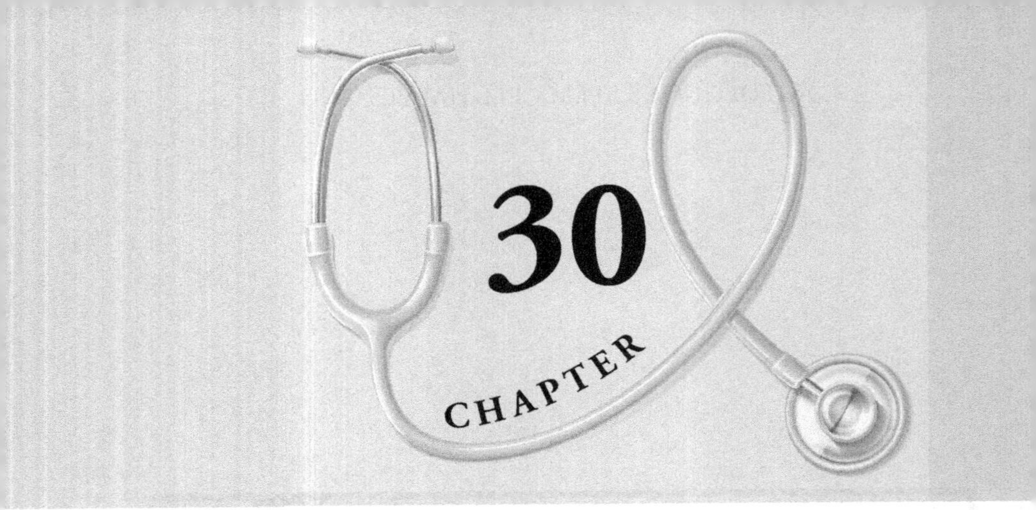

30 CHAPTER

Harvesting Stem Cells begins

"Ask, and it shall be given you;
seek and ye shall find;
knock, and it shall be opened unto you." (Matt. VII. 7-8)

It's Monday 12 March 2018. We drove into Auckland Hospital to the day stay ward to receive the **high dose of chemotherapy, Cyclophosphamide,** that precedes harvesting the stem cells. This is a much stronger chemotherapy dose than Patrick had had in the past five months of induction therapy. This process was to kill off as many other cancer cells it could that hadn't responded to the induction therapy.

With his head shaven and ready for anything we arrived first thing in the morning. Between blood tests, fluids, chemotherapy, and more fluids, it was a very long day. The stronger chemotherapy trashes the immune system so Patrick had to be extra vigilant and careful. Our children were all unwell with colds or sore throats so they had all stayed away.

Patrick was pretty good that night, he felt a little nauseous but wasn't too bad and managed a light meal. It wasn't until he woke in the morning that the vomiting began. I felt so sorry for him. He couldn't move without wanting to throw up and that lasted the whole day and night. He took all the pills they had given him for nausea etc, but they really didn't help. Bless him, that was a tough 24 hours.

48 hours after treatment, he was starting to feel better and managing to get around a little. He had stopped throwing up but still felt off and very tired. By day three he was functioning. Tired but not nauseous; he could eat but he wasn't interested in food. This actually went on for weeks as he didn't desire anything to eat. He ate because he was hungry and he could taste the food OK but was disinterested.

Now it's Friday 16 March 2018, four days after the high dose chemotherapy blast, and time for him to start injecting himself with Filgrastim. This is for the **Mobilising** process, to stimulate and increase new healthy stem cells. Amazing eh? Quite incredible. So these injections, which he injects just under the surface of the stomach, actually ignite the production of new healthy baby white blood cells!

Patrick is an old hand at injections, he loves all that sort of stuff. He used to inject me with B12 injections twice a week which is a lot more difficult as it goes deep into the flesh, so it was no bother to him to inject himself. He didn't really notice anything for the first few days. He was to inject for five days and then go into the hospital for blood tests to see how he is doing. The tests show if he is producing the new stem cells, and if so how many.

On the morning of the fifth day of injecting, Tuesday 20 March 2018, we woke up and Patrick was pretty miserable. He had hardly slept due to the pain in his body, and said that areas around his bone had been aching constantly. This was the day we were booked for our appointment at the hospital to take bloods and see if the stem cells were available yet for the harvesting. If they were, we would go the next day to have them harvested, if not, he needed to keep injecting, and we would go back to test again the following day to see if they had produced yet. It can be quite a process.

This morning though, with Patrick complaining of his pain, I was so delighted I got up, danced, sang, turned around in circles, clapped and laughed. Patrick looked at me like I was mad. "Patrick that's brilliant!" I yelled, "Don't you remember what the nurses said. If it aches it is a good sign the cells are producing. "Yay it's working, you're doing amazing. Yahoo!" I yelled as I continued to dance and twirl and laugh with excitement. "So sorry you're in pain Patrick, but I am delighted for you." I laughed.

Patrick just lay there looking up at me open mouthed. He didn't speak and it was a bit odd. I could tell he wanted to join in but the pain left him unable to. He understood me being happy but couldn't muster a smile so he just stayed neutral so as not to ruin the moment. He lay so still just watching me, almost in disbelief in the contrast of what he felt to my reaction. Another moment I will never forget!

Secretly I had been worried, as up until then he'd had no pain and I was concerned the injections weren't working. I have found out since that you don't actually have to experience pain to be producing stem cells. Some people don't have pain and still do well however if you do experience pain it is definitely a good sign.

Driving into the hospital for the blood tests I was still so happy, at least we had gone through this past week of him being unwell for a reason. It was working! Poor Patrick was moaning and groaning all the way to the hospital and he refused to take medication to help with the pain as he didn't want to upset any part of the process. We had been told it wouldn't but he was being over cautious. Fair enough!

The trip reminded me of when I was in labor with my second son. There I was, a passenger in the car driving to the hospital as Patrick is now, groaning in pain as my dear boy was getting ready to come out.

I said to Patrick "Now you're getting a bit of an idea of what it's like to be in labor, you're giving birth to millions of stem cells right now!" Because that basically is the process. Millions of stem cells get generated and crowd the bone and the pressure causes the pain. Go figure. So all the way into hospital he was miserable, and I was delighted the babies were coming.

When we got to the hospital they took the blood tests and then we were told to go away for two hours while they waited for the results. We walked down to the lovely rose gardens next to the hospital and had a cup of coffee at the cafe there to fill in time. Then the call came. At least **two million stem cells waiting to be collected!** We were so thrilled I literally danced all the way back to the hospital singing and laughing again. Brilliant! We thought this was an excellent result.

Without these stem cells, Patrick's stem cell transplant could not go ahead. This is such an imperative part of his treatment plan. This was such a good sign, two million plus cells on the first blood test check. Two million stem cells is the minimum requirement for stem cell transplant and Patrick had enough to start the collection process rolling already.

That same afternoon we had to stay at the hospital to have a small operation to put the **PICC line** into Patrick's neck due to his veins no longer being viable. This was to get him ready for stem cell harvesting, tomorrow! This small operation could not be booked in advance as we didn't know which day the stem cells would produce. We had to wait a number of hours until they could fit us in but we didn't mind at all, we were just so delighted everything was going to plan.

The operation itself took about half an hour. They put a double line tube into Patrick's neck that ran down to his heart area. On the outside, at the neck, are two plastic openings attached to the tubes and these are used for the harvesting process. One tube is for the blood flow coming out, so the harvesting machine can connect to it and remove the stem cells, and one is for returning the blood back into the body.

Patrick was pretty good after the op with just a light anaesthetic given. He was not allowed to drive after though of course, which was just as well as he slept most of the way home. I'm not sure if that was because he was tired or if he just wanted to forget he had this 'bulky awkward thing' sticking out of his neck.

The poor boy then hardly slept that night as it was so uncomfortable lying down in bed. He tossed and turned, and it was a terrible night. Meanwhile we were hoping more stem cells were still producing as Patrick had the production process moving along with injecting his stomach again. We were still rooting for five million cells to have some frozen and stored for possible future use.

We were booked in the morning 21 March 2018, to go to the stem cell retrieval place for **harvesting the stem cells.** It is the same place where people donate blood. We knew as we pulled in that this could be the first day of many that we could be coming here to collect all the stem cells we needed. Patrick would keep injecting to get as much as he could, and they would keep removing and storing them, until we got to the required five million to do two stem cell transplants. I was pleased to see a really nice cafe was next door, at least we could get a decent coffee today and some healthy food, as we'd heard the retrieval process usually takes all day.

The place itself was amazing to see. We had to go past the blood donor room and it was so heartwarming to see so many chairs all lined up where people came, solely out of the goodness of their hearts, to donate blood.

Our room was a small one out the back with two beds and a large boxed machine. Pretty much that was it. Oh, and a TV on the wall. The nurses that were performing the stem cell retrieval were so lovely as they talked us through the whole procedure, and took a further blood test from Patrick to see what his stem cell count was now for today.

Part of me was in fear that he might have gone backwards, he had not been in as much pain today as the night before. Could it be that some of them had died? The girls asked us how many stem cells they had counted yesterday and we proudly told them two mIllion.

They both paused, looked at each other, then turned and smiled hesitantly. “Oh that’s good.” one of them said.

I immediately picked up on it. “What do you mean that’s good?” I asked abruptly. “Isn’t that really good?” Again the hesitation and now a slooow answer “yes… but you need five million right? That’s not easy to achieve. Don’t be surprised if you have to come back tomorrow for more.”

We could tell they really didn’t want to burst our bubbles bless them, but they had to be honest. One of them tried to give more encouragement. “Don’t worry, she said, you’re doing really well, lots of people don’t even get to two million. Children produce them really easily, but it’s much harder for adults.” But it was too late, the bubble had burst. Oh well, like I’d thought earlier, at least there’s a decent cafe for the days ahead.

They started getting the procedure rolling, ready for removing the stem cells, while we waited for the results. The doctor finally came in, beaming. “We have your results Mr Henshall, nearly nine and a half million cells!” We all chorused our own words of delight including the two nurses. How brilliant was that! What a clever boy! The doctor continued. “Yes, that’s an excellent result. We will be able to get all the stem cells today no problem.”

Patrick piped in quickly “Well if I have that many, is it possible to freeze as many as I can, in case I need even further stem cell transplants in the future?” Gosh, nine and a half million cells would be easily enough for three stem cell transplants if needed over the years ahead.

“That is exactly what I was about to say.” the doctor replied. “We will get as many as we can today, so don’t worry.” He was delighted for Patrick. Honestly, once again, such lovely, kind, friendly people, all of them.

The doctor then proceeded to do some calculations relating to the way the machine runs, and the amount of stem cells to retrieve, to set the pace of the retrieval to the time we had in the day. You can get a little dizzy with the procedure so it can’t be done too quickly, but it is measured as you go, and if you can handle it, they speed it up a bit. The nurses set the calculated statistics into the machine to set the flow. The machine had two tubes coming out of it which they then connected to the PICC lines in his neck, and away we went.

Patrick was handling it all very well with taking the odd sugary drink, Citrate, which they supplied if he was getting a little dizzy. This is an anticoagulant which prevents blood clotting through this process.

We patiently settled in to wait out the process. One tube was collecting the blood from Patrick's bloodstream and sending it to the machine, where the machine then separated the stem cells from the blood, and then the blood flowed back through the other tube to the PICC line in Patrick's neck, returning the blood back into his bloodstream. Amazingly by 2.30pm we were done!! How fantastic was that? We'll be home before the traffic!

Another doctor came in and told us the procedure from here. The stem cells would be taken away to be tested for quality and counted, checking for how many healthy cells Patrick actually ended up retrieving through this process. The cells would be then sent back to where we were, right there, where they had freezers that would store them for him for up to ten years. The doctor said he would call Patrick himself that night, probably around 7.00pm, to confirm they were safely frozen and let him know how many they had managed to get.

So I just want to write here about how important this is. This is the best time and opportunity for Patrick to obtain new healthy stem cells. Now that he has had his induction chemotherapy for five months it has enabled him to be in a position to collect the stem cells, it is also the best time to reproduce them. Apparently after you have been on, say Lenalidomide for maintenance treatment, or when you are in relapse, being after remission, when the cancer comes back, it is usually a lot harder to get new healthy stem cells so the fact that he has produced possibly enough stem cells for three stem cell transplants takes the worry out of that, and gives him a great opportunity for help in the future. So we crossed our fingers that all had gone well, left the clinic, and waited for the call.

I was in the garden when it came. It was Patrick's turn to come out to me singing and dancing with joy. **Eight and a half million stem cells collected** and frozen in that dear wee freezer for his future life!! It couldn't have been a better result.

You know we were so happy, crazy really. Here we were caught up in the middle of a nightmare, yet we were so happy to have all these stem cells for all these transplants. Really, if we had a choice, we would never do a stem cell transplant as they sound so horrific to go through, yet here we were dancing with joy that he possibly had enough for three stem cell transplants now. Is that an oxymoron?

Anyhow, it felt the last six months of crap was really worth something at least. It was good to get some bloody good news and we were up for celebrating! I was so proud of Patrick and so happy for him too. It's like being given a longer life span really. We had enough cells to do possibly three stem cell transplants that could keep improving his overall survival.

We were not naive. We knew that the first lot would be used shortly, and that Patrick may not get a chance to use the rest. If the cancer comes back with a vengeance, often you do not get the chance to do another stem cell transplant… but hey this was hope. If there is a chance we'll be ready. Yahoo!!

Now, the last thing we were waiting on… the results of the bone marrow test!

Romance on Chemotherapy - Medial Subconjunctival Hemorrhage

"You can't have everything.
Where would you put it?"
- Steven Wright -

We had a few week's break after the stem cells were removed. This is standard to give the body the opportunity to recover from the heavy dose of chemotherapy. What a seriously welcome break that was, enough to recharge a little and start to catch up on things around home and work before the actual stem cell transplant process. We had in the end devoted pretty much nine days solid to the harvesting process where nothing much else had got done.

Again I wanted us to use some of this time to have a break away once we had caught up with things generally. I made another attempt at broaching the idea with Patrick. Although we had caught up on ourselves now and were a lot less exhausted, I still welcomed a bit of fun time away, a relaxing time away… and actually, also an intimate time away. I had no idea who Patrick was going to be at the end of stem cell transplant. What condition he would be in? Would he permanently be marred by this process? Would I get my man back again or could this be our last time spent together the way it has always been? We both also wondered how he would be afterwards in the 'you know what' department! I thought a nice intimate time away for the two of us would be very special, just in case!

In regards to romance, I'll put this in here. Patrick was very relieved to discover after the fifth month, and the end of this round of drugs, everything was still in perfect working order. In saying that, we had rarely had sex for five months! I hope it's OK I talk about this, that's the point of this writing right? To talk about the way it is. Sex is such a huge part of our lives whether we talk about it openly or not, so it needs to be mentioned, right?

It had initially been Patrick's decision to not have sex during treatment. He found the chemotherapy so lethal he didn't want it near me, hence his insistence on washing his own clothes, and washing them separately to everything else also.

As time went on, during treatment he was too exhausted to be bothered sexually anyhow, however even on his weeks off chemo he was not convinced the chemo was out of his system. We pretty much only 'engaged' almost two weeks after his last treatment in a cycle. Just a day or two before the month's treatment would start again Patrick felt that the safest. Articles we had both read suggested we needed to be cautious so we had resigned ourselves that this was the way it was to be for now and got used to it.

As I said earlier, goodness knows where stem cell transplant was going to leave him. It felt like right now I was trying to grasp on to what we had before it was taken from me… however, yet again, Patrick wasn't interested in going away… at all.

In the end I gave up on us going away together and decided that I would go on holiday without him, at least I would have a break and relaxing time away from it all. I was fortunate that my brother was going overseas and his lovely home in the country was going to be empty for a week. Although it is in the country it is only 30 minutes from Patrick's, and from my office so I grabbed the chance and went and stayed there for the week. I was still working part time, but it was nice to be away, it felt like a break but even being so close Patrick wouldn't come away with me. He seemed dead set against anything to do with us having time out.

When I look back, I am sure this was part of his depression resulting from the medication. He had no zest or 'get up and go' in himself. Gosh if I'd been through what he had I probably would have felt the same way.

So I went away on my own. That week away without Patrick really helped me to disassociate a little more from the intense commitment I had in going through this with him. The switch earlier in myself was starting to unfold. I realised I had gone through every step with him, almost every breath of it with him. As well as taking on the responsibility of everything else, and it was too much. Going away on my own was the first step in saying to myself "too much, too much".

Feeling this at a deep level I started to give myself permission even more so, to back off. I didn't know at this point what that would mean but I knew I needed to do things differently going forward. Taking care of not just Patrick and everything else, but myself too. I was reminded again that no one else was going to do that but me right now, so I needed to step up for myself!

I knew we had this whole stem cell process coming up, and I wanted to be there for him 100% through that, however, after that, I realised I needed to take a step back and take care of myself more. I shouldn't accept being exhausted. Permission to be OK!

The following weekend was Easter and everyone was away… except us. Yep, even on a four day public holiday Patrick had still refused to go away. On the Monday I needed to go to Warkworth to check on the Airbnb after guests had checked out and I managed to convince Patrick to at least come up with me for the day.

It was 1 April 2018. We had such a lovely memorable time. This was Easter Monday. It was a beautiful day and still warm enough to swim, although now officially the end of our summer. We decided to go for a drive to Pakiri on the north west coast of Auckland and took a picnic and our dog. Honestly New Zealand's beaches are amazing. Pakiri is a huge beach and we hardly saw a soul, even though it was a public holiday. We had an awesome swim and a picnic on the beach afterwards. For this brief time we didn't have a care in the world. It was all very romantic and special and some fun time for just us. Finally! It was just one day but I grabbed it and was thankful. It was a nice memory for us to hold on to at least.

Patrick's hair is actually starting to grow back. It was 20 days after his high dose of chemotherapy and his hair wasn't falling out yet! We were seriously starting to wonder if he was going to be one of the very few percentage of people who didn't lose their hair in this process; how ironic would that be after he'd shaven it to prepare. This wasn't to be though. The following week Patrick was in the shower when he noticed, as he was washing his head, that the slight bit of regrowth he now had was falling out; we both felt very flat about it. Somehow to me he officially publicly became a cancer patient with the visible stamp of chemotherapy for all the world to see. Patrick felt it too and it was a flat day. That's the mind for you. Everything we had been through so far was far more significant of an indication that he had cancer. He'd been bald already now for three weeks yet this simple sign of his hair actually falling out, well it seemed such a huge notice board saying you've got cancer! It really played on both of our subconscious causing an unexpected huge impact, however by the next day we both woke knowing that was the least of our worries and we moved through what had been a shock to carry on with renewed spirits.

The next surprise came on 22 April 2018. Patrick woke with his left eye all bloody. On going to the hospital it turned out to be a **medial subconjunctival hemorrhage.** It's a harmless condition and apparently there is pretty much nothing you can do about it. It worsened over time. Patrick's eyes had been incredibly dry since his high dose of Cyclophosphamide and his eyelids were very heavy with it. He would often have to spend periods of time throughout the day resting with his eyes closed as he couldn't cope with the heaviness. We wondered if the **Cyclophosphamide** had caused the hemorrhage although no one seemed to really know. It was an added complication he could have done without. Patrick wore an eye patch when going out so he didn't give everyone a fright when they looked at him!

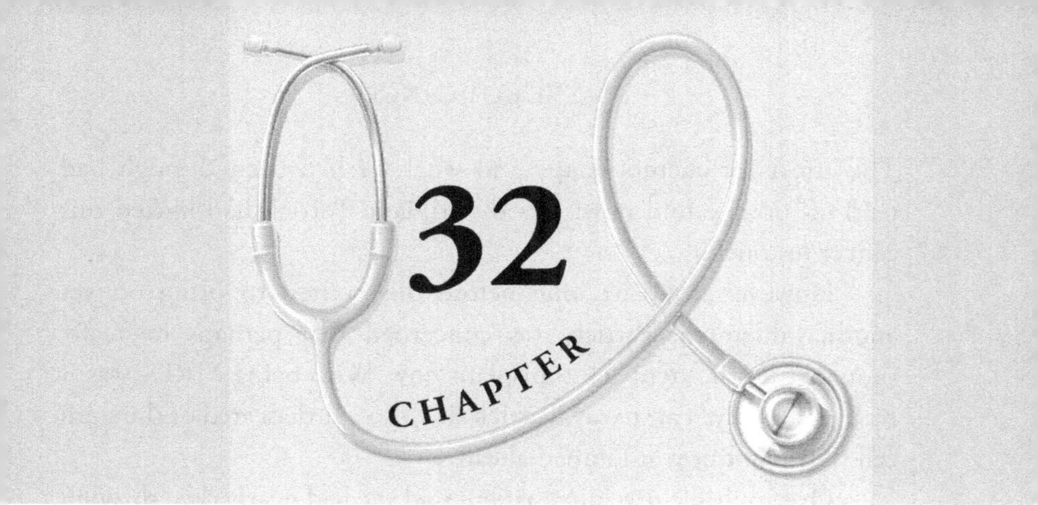

MRD-!

"You create your thoughts,
your thoughts create your intentions,
and your intentions create your reality."
- Wayne Dyer -

Patrick's bone marrow results arrived 23 March 2018 - it had taken two weeks for the results to come through. Patrick always had results sent to him, or accessed them online, so he was aware of them before he saw or spoke to a doctor.

The bottom of the report has the haematologist comment: Flow cytometry reveals a small population of normal plasma cells (0.019%). No abnormal plasma cell population could be detected. The sample is therefore negative for residual disease to a detection threshold of 0.0002%.

We were so delighted to see the results. **As we read it he was MRD-!!**

FANTASTIC NEWS!!

We were beside ourselves with joy… dancing, laughing and relief, all mixed up in one. We spent a week celebrating in little ways.

The efforts of chemotherapy and what we had been through had paid off double fold now! Bloody brilliant! Patrick had kicked this cancer to touch!

However it wasn't long before this started to bring on yet another dilemma. Patrick was concerned that perhaps he really shouldn't do the stem cell transplant now. With being MRD- was it really necessary? Fair to say, Patrick was also a little scared of the stem cell transplant now it loomed ahead.

One multiple myeloma patient said she had nearly died through it. Two of Patrick's friends had received stem cell transplants. One was still recovering a few years later, and the other, some seven years later said he had to find a 'new norm'. What does that mean? We had heard so many horror stories over time… then again we also heard from a multiple myeloma patient that she found it relatively easy in comparison to what she had thought. We were both in great trepidation of what lay ahead and I'd booked three weeks off work to support him through it. There was no way he was going through this on his own so with my new resolve I cancelled work so I could cope better through it all.

So it is understandable and reasonable to question if it's worth it when he was already MRD-. It was such a contrast to earlier when Patrick had found out about the 1p32 deletion and was pushing for double stem cell transplants! However, I suspected the report he'd read on the negative aspects of a stem cell transplant for 1p32 deletion patients was still playing at the back of his mind, despite the reassurance received from specialists.

I could totally understand where he was at in his quandary. We were so thankful that with our wonderful NZ medical system the stem cell transplant process is so readily available, and free… not to mention the specialists' personal desire to do everything they can to assist you to good health. We were both constantly grateful so we didn't want to come across as unappreciative in this process.

However the questions needed to be asked and it turns out they were valid, and not the first time of course, that this type of query has arisen. Patrick's stem cell transplant specialist Dr Richard Doocey at Auckland hospital, was overseas at this time attending a conference in America where the latest and greatest treatments, studies and findings were being presented on multiple myeloma. Patrick emailed him telling him of his results and his dilemma as to whether he really needed to put himself through a stem cell transplant if he was now MRD-.

Dr Doocey replied that Patrick's MRD result was great news but still the preferred management strategy is an upfront stem cell transplant rather than delaying it until time of relapse. He advised that this was validated in clinical trials and was also the recommendation of the USA Specialist we'd spoken to earlier. Apparently he was at the conference and Richard had taken the opportunity to speak to him of Patrick's situation. Richard knew Patrick had contacted the Specialist earlier for advice around his personal case and so he knew the Specialist was aware of Patrick's circumstances and 1p32 deletion.

How kind and thoughtful was that for Richard to put himself out to do that!! And sorry, maybe I'm naive, but unbelievably this Specialist, and I'm going to say it again, who was an internationally recognized clinician scientist with expertise in the field of molecular genetics and treatment of multiple myeloma, remembered Patrick and his case and details from when he had contacted him… and so did his wife with whom he'd apparently discussed it and who was also at the conference; she was also a specialist in this field. So all three Specialists agreed that the best course of treatment was the stem cell transplant even though Patrick is now MRD-.

Patrick would repeatedly ask me what I thought he should do but I had decided to stay out of it. I always replied with the same answer. "I have no opinion on it. It is solely your decision." And that was the truth, I honestly had no opinion. How could I? It was his life, his health, his decision. I honestly had no opinion. It seemed a difficult decision and one only he could make.

Patrick still wasn't convinced he should do the stem cell transplant, and consequently wrote to his specialists at North Shore Hospital, Dr Henderson and Dr Simpson, on 5 April 2018. He hadn't been able to get them by phone so he wrote saying he did not want to do stem cell transplant and was prepared to come off the Kiwi Trial.

Dr Henderson and Dr Simpson both promptly made appointments with Patrick to discuss this. Just here, how's that, these two top NZ specialist's taking that much care in their already full busy workloads, to arrange appointments to discuss Patrick's concerns.

On seeing Patrick, Dr Henderson totally understood his dilemma, but he also recommended that he should proceed with stem cell transplant. So the last specialist Patrick had to speak to was Dr Simpson, the specialist in charge of the Kiwi Trial before making his final decision. He certainly was covering his bases. We had an appointment to see him about a week before the stem cell transplant was due to take place and at this stage nothing had been cancelled. Patrick had kept everything open while he was taking his time to decide what to do.

David, in his usual patient and kind way, took the time to explain what he saw and why he also thought Patrick should definitely do the stem cell transplant. Firstly, although Patrick was MRD- David pointed out that apparently he was not yet in 'complete remission', only 'remission'. It was obvious David had already reviewed all of Patrick's recent blood results as he went on to say that to achieve complete remission Patrick needs to be immunofixation negative. I had to google that later, to find this relates to the Immunoglobulins (Ig), also known as antibodies. David was concerned about one of the tests taken that summarised:

"Immunofixation still shows a band in the IgA heavy chain lane in the beta-1 region which was previously reported as an IgA lambda. The

corresponding free lambda light chain was not visible by immunofixation but visible by immunosubtraction. This finding is relevant. There is marked suppression of uninvolved immunoglobulins (immunoparesis)".

David explained in layman terms that this result showed that there was a small protein visible, meaning Patrick was not immunofixation negative yet, therefore not in complete remission (CR). FYI CR was defined before MRD testing became available. It was an important measure. He then went on to say that in addition, Patrick's Serum Free Light Chains (SFLC) were not quite normal, with a falling ratio despite the lambda light chains not going up. We are so thankful that we have great specialists watching out for us and picking up on these details.

We were both very surprised though and a little in shock as we hadn't expected to hear this. It took a moment to take in what David was saying. We had naively thought 'complete remission' came with MRD-. David quickly filled the silence that had fallen in the room informing us that MRD is still a more important measure than whether someone is in CR or not, so we should still feel very happy with the fact Patrick is MRD-. He said it wasn't dreadful news, but it definitely supported further treatment, and it would be a shame to stop here when Patrick was responding so well. He highly recommended Patrick proceed with stem cell transplant and then went on to explain how important it was to get the deepest remission possible. The deeper the remission the more chance of keeping the cancer away. The longer the remission the more time and chance for improved treatment options, and apparently the better the chance of fighting the cancer second time around also. After listening to him it became so clear to us. We looked at each other when David had finished, and then we both turned to David simultaneously answering "OK!"

David stopped for a moment, appearing stunned and a slight smile appeared. "I thought it was going to take a lot more to convince you." he said. I spoke "You've made it so clear David and to be honest, we had thought Patrick was in 'complete remission'. Knowing all this now it seems a no brainer he has to proceed." Now I had an opinion, and it was very clear! "You will get no more fight from us, don't worry."

Fortunately Patrick felt exactly the same way. So that was that. Stem cell transplant, here we come.

Just making a note here how incredibly caring our specialists are. Both Dr Henderson and Dr Simpson are in charge of huge departments at North Shore Hospital, yet took the time to make sure Patrick was fully informed and understood what they knew to be his best chance for longer remission and hopefully as a result, overall survival.

I can only say here how wonderful it is to be able to fully trust your specialist team. In dealing with this dangerous life threatening disease, we were learning more and more that we could let go of wondering and could leave it to the experts. All we really needed to do was concentrate on getting through it and getting Patrick well again. We walked out of the haematology ward that day in silence together. We stayed silent all the way home. When we got home I went to our room and had a quiet wee melt down.

Oh wow! What were we in for? I realised now, secretly, these past few days I had felt so light at the thought Patrick may not go ahead with the stem cell transplant. I had been thinking that maybe now it was all over. No more treatments, or upside down life. This was now flipped; we were now about to go through one of the biggest processes we could imagine, with little knowledge of what that would entail. The biggest concerns were all flashing up at me. How long will it take for Patrick to recover? Would he recover well? Will I get my old Patrick back? They say after stem cell transplant you are never the same again. Patrick's friend's comment "you find a new norm" was constantly in my head. What will that be? Yep, I didn't want it for Patrick, and quite honestly for myself too.

I noticed how I was no longer in fear as I had been a few months earlier. The sessions I had given myself around my fears were holding me in good stead however I felt I was about to lose my man as I knew him and I felt sad and lost and lonely. No one can help, no one can take this away. I realised I'd fallen into a false sense of relief that Patrick may not have the stem cell transplant, and my mind, body and soul needed to readjust to the fact he now definitely was. There was nothing anyone could do. We just have to do this, and get through it.

Fortunately my school of philosophy training, my meditation practice, and my knowing kicked in. You just have to stay present, everything will be OK in the moment. It's all there is, and it's real so get present girl. Be the observer, and go on this interesting journey of discovery, it will be what it will be. So long as you stay present you'll get through it. I knew this was true so again I pulled my socks up and onwards we go!

Pre-Stem Cell Transplant and Admission - 'Melphalan'

"Life begins at the end of
your comfort zone."
- Neale Donald Walsh -

Tuesday 1 May 2018 - **Pre-admission.** A pinch and a punch for the first of the month. Let the fun begin!

We arrived at Day Stay on Tuesday 1 May 2018 at 11.30am. We were here for the day, to allow all the pre-checks to be completed before checking in to the hospital for the stem cell transplant on Wednesday.

We met with Susan, our fabulous point of contact at the hospital since Patrick's very first appointment there with the specialist. She sat us down and explained all the tests that he was about to do today. She went into some detail about the stem cell transplant process, what Patick could expect over the time period, what the ward was like, and asked if we had any questions. She was fabulous and this helped put our minds at ease.

She kindly took us to the ward Patrick would be in. The **Motutapu Ward**. She thought it would be nice for us to get an idea of what it was like before actually arriving on the day. She was of course right. This ward was recently renovated and opened in August 2014; it is a purpose designed facility and outstanding for patients with blood cancers.

Right away you could see this was no normal ward. As we came out of the lift we were met with double glass sliding doors and as we went through those we were faced with a reception desk. Here, everyone that comes and goes is approved and monitored. It was so white and pristine and as we wandered from reception through the corridor we managed a peek into the rooms where the odd door might be open. They seemed spacious and light but we didn't want to linger and look as the rooms all had patients. The ward was full so we could not get to view any room properly however the feeling was that they would be comfortable.

Susan showed us around the facilities. There was a gym that apparently everyone is encouraged to use. She showed us the ward kitchen which looked great. It was small but with all you needed including pots, frying pan etc. Susan talked about how often caregivers would use the kitchen to cook meals for patients as patients are often very fussy about what they can and can't handle to eat. She also showed us the large freezer inviting me to prepare meals for Patrick at home and then store them here. She suggested that it would even be a good idea for meals for myself. I had managed to pre-cook and freeze a few meals over the past couple of weeks at home, intending them for Katelyn so she would have healthy food to eat if I couldn't be there. Hmm, I hadn't thought about myself or Patrick.

Susan then took us down the lift to show us the nearest cafe, and the shops that were also there. I knew she was doing this partly for me and I really appreciated it. Then we went back to our meeting room as a centre point to begin our tests for the day.

Susan gave us a printed copy of the Pre Admission schedule. First listed was the **pre-admission tests** Patrick was to do. **Preadmission: Tuesday 1st May**: Blood tests at 11.30am, Insertion of PICC line at 12.30pm, ECG and CXR at 1.30pm, Pentamidine Nebuliser at 3.00pm, Pre Admit in DSH at 3.30pm.

We noticed that on the schedule they have put **Day 1 Wednesday 2 May (if there is a bed)** as being his admission day in Motutapu Ward where he will receive a very **high dose of Melphalan with fluids.** They then have the next day as **Day 0. Stem cell return**.

I know that seems odd but the Day 0 count is the counting system for the stem cell transplant process. It always begins at Day 0 which indicates the day of stem cell return, a bit weird but that's the way it's done and we're not sure why it's done like that... but as I describe the stem cell transplant going forward I will use their system otherwise it will get very confusing.

The first step today, on our pre-admission day, was to have Patrick's **blood taken** in the Day Stay ward, then we went across the hospital to have his central venous catheter (CVC) put in. This will stay in for the duration of his hospital stay and is used for administering the chemotherapy and other medications, and the infusion of the stem cells themselves!

Luckily for Patrick the CVC line wasn't put through a vein in his neck, they put it through a vein in his upper arm which was so much more comfortable for him!

Then we went to another area in the hospital for an **X-ray** and then another area for an **ECG**, then back to day stay to have the **Pentamidine Nebuliser**. This is an antibiotic that is given with the aim of preventing a specific type of pneumonia called pneumocystis carinii pneumonia (PCP). Why they use such big names I'll never know.

I couldn't be in the room with Patrick for this because Pentamidine is a very strong drug. The procedure is done in a single room that is well ventilated, away from other patients.

Pentamidine is given via a nebuliser. First you are given Ventolin through a nebuliser with a face mask. This helps to open up the lungs so the Pentamidine can infiltrate your lungs better and it also stops the tubes in the lungs from spasming during the Pentamidine administration. It is important apparently to seal your mouth around the mouth piece and to breathe in and out through your mouth only so that your exhaled air goes out through a filter! Sounds like lethal stuff. They discovered this product helps with avoiding pneumonia in people with poor immune function! Another amazing medical discovery.

Patrick went into the room for about 20 minutes and came out with his face all bitter and twisted trying to get rid of the awful taste it had left in his mouth which took some time to dissipate. We then waited for the resident doctor to give him a **physical** 'once over' and then **final approval was given for admission into hospital for stem cell transplant.** After that we were free to go home... it was 4.30pm. All that in one day! We had managed a fifteen minute break in between for a cuppa and snack to eat. It was a pretty full on day and we were now quite familiar with Auckland hospital! The long and short of it was that he was now ready to be admitted and we had just found out a bed was free for admission tomorrow.

You often don't know if a bed will be free until the day before, it just depends on when patients definitely check out, though they have a rough idea. The CVC line apparently doesn't get put in until they are pretty sure a bed will be free.

We had been crossing our fingers and toes that not only a bed will be free but that Patrick would have his own room but unfortunately at this stage that couldn't be confirmed. We were assured that even if Patrick started out sharing, within a few days he would get his own room. I was trying internally not to be selfish. If he had to share, I'm sure it was because someone needed their own room more than him. It's part of my phobia with hospitals, I've always had a fear I'd end up in a ward with three others really sick and having to endure all their sickness as well as my own. I just didn't know how I would cope with this type of situation.

I've never been a good nurse. I'm good at delivering meals, drinks and emotional support but I can't stand all the squeamish stuff that I won't even mention 'cause it's too much'. So yep my fingers and toes were crossed real tight!

We left the hospital quietly together, both exhausted and lost in thought of the events of the day. My thoughts were still back at the hospital. While we were waiting for the resident doctor to arrive earlier, we started chatting to a lovely lady who was having a blood transfusion in day stay. Very soon, as happens in this environment of care and concern for each other, we learned that she had AML. Acute myeloid leukemia. She had been told on diagnosis she had no more than a year to live and that there was nothing they could do for her. Apparently there is no real treatment other than stem cell transplant that could help and she didn't qualify for that, she was too old! What's that about!?? As we spoke I did the calculations and I'm sure she was already on borrowed time.

She talked openly of how she had been admitted many times into emergency by ambulance in the last few months and it was no longer safe for her to live on her own. She had to move to Auckland to live with her daughter. It was so surreal. She looked fine and she didn't look old… maybe late 60s. She looked maybe a little thin and tired but she was so calm and accepting, and full of gratitude for every day she survived, without a complaint in the world. It just was. I found it hard at first to really grasp what she was saying. In fact I don't think I fully did until we left the hospital and it had time to sink in.

This lady probably wasn't going to see the next couple of months, she had maybe a few weeks, or even possibly days. Bless her… and all she had was gratitude.

Why couldn't she have that stem cell transplant? Honestly I don't know, but I felt it wasn't fair. It should go on attitude not age, she was worth saving. An inspirational woman like that was worth giving it a go. She spoke of how lucky we were having the transplant and Patrick looked at me a little guiltily. Here he was where he had almost turned it down!

When we left I knew I probably would never see her again and felt really sad about that. All the problems of the world seemed annoying and insignificant right now. This was real life with real problems… yet this woman didn't allow herself to see it that way and instead looked for the blessings. She was a true inspiration in just that short time to both Patrick and I.

As I drove home my thoughts were still with her, my heart was still with her, and I thanked her in my own heart for the gift she had just given me. Another level of gratitude to open into. Our problems can always be insignificant if we allow them. She showed us her courage so clearly today. How dare I complain about what we are going through, I felt ridiculous for doing that now. What perfect timing, as we entered into stem cell transplant and weeks in hospital, to have this wonderful lady, and we didn't even know her name, show the benefits of letting go and just being present and thankful.

We went home exhausted from the day. It would have been so nice to have a home cooked meal waiting for us but we ended up with takeaways… although Patrick didn't mind as he knew he wouldn't be allowed any in the weeks ahead.

Really we weren't prepared. We didn't even pack for the next day, I'm not sure why, we were probably just too exhausted. Over the last couple of weeks there had been so much to do to get free for the stem cell transplant process, and then at the hospital for prep, I think, looking back, we just hadn't had the time or space so we went to sleep early and woke early to get ready. I had the most important thing for me on the 'to do' list for the morning… knowing how to run Netflix on the main TV! Patrick was always in charge of the remote and I had no idea!!

Wednesday 2 May 2018 - DAY 1 - Admission to Motutapu Ward

We packed a few things for Patrick, and I packed a bag for myself too in case I decided to also stay the night. We had absolutely no idea what we were in for, so at least I'd be prepared if he needed me. I packed a small chilly bin of food for us and one of the meals I had at least thought to pre-cook and freeze. Katelyn had decided to come with us on her way to school to help get Patrick settled.

As we drove into the hospital I had a bit of a joke with Patrick. Apparently when you go in for a stem cell transplant you are guaranteed to lose about five kilos through the process so I made what I thought was a fun, light suggestion, that he might be lucky and lose even more! He didn't appreciate that, he knew that would mean he would be really ill. I hadn't considered that, but couldn't help having a laugh still. Patrick was always 'working' on his weight. Maybe I was just needing to lighten the sobriety of the morning, anyhow I was the only one who got it.

The lovely Susan met us at haematology reception and took us over again to the Motutapu Ward, this time for admission. After we checked in, and it was verified that neither Katelyn or I had colds or illnesses, Susan took us down the main corridor to his room. What a pleasant surprise. Woohoo… he had his own room! What a silly relief.

The room felt very familiar, similar to a private hospital room. It was a fantastic standard for the public health system and I was totally impressed. Patrick had his own private bathroom, plenty of wardrobe and cupboard space and a TV. A fold down bed was available for guests and overall, it was a spacious room. I was so happy Patrick had privacy and a bit of comfort through this ordeal.

Katelyn and I then went and unloaded the car bringing everything to the ward and proceeded to set up Patrick's room. Katelyn then left, not wanting to miss out too much on school.

It wasn't long after Patrick had got settled that this lovely smiley man came into the room announcing he was from the Leukaemia and Blood Cancer NZ and introducing himself as Donal. I'm so funny really, I had this internal attitude that it was nice he'd dropped in but we really didn't need him, we were perfectly capable of coping and support was not necessary. Looking back it was my stupid ego in the way.

I'm not sure if Donal picked up on that or if he did, he ignored it... and I will forever be thankful that he did. Donal ended up staying for about half an hour just chatting. He talked about what Patrick was about to go through and explained a few things he may experience and how he would be feeling. He talked about the gym and physio that he ran in the ward a few days a week, encouraging Patrick to attend. He also asked what our concerns were, and how he could help. Well that was refreshing.

One of my earlier concerns was how much it was going to cost to park at the hospital for long periods every day, but Susan had already kindly organized vouchers that would allow me to park in the haematology car park. Despite Donal being so lovely, I didn't want to appear ill-prepared. I wanted to be "Miss Capable", so when he asked if there was anything he could do, my immediate response was no. That we were all good.

Bless Donal again, he pushed through my blocks and came forward suggesting that with Patrick being out of work now, perhaps we would like some petrol vouchers to help with the cost of hospital visits, and he even asked if grocery vouchers would be helpful! I couldn't say no. In all honesty both would be very welcome.

Donal also talked to us about support groups available after Patrick had his stem cell transplant. Patrick was quite keen and I too thought it would be good for him. Donal gave him all sorts of information on a number of different types of support groups he would be entitled to… and one for me. Apparently there was a support group for partners of patients!

Again, my immediate response was more of 'I don't need that'… again Donal kindly pushed through and gave me the information on it. FYI… by the end of stem cell transplant I was keen to go! It was unfortunate it was on a day I worked with regular clients so I couldn't and it was also a fair distance from where Patrick or I lived. Finding the energy and space to get there also seemed difficult but I could have done with it, and looking back I wish I had found a way.

Donal eventually left, assuring us we would see more of him, and leaving his details in case we needed anything. Unbeknown to us at the time he would come to mean a lot to both Patrick and I, in fact he still does. He became a foundation of support. In a way he didn't probably do a lot, we just knew he was there, he was available, and importantly, that he cared.

Pretty much after Donal left there was no mucking around. Patrick had a drip of saline hooked up and it all began. The saline was administered for approximately two hours to get him fully hydrated ready for the Melphalan.

By 1pm the chemotherapy commenced. **Melphalan** was the chemotherapy administered and it was surprisingly all over very quickly taking between half an hour to an hour. One hour to cause so much destruction to the body. One hour of time to kill off any of the remaining stubborn cancer cells and pretty much destroying his entire immune system with it! The process shuts down the bone marrow production completely and a few days later the immune system breaks down as a result.

This was a seriously incredibly high dose of chemotherapy. It completely stops new white blood cells from being produced. This then leaves Patrick fully exposed with no immune system to fight bacteria or infections hence the reason for him being confined to the

Motutapu Ward, which has been specially designed solely for stem cell transplant patients.

High security was enforced to ensure bugs don't enter and endanger patients. No flowers are allowed and no children. Any sign of illness and you are not permitted entry… in fact you need to sign a form every time you visit to state you are in good health. Hand washing is required as you enter. I think it's important to note here though that visitors are allowed, as we had thought it was only direct family permitted to visit.

After the chemotherapy was administered, the nurses then hooked up the line for saline. Fluids, fluids and more fluids were continuously fed through his line until the stem cell transplant took place at 2pm the following day. This saline fluid was to flush out the Melphalan. It is so toxic and the dose so high this amount of flushing was required. This will also 'hopefully' aid the body in accepting the new stem cells.

Poor Patrick was constantly going off to urinate. For a time, before and after the chemotherapy, he had to urinate directly into a bottle so they could ensure he had passed the required minimum amount of fluids. Once the volume passed was considered enough he could then just go normally, but he was still having to urinate about every three quarters of an hour right through the night and the next day.

The other thing we had to keep an eye on was keeping his mouth cold. Melphalan can cause serious and numerous mouth ulcers as the body has no ability to fight off bacteria. Patrick was told that keeping the mouth constantly cold for six hours after treatment can significantly help avoid that happening. This is known as Ice Therapy.

Basically you have to keep sucking on ice or ice blocks for six hours. We went through five buckets of ice and four lemonade ice blocks in that time and I stayed diligent making sure he kept on to it. He was pretty tired from the chemotherapy and wanted to sleep, but I wouldn't allow it, he had to keep sucking ice. I took on the job as a great prodder, encouraging him to keep going and filling up those jugs with ice and fetching ice blocks, so there was no excuse. It got pretty tough for him after a while but he persevered.

I finally left him at 8pm with one last cup of ice to get through for good luck! He promised he would. We had decided there was no point in me staying the night, in fact, I would have been in the way. The side on which Patrick was hooked up to the drip was the side the fold down bed was on and he would have found it very hard navigating around the fold down bed to get to the bathroom every 45 minutes with his drip line attached. The nurses would also be coming in at least twice through the night to check him and change his bag so I would have gotten very little sleep.

Patrick was feeling pretty good in himself. He was drugged up with a lot of anti-nausea tablets which we knew were definitely required. A couple of times he asked for them to be topped up as he would start getting queasy but other than that, and being tired, he was doing well. He even managed to eat the hospital dinner that night preferring something more bland to what I had brought in.

When I left I made him promise he would call if he got worse or if anything went wrong. It was very hard to leave him and I stood over him, looking down on the bed as he smiled up at me. I felt overwhelmed with emotion at how incredibly brave he was. I said to him "You're so amazing Patrick, so brave. I think I'd be an absolute mess by now feeling sorry for myself and yet look at you." I bent down and gave him huge hugs as the tears of love formed for this brave man. He started rocking me and singing to me "I've got you babe…" making up some of his own words as he went. Very romantic. Honestly what a man.

I tore myself away and headed for the car, a warm bed and my dog to cuddle for the night. Home was bliss. I highly recommend it!

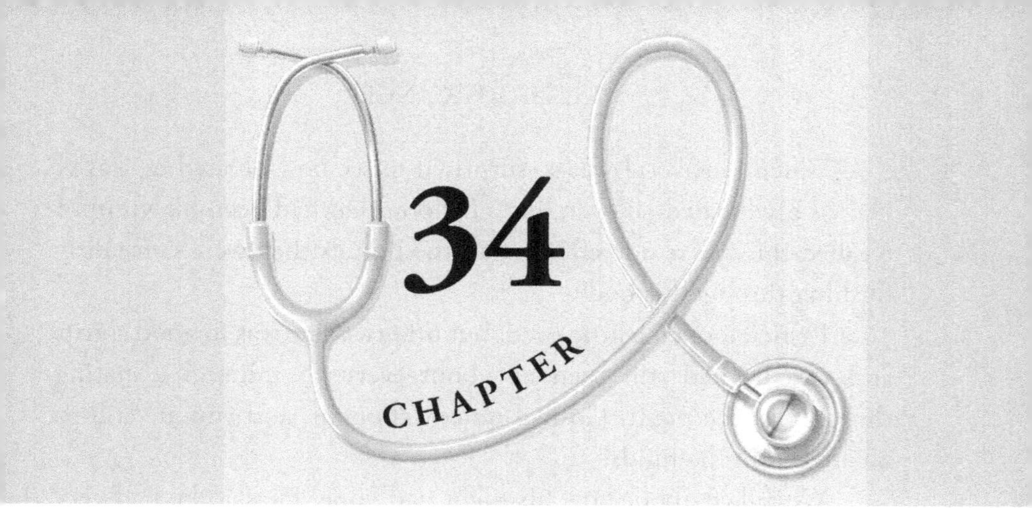

Stem Cell Transplant Day 0 and 1

"By the mile it's a pile,
by the yard it's hard,
by the inch it's a cinch!"
- John F. Demartini -

Day 0 - Stem Cell Transplant

Rising early the next morning, I walked the dog, got the house organised and headed into the hospital as soon as the peak traffic had died down. Patrick's stem cell transplant was taking place in Auckland Hospital, which is right in Auckland City itself. It's a mission to get there from the North Shore especially in peak traffic when the trip can take up to three times as long as normal. I did feel a little guilty for not staying the night with Patrick even though I'd spoken to him first thing this morning and knew he was OK. I was very keen to see him.

When I arrived I was so surprised to see how bloated he was… like visibly bloated all over, like a balloon that had been blown up. I recalled this was a side effect of all the liquids they were constantly flushing through his body.

Patrick looked a little tired, but otherwise he was in good spirits and said he had still been up about every 45 minutes urinating throughout the night. Gosh, I quietly thought, and you are still so bloated from the fluids!

We talked about how his night had gone. He said he had very little sleep between urinating and the nurses checking on him through the night. When getting up to urinate he would also often gargle and brush his teeth. Another suggestion to help avoid infections in the mouth. Anything to avoid the horror stories of mouth ulcers that can occur with this heavy dose of Melphalan.

Patrick tried to explain how he was feeling internally. Screwing up his face, he said he felt out of sorts from all the chemotherapy, it seemed hard for him to describe how he felt. Otherwise, he seemed in pretty good spirits.

Today was the day Patrick's stem cells would be transplanted back into his body. We really still had no idea exactly how this was going to occur, we were just going with it. The morning passed with nurses coming and going checking his blood pressure etc, then finally Susan herself arrived with the two lovely nurses that had been at the blood donor centre where he had his stem cell collection. They had been so lovely that day, that we were both delighted they were with us for the return of the stem cells process. To be honest, any nice familiar faces were really welcome and it was definitely helping to put us at ease.

They came into the room wheeling an R2-D2 type of machine. I was so surprised. I hadn't known what to expect, but not this! In one breath it seemed antiquated or retro, and in the other breath quite spacey and modern… anyhow I was quite fascinated which was a nice distraction.

As they started to check Patrick's vitals, his drip line etc, Susan asked if we minded if a couple of new nurses from the haematology ward were present for the process as they had not seen it done before. We were more than happy to help out and so, of course, welcomed them too. When they arrived they turned out to be two nurses we had encountered in haematology on our previous visits there, so it became a bit of a party.

It was time to get started. Susan went out for a bit and returned wheeling a large tray of warm water on a stand. The focus then went to R2-D2. It was here that Susan mentioned how many frozen cells they had in the container for the transplant today. She was advising the harvesting nurses so they could assess how to set up the infusion that there were approximately four million... wait, what?!!!

Patrick and I both looked at each other. We had expected the eight and a half million stem cells he had harvested to be divided into three lots, not two lots of four plus million. This was one of the reasons we had been so delighted with getting so many... enough for potentially three stem cell transplants if that was ever warranted.

Patrick immediately raised the question and Susan responded. She explained that with your first transplant you want to be sure it works and the more stem cells you use the more chance you have of it working well. That is why they chose to split it in two rather than three ways. It was considered four million stem cells would give a much better chance for a successful outcome. We felt we couldn't argue with that, we knew how important it was to get the best result possible with the first stem cell transplant. It meant longer progression free survival and possibly longer overall survival. Although neither Patrick nor I spoke of this together in the room the unspoken exchanges between us confirmed our acceptance of this to each other. We were happy to go with it, not that we really had any choice at this stage.

As Susan started to open the lid of R2-D2 she explained how the frozen **(cryopreserved)** stem cells were in an encapsulated casing inside an outer container. The casing contained dry ice to keep the stem cells frozen on their journey to Patrick. In the second photo following, you can see the first layer of R2-D2, the encapsulated casing.

When Susan took the next lid off it exposed the interior of the container, where you could see the dry ice emanating a fog from inside.

Susan explained that this was the middle container which was externally surrounded by sponge to protect it from moving around, then inside this white container was a crate that held the stem cells, which were also held in another container!

You couldn't see the crate inside the white container due to the dry ice fog, but Susan put her hand in and pulled up the stem cell container from within the crate. This is shown in the fourth photo following and you can see this flat metal container is frozen over.

Susan then opened up this flat metal container, and voila, there they were, four million stem cells frozen in a plastic bag. A picture paints a thousand words.

Once the label on the bag was checked and the stem cells were identified as definitely Patrick's, Susan then placed the bag into the tray of warm water she had wheeled in earlier, and they began to defrost. A very simple process, but I understand it was very important to have the temperature of the water just right at 37°C/98.6°F to match that of the blood in your body. It would have taken about five minutes I'd say… nothing high tech here!

From there the defrosted stem cell bag was hooked up to Patrick's CVC line by the two nurses that had been in charge of the harvesting. They then set up the appropriate flow for the stem cells and from there, honestly again it was all over so quickly. I didn't time it, but I don't think it would have been more than an hour and the infusion was complete. Patrick had been continuously checked through the process but really, he felt fine and was stable which, as he said, wasn't surprising as it was just his own blood being put into his body. He was instead having a great time surrounded by all these lovely women and I myself was too fascinated to be nervous. The whole room was really relaxed and it was such a relief it was all going so well!

We had been warned there would be an odd smell in the room through this process, a smell like garlic or asparagus, which could last up to 24 hours after the stem cell infusion. Weird huh, but it was true. Apparently this is due to a preservative called DMSO **(Dimethyl sulfoxide)** which is used in the original freezing process. It was unpleasant but honestly, if this was the worst thing we had to deal with right now, then it really wasn't a bother at all.

By early evening Patrick found himself getting very tired. He managed to eat the dinner that had been brought to him but following that he really just wanted to sleep. I was pretty had it too from all the excitement of the day so I left about 7pm with Patrick apparently falling asleep not long after.

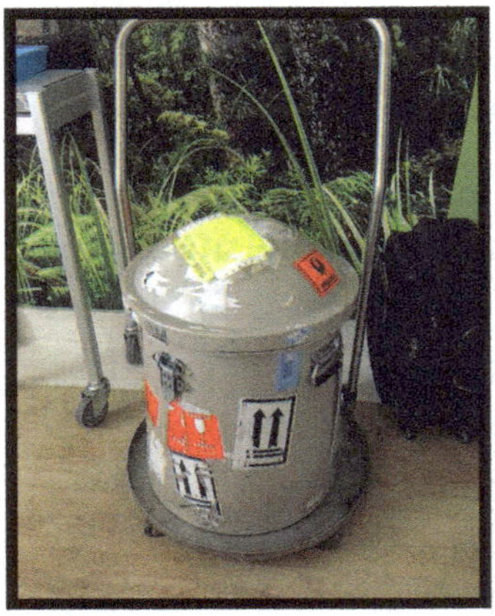

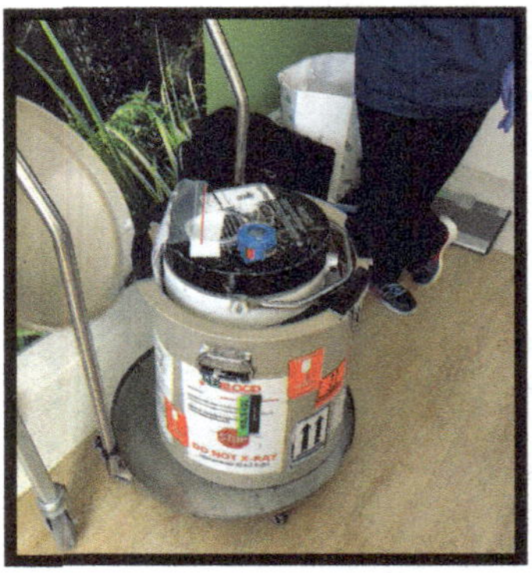

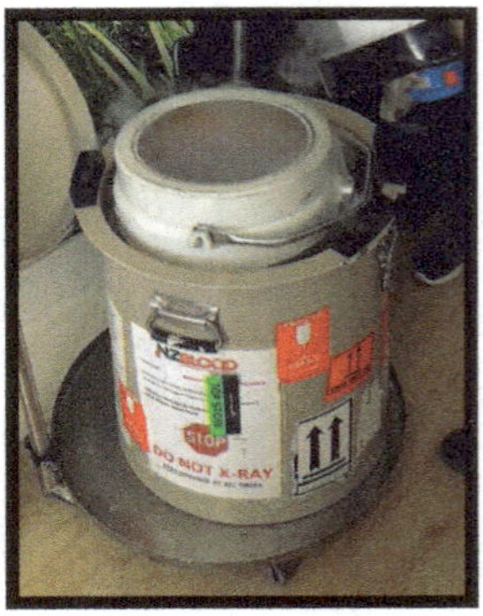

Stem Cell Storage

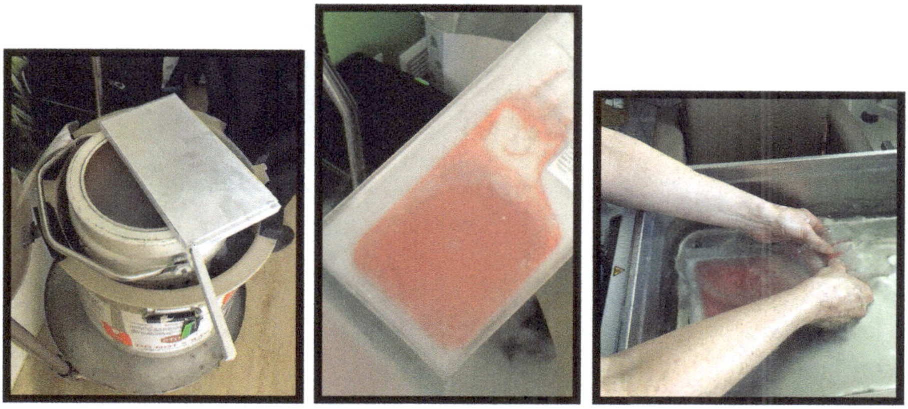

Defrosting Stem Cells

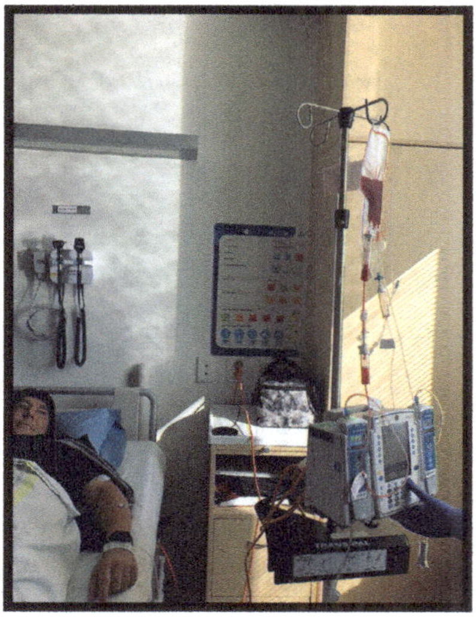

Stem Cell Infusion

CHAPTER 35

Angels

"It is very rare or almost impossible
that an event can be negative from
all points of view."
- The Dalai Lama -

DAY 1 - Friday 4 May 2018

The next morning I woke and rang Patrick straight away to see how his night had been. He sounded so groggy and tired and the night had seemed a repeat of the night before. He had still been up constantly to pee, though now about every hour, and he was feeling really shattered.

Patrick's daughter Jasmine was going to visit him this morning, which for me was fabulous, I didn't have to rush in myself. I had a lovely walk on the beach with Indi, popped into the supermarket to get a few things that he wanted, got his washing done and had a leisurely breakfast.

I didn't arrive until just after lunch. Patrick was asleep when I arrived so I sat and read until he woke about an hour later. It seemed the morning with Jasmine had spent his energy and we just had a quiet afternoon together. He was still in good spirits though feeling 'off' still, and peeing a lot. So far so good, we were coping OK!

I had brought some food in for his dinner only to find that he wasn't allowed to eat it. It was a precooked chicken meal I purchased at Farrows as a last minute thought of something he may like but it turned out he wasn't allowed to eat anything that was reheated, particularly chicken I suppose. Bacteria was a huge problem to watch out for so he had the hospital dinner and relatively enjoyed it.

Dinner had come early and I left straight after as Patrick just wanted to sleep. Everything seemed to be going smoothly, he had been regularly checked all day by the nurses for blood pressure etc, and all seemed to be going to plan. I felt absolutely fine leaving him, knowing he was stable and in good hands. I was thankful to get away early as I still had an hours drive ahead of me to Warkworth to prepare my home for an Airbnb booking the next day. It was 11.30pm when I finally got back to Browns Bay and fell into bed.

DAY 2 - Saturday 5 May 2018

By day 2 Patrick was lethargic, feeling flat and still constantly peeing, but now an added complication of diarrhea. When I say diarrhea… I mean diarrhea! This was difficult to manage and while he adjusted, it was a tough first 24 hours. He was also no longer able to face the hospital food, hence the orders for very specific foods started coming through!

I'd got up early, walked the dog and shopped for the food that he wanted. I was at the hospital by 10.00am and parked in the oncology car park. I had a number of bags with me to take to the ward… the new pillow we had bought the week before that I'd kept forgetting to take in, washing done from the day before, a bunch of bananas and the immunity drink he likes. Two bowls so he can have his own cereal when he wants in the morning, or for us to have soup at night, some soup and cereal and milk. I looked at it all and thought to myself, you're going to have to do two trips girl!

Twice now in the mornings visiting, I'd loaded up with things to take in to him and found it all way too heavy before I'd even got up the hill from the carpark to the hospital. I'd arrive with aching arms and back and I told myself the last time "Don't do that again, take two trips!" However I lifted the pillow and the clothes and thought them very light, so decided to pile up with the food and bowls and take it all at once yet again… oh dear, big mistake. Those bananas were heavier than I thought… and the bowls! As I got to the top of the hill I wondered why my handbag was so heavy, oh yeah my iPad is in it. I put it all down and had a rest. I realised how low in energy I was just from climbing that small hill. After I finally got home last night from preparing my house for Airbnb, getting to sleep late and waking early, it seemed to have exhausted me without me realising that until now! I picked up all the bags again and got up the next incline on the hill, to the main haematology entrance, only to find the doors locked. It's Saturday.

I was surprised they were closed. It's an international city hospital; I don't get why the department is not open 7 days a week! People are queued up waiting for treatments and on waitlists and the facilities are there sitting empty and useless all weekend. If I was running the hospital this is the first thing I'd introduce, seven day working weeks. It only requires more staff, more funding… although I wonder how much extra it would really cost if we could then treat people quicker so they get less sick.

I had put my bags down on the bench seat outside the haematology doors. I looked down on them and reassessed my position as my arms were already killing me, and I now had to get around to the front of the hospital. I decided to lift the food bag with the banana and plates up to my chest somehow so the weight didn't drag so much on my arms and back. I maneuvered the other bags around this one and headed on. Just as I was crossing over a driveway, only about a dozen steps on, I felt movement from the food bag and looked just in time to see one of the bowls go flying out of the bag. I watched it as it flew in the air and came down with a crash on the road. There was nothing I could do, my hands were full of bags and I just had to watch. It's a weird feeling when you see something happening that you can normally try and prevent, to reach out and grab, or soften the fall, yet all I could do was stand there and watch.

It reminded me of the time I drove my car into one of those huge supermarket windows; I had been forced to swerve off the road by someone pulling out in front of me. I had my foot on the brake as I headed towards the supermarket and in front of me was a huge glass window pane. I was slowly pressing down on the brake, trying not to spin the car out with sudden braking, which I successfully did, but alas I stopped right on the window. Just nudged it enough and there I was sitting in the car, just watching, with nothing I could do as the window shattered into hundreds of pieces and fell tumbling in front of me. All I could do was resign myself, totally defenseless to stop it.

Something happened in that moment as I stood in the middle of the driveway in the hospital grounds, watching the bowl shatter on the road. Why didn't I take fewer bags? Look how defenseless and useless you are. And then it really hit me how defenseless and useless I am in this whole situation. Right here in the hospital car park, totally defenseless and useless to help Patrick. I can't even get his things to him OK. I just stood there, looking down at the smashed bowl, hands full, overwhelmed with emotion, tears began running down my face, and I seemed frozen in time just thinking what now?

And that's the way it is. I didn't know what I was walking into today at the hospital. How would Patrick be today.? What will we do? How will I handle it? How can I help him? Will he be able to handle his day? Was he going to be alright? Was he going to survive? I felt defenseless and useless and a vulnerability formed in that moment, one I hadn't allowed for quite some time through this. I felt my body soften and open into it rather than fight it. This was the reality and I needed to accept it. We are at this stage that yes, he is very vulnerable and yes, we are defenseless. We are now at the mercy of his doctors and nurses and his body's ability to handle all of the monstrosity of drugs poor Patrick has received and the process his body is going through.

All of this of course was probably thought through in split seconds, though it seems even now like it was minutes that I stood there looking down at the pieces. I'll never forget the sound of a man's voice next to me and I looked up to see a lovely guy with a fluorescent green work vest on, asking me if I needed a hand. "I can clean this up for you if you like." he said. I looked at him and his truck and he had obviously stopped, seeing my predicament. He wasn't a hospital worker so he must have been there doing some outside job. Wow! How kind was that? It still brings tears to my eyes as I write this.

I put down my bags and said "Oh it's OK." as I started to pick up the pieces. Then another man came over who was working on the road further down, I'd passed him on my way up. He was carrying a shovel and broom. "I've got the rest." he smiled at me. The first guy reached out his hand and said "Here give me the pieces, I'll put them on my truck with my pile of other stuff." And there it was. I was so humbled by their help and accepted. Complete strangers going out of their way for silly me and a silly little broken bowl, they were my angels. I wish I could see them again to tell them they were my angels from heaven that day.

I can't say enough how much support means when you are going through something like this. I can't even find the words right now to explain it. I felt so vulnerable standing there defenseless, and that is what support does, it helps the vulnerability and it helps the feeling that you are alone and may not be able to cope. But then with support, little by little, you can see you will get through it as someone will be there to pick up the bowl, to help clean up the mess, to help you cope and smile.

When I got into the main hospital side entrance finally, I ran into one of my dearest friends, Bronnie. Bronnie is the friend of mine who was taking her children on holiday to Hawaii for the ten year anniversary of the death of her husband who had passed away from cancer. She was there with her lovely new partner, Westy, apparently visiting his mother. Another angel to run into that day as she told me their story....

Bronnie's mother-in-law, Patsy, (Westy's Mum) is 86 years old and still driving. She unfortunately had a car accident a month earlier and broke 27 bones in her body. Every rib was broken, an elbow, two bones in her neck, two in her lower back, and her sternum. Due to her age and condition the doctors felt they could do nothing for her and they gave her approximately two days to live.

Patsy's seven children had come in from all over, including Australia and Hong Kong, to say their goodbyes... but Westy's Mum didn't want to die, she wasn't ready, so here they are a month later visiting her in hospital.

The hospital had made no intervention, not one operation to assist in her recovery from such a horrific accident and such extreme damage to her body. Yet this slight woman, Patsy Turnball, weighing 39 kilos, miraculously, with her will to survive and the emotional support of her family, mended every single one of those bones on her own. What a miracle... and what a story to hear on this day. So inspirational, so motivating, so full of hope and strength in the possibility of the body and how it can heal. It's awe inspiring. What spirit and determination and power coming from this dear wee, slight 86 year old lady!!

Bronnie was an angel that day, sharing this story with me. It lifted me up and carried me to Patrick's ward, feeling... actually knowing, that anything is possible. If Bronnie's Mother-in-law can do that, wow, there is so much hope for his recovery.

FYI... six weeks after her accident, Patsy walked unaided out of the hospital to a new apartment that had been arranged for her in a retirement home, and she left that hospital smiling!! Hard to believe she was initially only given two days to live!

The last picture you will see is Patsy three months later looking amazing. Yep right there - an incredible woman! I went into the Motutapu ward feeling so inspired. What a flow of emotions I'd experienced this morning. I was feeling raw with my heart wide open, but it was a beautiful thing.

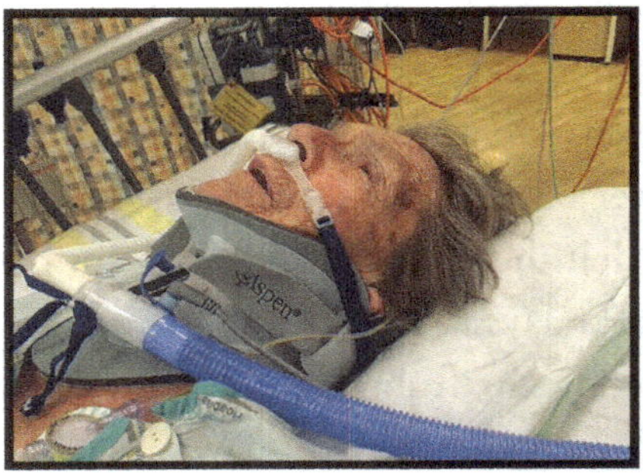

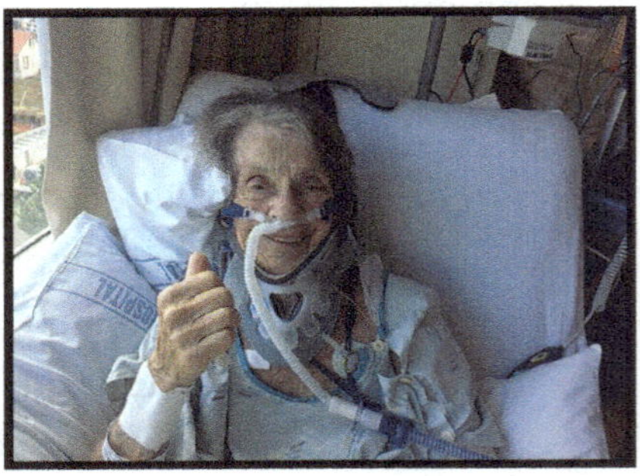

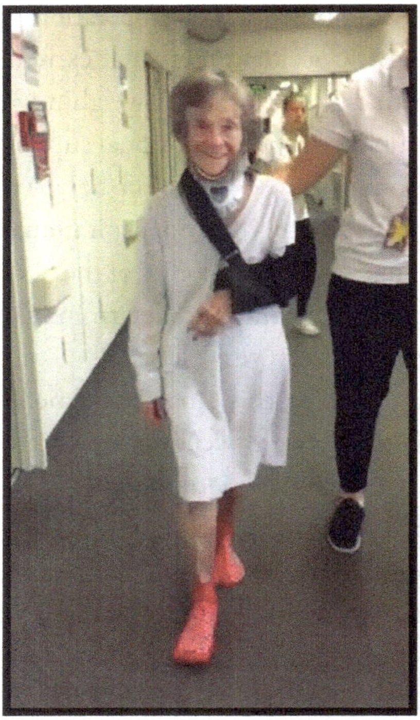

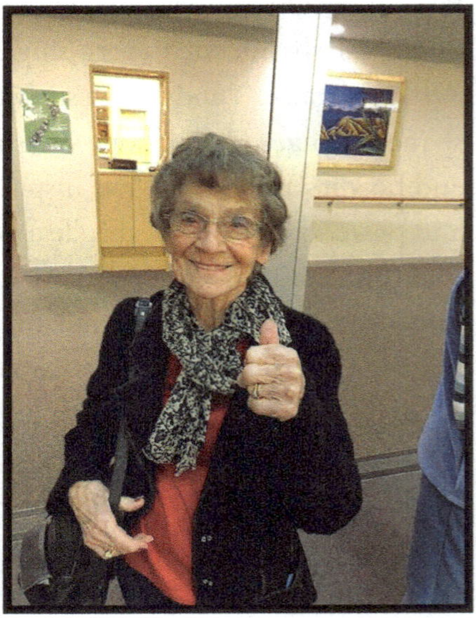

My dear Patrick was still looking bloated, even though, apparently on weighing in this morning, he had lost a couple of the kilos. Patrick had put on six kilos from the saline fluid he had accumulated from the constant flush he was given after the Melphalan treatment. He was really tired and it seemed moving around was not easy for him with the nausea that had worsened. Thank God for the drugs, they were keeping it just enough at bay that he could get around slowly without throwing up. He described it as just on the brink! He was still managing to eat and said he'd had a good breakfast that morning.

The poor boy proceeded to tell me about his awful night with diarrhea. Apparently he had a couple of accidents and had spent half the night on the toilet. He was embarrassed and I could tell he felt very vulnerable with the position he was in. I so felt for him. In the short time since I had arrived he had already gone again… and he was cold. Patrick grabbed the hoodie I'd brought in for him and threw it on over his long sleeved icebreaker top. It was then that it hit me how much he had been wearing these last couple of days. Trackpants, socks, his long sleeved merino top and yet I was really warm in the room. When I asked him he said that, yes, he was cold. He said that particularly at night he was really feeling it. I'm not sure if that is because the beds are so basic with no real blankets to speak of or if it was his body reaction to all the drugs, but he was cold. I was warm when visiting so somehow with the treatments his body temperature had dropped. Mental note to bring in a couple of nice warm rugs tomorrow!

It was with great surprise that he then said he wanted to go out for a walk and that he was allowed. The doctors had been and said his white blood cells and platelets were still at a level that he could go out today, they had not dropped to rock bottom yet. Patrick figured that so long as we stayed in close proximity to toilets, he was good to go!

One of the most fantastic things about Auckland hospital was its proximity to the Auckland Domain and Winter Gardens. Literally just a short walk, as it is right next door. The world opened for Patrick who had seen only the hospital these past five days. I tried to experience it through his eyes seeing the green fields, hearing the kids playing sport, the vast expanse of fields and trees and lakes that lay before us. What a treat. It was cloudy but very calm and not cold at all. We began our slow meandering walk around the grounds. It's a place Patrick has always loved and visited often with his parents and siblings when younger, and then took his own children, so it was quite lovely for him to so easily be here today.

I wondered whether this had been planned when they built the hospital. Was the park here first or did they build the hospital here because of that, thinking it would be therapeutic for patients and caregivers? If so, they were so spot on. If not, what a fantastic benefit anyhow.

We wandered up as far as the Winter Garden glasshouses and had a look through them, then down to the cafe where Patrick surprisingly ordered a banana smoothie… after going to the bathroom! Sitting at a table by the pond with the waterfall, listening to the birds in the trees and watching the tui on a branch above our heads, chirping away, it was so peaceful and pleasant. It was such a treat for us both to spend this time together and somehow it felt romantic. We then continued to walk around some more of the gardens before he tired and we headed back.

It wasn't long after we were back that lunch arrived. Patrick was already lying down ready for sleep but he sat up for lunch, took one bite and that was it. I could feel a shift in him. He had gone to the next level, I knew, in just a short time this morning. He was put off by the food in front of him, which actually looked not too bad. I cleared the food away immediately asking what else I could get him instead, but he wasn't interested.

"I just want to sleep, sorry darling." he said as he laid down and turned on his side. He was always apologizing for needing to sleep, poor thing. I gave him a hug and a kiss and left him to sleep for the afternoon, bless him. It had been such a lovely morning though, an unexpected surprise to have not been sitting in the hospital room looking at the four walls... and instead we had this romantic morning spent walking hand in hand around the gardens. I left with my heart further opening feeling warm inside now, allowing the love to flow.

To be honest, I had slept so badly last night, I was pleased to be heading home and decided on the way home I really needed a good afternoon nap myself. I had woken about 3am and I'd swear I'd heard Patrick walk in the room and say my name. Then I worried maybe something was wrong and kept checking my phone. Thankfully I talked myself out of that, however I was left feeling so alone. It would usually be Patrick I would wake and talk to if I was worried or afraid but now it was him I was worried and afraid for.

While driving back from the hospital feeling so tired, I listened to how I felt and decided I needed to take the whole afternoon to rest, and then go back in the evening. Guilt kicked in about leaving him on his own for so long, so I decided to ask for help. Bugger it, I needed it right now. Katelyn, Patrick's youngest daughter who is 16 years old, had just come home from her mother's the night before. I rang her and asked her if she could go to the hospital to see him mid-afternoon, so I could have a good rest and then return in the evening and to my delight she said she would.

When I got back to Patrick's I just crashed in bed and fell into a deep blissful sleep and woke up late afternoon. I phoned Patrick immediately to see how he was. He insisted he was feeling a lot better and that I didn't need to go and see him tonight, that Katelyn had just left and he was doing fine. But it was Saturday night. I sat there on my own thinking to myself, what else would I do? What else would I rather do? It really hit me in that moment... that was all I wanted to do, be with him. Not because I had to, I just wanted to. I wanted to be with my man who was all alone in hospital.

I hung up and had a really good cry. What was going on? I cried for ages not really knowing why at first, but as I released I realised it was love, that was all. Simply love. I loved this man, and he was going through the toughest time of his life, and I just wanted to love him. I really feel some of that got lost along the way. So much doing, worry, and unknown to get through. Caring love was there but the intimate love seemed to have slipped away in the doing. The combination of the day's events with all my angels and now, certainly adding up to one big love. I embraced it. It was raw and real and warm and cosy. I sank into it as I got ready to go back to the hospital.

Something else hit me as I was getting ready. We had been so busy completing things before needing to go to hospital and then so busy with all the treatments and adjusting to the effects the whole thing had been a whirlwind, and finally now it had all stopped. There was nothing else happening for him right now but to wait for his levels to drop. It was the first relatively calm time we'd had for a while. In this calm right now though, I realised, feeling a bit ashamed, that gosh Patrick didn't have any nightwear when he went into hospital! We did not once consider what he would need for hospital in the ten days leading up to his checking in. There was so much to get done around the home, for work, personally etc, and it all took so long. Patrick was still not himself from the high dose of chemotherapy he had received before the stem cell removal process so his mind was not sharp and it took ages to get things done. We just hadn't had a chance to think much ahead.

I realised there he was sleeping in his track pants and t-shirts and hoodie at the hospital. It had taken me until now that the light came on to realise this was not right. I had been bringing his clothes home to wash so he had fresh clothes to not only wear but sleep in. Finally, ding dong, it clicked, he needed nightwear. Patrick didn't own any nightwear, so perhaps another reason why I hadn't thought of it!

On Day 0 of being in hospital Patrick had asked me that morning to bring in his old brown slippers. They had been around since before I met him and were apparently about 15 years old. He's had a number of new pairs of slippers since but worn them out, somehow these old trusteds never got thrown out. I'd taken one look at them and knew they couldn't go in. On that day I'd realised how bad it was we hadn't thought of new slippers and a new dressing gown… it still hadn't come to my mind on that day he should have sleepwear! As I'd driven into the hospital, I'd messaged my trusty, classy girlfriends on my predicament of urgently needing slippers and a dressing gown. I had no time at all to go shopping around for them, I needed to be with him.

I immediately got referred by them to Citta as it was very close to the hospital for the dressing gown, and an online site for gorgeous leather, sheepskin lined slippers. Within half an hour I had picked up the dressing gown, and ordered the slippers to arrive the next morning. Where was I, that even at that point I hadn't thought of pyjamas! And dear Patrick hadn't complained once.

Looking back now, yes, I think we were still in a mode of just trying to keep up. I was on the treadmill addressing the most urgent things in front of me with no time or space to look around.

So yeah, I felt pretty embarrassed about this. I looked at my watch and saw I still had time to get to our local mall before going to the hospital. I whipped in and had him sorted with a couple of pairs of lovely fleecy pyjama pants, and a really cozy bedtime hoodie which he was so appreciative of when I arrived, bless him… so it took until the evening of day four to be organized for his stay in hospital. That's shocking for me, Miss Organised, Miss Capable but indicative of this crazy time.

When I got to the hospital we decided we would settle in for Saturday night at the movies in Patrick's room. This was the first movie we were to watch since he had checked in. You'd think we would have watched movies a lot to wile away the time these last days. What did we do with the time? I have no idea actually.

The first couple of days were spent with treatments during the day, but the rest of the time, nights and the other days up till now, I really don't know. They just went, coping with Patrick being so tired, diarrhea all day, peeing a lot, fighting off nausea, nurse checks, administering drugs and all with very slow movement. I really don't know how those days passed other than just coping with what needed to be dealt with next. So that's it, it was all a bit of a blur really.

We watched "The Clapper." A silly lightweight comedy but it was so nice for us to just have a wee laugh and do something light. I was lying on the lazyboy, Patrick on the bed, holding hands in the dark watching Netflix on his iPad together... a perfect Romantic Saturday night in!

When we had checked into the hospital for the stem cell transplant I hadn't imagined we would have these lovely wee moments together over this time. I had expected... well actually I really didn't know what to expect. I think I had thought he would be so ill that we wouldn't be able to enjoy a moment of his time here. This I suppose made this night a real treat, something very special, and I allowed myself to fall into the beauty of that and I know I will never forget it.

When it was time to go I was very emotional again. I had to stop as I was about to leave and sit myself on the bed with him to take just one more moment together. I all of a sudden started crying my eyes out and Patrick held me as I had my wee melt down moment with him. It was so hard leaving him again tonight, we'd had such a lovely time and the enormity of what he was going through was hitting me hard.

Through all this he never complained. Since our walk earlier in the day though, I could see the immense strain he was feeling in himself. There was definitely a shift. Earlier, just before we got set up for the movie, Patrick was sitting in his chair and we talked about him getting ready for bed first. "Yep, OK." he said. "I just need to sit a little longer to get the energy." He was slumped and looking like he'd had enough. I put my arms around him and he said "It's OK. I've just gotta get through this." It was said in a way of 'holy shit, I don't know how I'm going to, but I just have to hold tight to get there.' I just held him and didn't say anything, this was the first time he'd spoken of the difficulty… even then it was only half heartedly. Four days of constant nausea alone would be enough to wear me down, let alone struggling with the lack of energy and constant peeing and diarrhea… not to mention all that his body was going through with the treatments. It's hard to imagine. Yet he still didn't complain, he still remained completely positive in his thoughts and words. "It's OK. I've just gotta get through this." Unbelievable and heartbreaking in an odd and inspiring way.

So this was with me as I was saying goodbye. I could see he was into the next level with his treatment where it was going to get really tough for him. In typical Patrick style he picked me up very quickly, he never lets me dwell in tears damn it. Like the true gentleman he is, he then insisted on getting up and walking me to the lift. He saw me off with a lovely kiss and a hug. Such a brave and courageous man. Saturday night at the Motutapu Ward, Auckland Hospital.

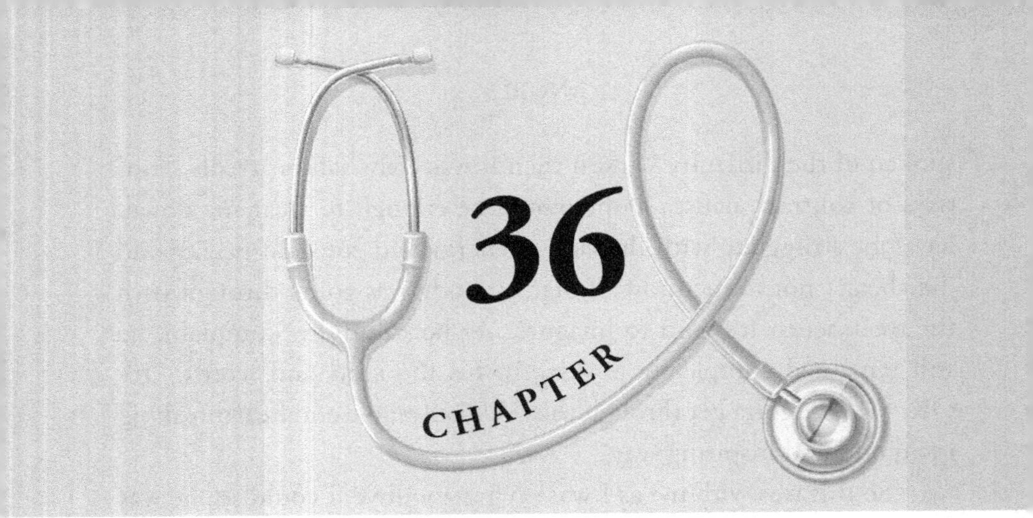

Stem Cell Transplant - Day Visits Home

"Kia kaha. Kotahi tātou."
- Stay strong. We are one. -

DAYS 3, 4, 5 and 6

From Sunday 6 May 2018 - Day 3 through to Wednesday 9 May 2018 - Day 6, Patrick managed to come home each day for 'day trips'! I would phone him at about 8am each day to get his status, as they would have his blood results by then.

Day 3 Patrick's haemoglobin was 116, platelets 141, and neutrophils 5.71, and no alarm bells with the rest. The doctors told him that as his immune system was not fully compromised yet he could actually go home for the day if he wanted to. What a fantastic surprise that was. He had to be super careful of course not to be exposed to any bugs, eat carefully, not be in public places etc, but he could come home. Yay!

Patrick needed time to get ready as he was still very slow getting around with such low energy, and nausea but by late morning I was picking him up. This continued for three more days, through **Days 4, 5, and 6**!

Each day, once I knew what Patrick's blood status was, I'd go in and pick him up late in the morning so he could come home for the day and early evening. His platelets and neutrophils slowly dropped from Saturday 5 May (day 2) through to Wednesday 9 May (day 6), but he was still in the safe enough zone to be able to come home. Platelet count went from 141, 148, 125, 100, 72, as the days progressed. Neutrophils went from 5.71, 4.75, 3.86, 2.95, 1.95.

The first day he came home I was so unprepared. A while back we had heard day visits could happen, but I think it had gone out of our minds as Patrick really hadn't been feeling great, but how awesome he could come home.

After picking him up I'd had to drive so slowly and carefully due to his nausea. When I got him home he just wanted to climb into his own lovely comfy bed and sleep, which he did for about three hours. When he woke we managed to find something he wanted to eat… tomato soup and Vogels! We sat and chatted in front of the fire for a bit, then it was time for him to go back already. The strangest thing to me at the time was that every day I picked him up after that he was that little bit better. Each day he slept less and by the third day the nausea had practically disappeared.

On the fourth day he could come home, Day 6, but he was only allowed out until 4 or 5 o'clock. His immunity levels were now very low with his platelets at 72 and neutrophils at 1.95. Apparently over the day they could drop to a more dangerous level, so they didn't want him out for as long. We pretty much knew he wouldn't be coming home the next day, and again we were about to enter another stage.

Yet Patrick didn't appear worse. When he was home that day he didn't sleep at all, mind you he had a bit of an extra sleep in the morning, just before I picked him up. However, not only did he not sleep he fixed the door handle to one of the bathrooms and tightened up all the others in the house, and fixed one of the blinds that had come away. He was eating really well and I said to him that I couldn't believe he was going back to the hospital. It's like all was normal and he should just stay at home. It felt like it was all behind us now… yet it was supposed to be the beginning of the worst stage!

Heading home after dropping him off, I was caught in peak traffic. In fact the whole trip into town and back took me nearly two hours. I had plenty of time to think and feel into where Patrick was at, and I started to worry. Why was he so good? Maybe the stem cells weren't taking, maybe this whole process wasn't working. He is supposed to be a mess, maybe something is wrong. I really was concerned and feeling sick to my stomach.

When I spoke to him later that night I was going to voice my concerns but as he spoke first it became clearer to me what was happening. Patrick told me that tonight he had started injecting his stomach again with a product that helped the stem cells go back into his bone marrow. Up until now it seems they were just swimming around in his blood. It sounded like the timing of this, with his blood count dropping to below zero, suggested we were definitely at the beginning of the next stage. This helped ease my mind. Maybe it is this injecting process that really takes him down, maybe it's all going to plan after all. Whew! OK Kushla, just brace yourself for what's to come now, don't worry, it's all going OK.

It turned out Patrick had been very lucky that his blood levels had dropped so slowly. You can see from the results they dropped a little every day, not everyone does that apparently, often it is a sudden drop. If it had been a sudden drop he would have gone into this next stage a lot earlier, injecting into his stomach. He would still have been suffering from the high dosage of chemotherapy he'd had as well as having to quickly cope with what was to come next.

He was doubly lucky also, I have since found out, to have had this slow drop to not only have had time to recover, but also because, as the doctors told him today, if your bloods drop slowly, you pull out of the next stage quicker, when they drop totally.

So wow, really, it couldn't have gone any better for him, and here I'd been worrying.

DAY 7 - Thursday 10 May 2018

The next day, **Day 7**, I woke up with chronic fatigue. I couldn't even get out of bed until late morning. I felt like a truck had run over me after a night out on the booze. It had all caught up with me.

I'd been running around doing way too much. Two trips a day to the hospital and back, getting in whatever food Patrick could eat that day, cooking food, looking after Indi and the house, worrying about him and it had all taken its toll. Unfortunately it turned out to be more than my body could handle and it was a good warning that I needed to pull back a little.

I phoned Patrick in the morning and for a change our conversation focused more on my health than his. I knew I just couldn't get in there that day and he told me not to worry, he had plenty of food and was doing OK. He still had diarrhea and his eyes also were annoyingly still very dry. He said he felt 'uncomfortable' and found it hard to describe that further. His energy was low, but otherwise he said he was doing OK. He was so lovely, making me feel very comfortable that I couldn't go in. Whew, a day for me. Other than walking the dog, I just rested and boy I needed that.

My youngest son Taylor offered to go and see Patrick after work since I wasn't able to get in. It filled my heart so much to receive this support. At least he now had a visitor for the day and I didn't feel quite so bad. Taylor organized some dinner for him and it was very lovely for Patrick to have him there.

Just a note here, Patrick did not have any mouth ulcers, nor did he get them… at all. The old ice trick had worked a treat!

Day 8 - Friday 11 May 2018

Then, get this, **Day 8**, when I phoned Patrick as usual early in the morning, he told me not to come in again for the day as he had too much to do!

What!? Although I was really pleased as it meant another day for me to recover from the fatigue I was very surprised. I asked "What do you mean too busy?" To which he responded "I want to complete my company's GST today and file the GST return!"

My first thought was that he was just saying he had too much to do so as not to bother me since I had been fatigued, but no actually, he really had things he wanted to do.

When I caught up by phone with him later in the day, he told me how he had spoken to his accountant for half an hour that day, then the IRD, then completed his accounts and filed and paid his GST return. He also listened to a magic podcast for an hour online. And then through all that organized two judicial serves that were done that day by one of his servers.

Yep. Right there, Day 8, sooooo amazing!! We never thought in a million years that was going to happen! On top of that he's doing magic performances now for all the staff! Over the last few nights he's apparently gone out to reception when all is quiet and done a few tricks for the nurses. They were all loving it and after the first night word got around, so he does a few tricks for the day staff every day too now… and the doctors are putting in requests as well on their morning visits. So he is very very happy in that regard. He loves his magic, loves performing, and loves making people happy, so even though he is feeling so lousy himself, giving back helps him feel so much better and puts him right in his element! It might be hard to get him out of there!

Patrick's platelets kept dropping and his neutrophils and white blood count were at zero over these two days. Pretty scary right! Completely at zero on 10 and 11 May. This of course was expected but what wasn't expected was how well he was. It was such a relief for us both. We had expected it would be horrendous about now and he was cruising through.

DAY 9 - Saturday 12 May

What's all the fuss been about? I don't know, it's **Day 9**. His levels have now finally dropped to their lowest low yet we are still here. We are still alive and we are surviving. Yes we are!

I have woken up Saturday morning 12 May 2018 so surprised I don't feel stressed. I remember Patrick on the phone at 9.30pm last night, chatting away sounding like normal Patrick. It's weird, I thought I would be nursing him in a terrible state by now. Honestly, what was all the fuss about? I knew intuitively we were over the worst already.

I noticed how free I felt from anxiety. I was no longer worried about what was to come and I am actually thinking maybe, just possibly, Patrick was going to be one of the ones who will get through this relatively easily.

Gosh, I don't mean to discount what he has been through already, it's been no picnic for him but really, I had expected disaster from all accounts and to literally lose my man through the stem cell transplant. Seriously. With all the talk about having stem cell transplants and that you are never the same again afterwards I think I didn't ever expect him to be able to function normally again in any form, or even find that new norm for quite some time… and here he was yesterday, doing his accounts! I don't want to count my chickens too soon but so far so seriously good!

After a break for two days I was so keen to get in and see him. I was already physically feeling a lot better and had received the food order on the phone in the morning, and the magic order too! (Every day from here on in Patrick asked me to bring in new tricks for him to perform to the staff.)

This day, however, I didn't stay all day and night, I'd learnt my lesson. I needed to pull back on these long tiring days, it was too much to handle. It was Saturday night again. This seemed to have rolled back around again so quickly and as much as I wanted to stay I knew I had to go home and give myself a chance to recover fully. Fortunately my other son, Chase, wanted to visit Patrick, so we arranged for him to come late afternoon, so I could get away. They had a couple of games of chess, which made it a pretty nice Saturday night for Patrick in the end.

Note on the blood results taken today that his platelet count was 17.

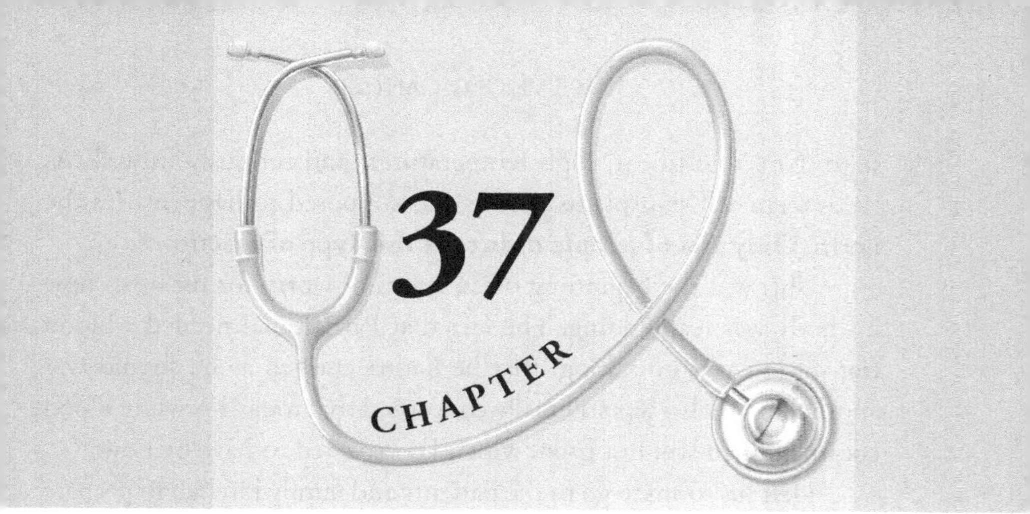

12 Days - A Record

"I am convinced that He (God)
does not play dice."
- Albert Einstein -

DAY 10 - 13 May 2018

On **Day 10** Patrick's morning blood results showed his platelets were less than 10. A dangerous level apparently, and at this point a platelet transfusion was required! That's a blood transfusion.

I had rushed to the hospital when Patrick phoned to tell me the results. We didn't really know how much of a problem this was but I started to worry this could intervene with his body starting to improve. Actually, I must admit I was a little more than worried at this point, although I didn't voice this to him.

Patrick was none the worse for wear for it. He seemed relatively fine other than needing the transfusion which is administered through the same CVC line that was initially put in for him the day before admission. But that was the thing, at this time he should apparently have been rock bottom… like in a really physically bad state. Not able to eat, high temperatures, and seriously unwell. As far as stem cell transplants go this was supposed to happen - it's the norm. **Only 1% of people didn't get this type of reaction.**

This was the beginning of 24 hours of worry for me as to how his body was really doing. The fact that Patrick had needed a blood transfusion was one thing, that he hadn't crashed as he should was another, but I also was still really concerned that today his white blood count still had still not risen, which I'd expected to have by now.

I left his room to go to the patients and family kitchen to prepare food. Walking through the ward I marveled at how high tech it all was, how pristine white it was, how clean it was, and how incredibly efficient the staff were.

Patrick had nurses enter almost immediately whenever he had a need to push the help button. The whole of the ward was so on to it and my thoughts went to how thankful I was that this facility was here for all the patients going through such terrible experiences, with such scary life threatening health problems hanging over them and having such potentially life threatening treatments. Everyone there was living in hope that the stem cell process will give them literally a new life.

Then it dawned on me. Gosh, Patrick was one of them! Patrick's life was in danger with his disease. Patrick was having a potentially very dangerous procedure and Patrick was going through a really tough time. Patrick was having complications needing a blood transfusion. This ward had been created for him. What he was going through was just as serious and demanding as everyone else here and he was one of the many I had been feeling so sorry for. We were one of them, yet until now I'd somehow felt detached from that. Somehow I'd felt that we were like the least deserving and that our situation was nowhere near as serious as others in the ward.

Funny how I'd put us separate; feeling sad for everyone else, but it was like we didn't fit in. Frauds almost for being there. Was it Miss Capable, feeling we would cope, no problem? Was it our positive attitude and manner with everyone that seemed to deem we were OK? Or was it that dynamic that when you are in a scenario you get conditioned and adjust and so you don't realise how serious it is.

Maybe it was the fright of the unexpected blood transfusion, but I certainly came to ground and was quite emotional to realise everything around me was for Patrick! It just goes to show how you can get so caught up in the doing, you sometimes can't see the wood for the trees.

DAY 11 - Monday 14 May 2018

Finally, **Day 11**, Patrick's morning blood results were showing that his white blood count levels were now rising. He was out of the woods. Yahoo!

Platelets 21, white blood count 4, neutrophils still not registered. This was the moment we had been waiting for, he was already on the way up and out of there.

This was such a significant moment. I was having a cup of tea in bed and was on the phone with Patrick when Susan came into his room with the results. It was such perfect timing. This is it! He's done it! He's through the worst of it. We were so delighted. Wow! It was going to be OK. I shouldn't have let my mind get in the way yesterday with all that worry and instead just trusted!

When the doctors arrived to see Patrick they told Patrick that he is in the 1% of people who didn't get a temperature and go through that truly difficult stage! How lucky is that? Quite unbelievable really.

He's been in the rare category all along, but this time was different. This time we were ecstatic, it was for a positive reason! The doctors also told him that his results indicated he was doing so well that he may get out as early as this Thursday, which was only 3 days away! Once the patient's white blood cell count gets to a reasonable level and the patient feels well enough, there is no need to be in hospital any longer.

When I visited that day, gosh we celebrated! Well, as best we could without a drink or party! I did a wee dance and we whoop whooped. He was on the mend!

I had a client booked for that night. I couldn't let work wait any longer or my business would seriously suffer but I went to work feeling so light and happy, feeling ready to start getting back a modicum of normal life.

Day 12 - Tuesday 15 May 2018

You can imagine my shock when this morning I rang him for his results. He'd had them through already, and the doctors had done their rounds. "You'll never guess when I'm coming home?" he said questioningly.

"What, when??" I quickly replied, just wanting that answer!

"Today!" he laughed. I won't forget that moment, right there. It was **Day 12**, and yep, apparently a record! Patrick's blood results had continued to rise.

Patrick went on to tell me that the head specialist who visited him this morning was staggered with how well he was doing. Apparently he said that if he manages to stay out of hospital once he goes home, it will be a record in his ten years working there.

I have to admit I did start reeling a little. The reality of him suddenly coming home was fantastic, but I started getting overwhelmed about how I was going to manage it. Patrick had a house inspection at 8.30am this morning; Patrick rented his home on the North Shore of Auckland, and I'd agreed to have the house ready and be there for it, I then had a client at 10.00am. I couldn't be at the hospital until 12.30pm at the earliest and I would not be able to organise anything for Patrick's homecoming during that time.

When I voiced this to him he told me not to worry, he said that would be perfect timing. He needed time to change, get drugs arranged etc anyhow. He was so keen to get home and I wasn't going to hold that back from him. Gosh, what a panic it put me into, but I could see a way through to achieve it all. This is just what you have to do right, it's not like you have a choice in the matter.

When I arrived at the ward at yes, almost precisely 12.30pm, he was still waiting to be discharged. He looked at me as we sat together in his hospital room and said, "You know what? I know this may sound silly but I think this good result is because I wasn't meant to get this cancer. I think this is a huge mistake that has been made and 'they' are trying to fix it up."

I just looked at him. I gave him the space to continue and he did. "The way everything has gone so well so far, I think it's been some huge mistake and maybe 'they' are going to make it right!"

How profound. My eyes welled with tears as I replied "Oh my god that's so not silly at all. You may just be right Patrick." And it was left right there, a possibility. I knew Patrick's reference to 'they' was God, the universe, whatever you want to call it. That someone or something had made a big mistake giving him cancer, an error on their part, and they were attempting to put it right! Well that would be awesome. Really though, why has he done so well? I knew one thing, that although we didn't know the answers, I was extremely thankful.

You know it's quite staggering, right through this whole ordeal, right up to Patrick's release day today, he did not complain to me once. Not once. Although he has done well, we know it was not a walk in the park and it still isn't. He has a long way to go still for full recovery yet not one complaint. I find that staggering and you do have to wonder how much his attitude has contributed towards his early release.

As we seemed to still have a bit of a wait for the release papers to come through he decided to put his feet up and dozed a little. As I watched over him I went back over the past 12 days honoring what this great man had been through. The diarrhea had been particularly difficult for him to handle. He could never be far from a toilet, and his upset stomach was constantly unpleasant, nausea included. He would want one thing to eat one minute, then change his mind five minutes later.

Hospital food would be delivered and some days he couldn't even lift the lid, the smell was too much for him. Every day I was off to the supermarket, getting the food he thought he could eat. In the end it came down to bananas and an immunity drink. If you have ever suffered from nausea you will know what I mean, but if you haven't, imagine being constantly sea sick as perhaps a good example.

His eye lids ached from the dryness in his eyes his whole time there. Something the doctors and nurses could not understand, but it had definitely only started since his high dose of chemotherapy before stem cell collection. Moving his eyes around and keeping his eyes open during the day gets more and more painful as the day goes on, until he just has to close them and rest them, even if he doesn't want to sleep.

The many nights he had spent with so little sleep constantly getting up to urinate had been exhausting for him, not to mention the extreme tiredness he felt from the further high dose of chemotherapy he had received when he arrived in hospital and from just the whole process in itself.

As I sat there looking at him I marvelled at how, even in this state, Patrick had found the gap. The gap of positivity, the gap where we find gratitude, kindness, sharing and caring… and he had taken that gap and gone for it… with a little bit of magic to help him along! Literally!! It started, as I said earlier, with a trick or two for the nurses at reception at night then it expanded to something for the nurses during the day. He was getting such delight from it that every couple of days I was ferreting around in his magic boxes bringing new tricks in for him to do.

On his second to last night, Sunday night Day 10, I had phoned him about 8.30pm. I had left early in the evening, so I wanted to see how his night had gone. He answered quite abruptly saying "I can't talk right now, sorry, I'm about to do a performance." Well that stopped me in my tracks. A performance? Was he exaggerating? I did a big pause and decided to drop it till later as I could hear he was rushed and said goodbye.

It was over an hour later and I had not heard back from him, so I decided to call again. He was in bed utterly exhausted but deliriously happy. Apparently Patrick had discovered on going out to do a bit of magic for whoever was interested, that tonight there were about ten staff, a number of patients and a couple of caregivers who had all come out at the mention of magic, to see him perform. Word had really got out! Lucky for him he had about half an hour's worth of magic on him, so a performance it truly was.

He was obviously so delighted that he had been able to offer something back and bring a smile and a laugh to not just the nurses but the patients and their carers too. He proceeded to tell me all the tricks he did, the reactions, and of how much fun it was for everyone.

He said he hadn't called me back as when he'd finished his performance and got back to his room he was dripping in sweat from his efforts. He'd had a shower and just fallen exhausted into bed just as I'd rung. It had completely wiped him out, but that was not considered at all. All he could think of was the joy he'd brought to everyone that night. I was so happy for him and so proud of him right there… need I say more?

Patrick definitely suffered the next day… Day 11. He was shattered. The following night he didn't go out to offer magic at all as he couldn't muster enough energy to. In a way it worked out perfectly as it turned out that was to be his grand finale as he was now going home today. It left a lovely memory for him.

My thoughts were interrupted and Patrick woke as the door opened and in came the lovely Donal from Leukaemia and Blood Cancer NZ. He was at the hospital twice a week running the physio class and had come to see if Patrick was joining them that day.

Patrick was pretty exhausted from the events of the morning in getting ready to leave and knew he would still have to find the energy to get home so he politely declined. Donal proceeded to tell us how disappointed everyone would be. He turned to me and told me about the last physio class he attended. Apparently one of the patients there had seen Patrick do a trick a few days earlier so he asked him if he would mind doing another trick for everyone there. Of course Patrick being Patrick agreed, going back to his room and returning to perform a few tricks that completely blew their minds.

Donals eyes were twinkling and the smile on his face showed me how delighted he was for everyone that they had such a great time that morning in his physio class, I think he had been hoping for a repeat performance today. Patrick had not told me about this earlier performance. It took me by surprise and deep within my heart I felt such pride again for him and his selflessness, bringing a glow of light, love and laughter to people who were going through sometimes unimaginably difficult times as they were here in the Motutapu Ward, level 11, Auckland Hospital.

We all had a good laugh at how much fun it had been for everyone. "What you don't know," Patrick then told Donal and me, "is that when I got back to my room the nurses at reception all jokingly scolded me for causing such a commotion. Apparently they could hear all the laughter and applause around the whole ward!"

So yes, it wouldn't surprise me if his outstanding attitude had something to do with his amazing ability to heal through this stem cell transplant… but in saying that, I am a little reluctant to do so, in that I don't want to take it away from those who have struggled deeply with recovery, sometimes not recovered at all, due to no circumstances of their own, but a body that is finding it too hard to heal.

You know before we leave the hospital, I want to mention this. Talking at times to patients on the ward, even those you meet in the corridor literally, or their carers, even the nurses, it often left me so humbled for the very very difficult road they faced, yet the resilience they all have in getting through it. I had spent a bit of time in the kitchen where carers were there doing just what I was, preparing food for their sister, friend, son, partner, or relative, whatever they needed or would feel like to eat.

One memorable story was a poor young guy who had been in the Motutapu Ward for three months. He had already had one stem cell transplant in that time and was now waiting for his second as the first didn't work. According to his mother, who was sharing their story with me while we prepared food in the kitchen, he apparently had an infection with a high temperature and had been very unwell for a number of weeks now. Until they could control his infection he couldn't have the second stem cell transplant, a transplant he desperately needed. Apparently he was at a life threatening stage now but the second stem cell transplant, however, had just kept getting delayed and delayed.

The boy's mother went on to explain how his father would stay with him during the day and she came after work with food for her son, and relieved the father. She would make him dinner, stay the night with him, and make him breakfast in the morning. Then she would go to work and the father would come to care for him again for the day. Every two or three days the mother would go home to shower, get new clothes etc, then back again. They had been doing this now for three months! This particular night I spoke to her, his uncle was there also. What incredible support and what a courageous family. No, I don't want to take anything away from these amazing people.

The other thing I want to mention was the outstanding care in the Motutapu Ward. We had yet to encounter one stroppy nurse, one impatient doctor, one form of lack of care or attention. It was all outstanding.

Gosh the difference this makes. Not once did I feel I HAD to be at the hospital for Patrick's 'care'. Not once did I feel I HAD to chase anything up. Not once did I feel I HAD to check on his treatment. Not once did I feel I HAD to check that his progress was being monitored appropriately. Not once did I HAVE to check IF they were doing all they could for him. Not once did I feel I couldn't voice an opinion and not once did I not feel welcome. Not once EVER! It was outstanding. I think there is something in the water, in fact I'm sure of it. In every department, ward or division dealing with cancer of both Auckland and North Shore hospitals. All I can say is what a difference it makes. All I had to do was get on with supporting Patrick with my love and affection, they were taking care of everything else. All Patrick had to do was focus on getting well. In my opinion every person in this field deserves a golden globe award for best performance as nurses and doctors.

PS… I can't confirm it, but I'm sure one day when visiting Patrick at the Motutapu Ward, I saw a patient go into a room who looked just like that lovely lady we'd met who had been told she was too old to be eligible for a transplant. It was too quick for me to be able to call out to her, plus I didn't actually know her name… but I'm pretty sure it was her and it brought me great joy that somehow she'd got that transplant after all.

PPS… By the time Patrick left the hospital he was the same weight as when he went in. He didn't lose a single kilo, let alone the five kilos that was expected. So much for my theory!

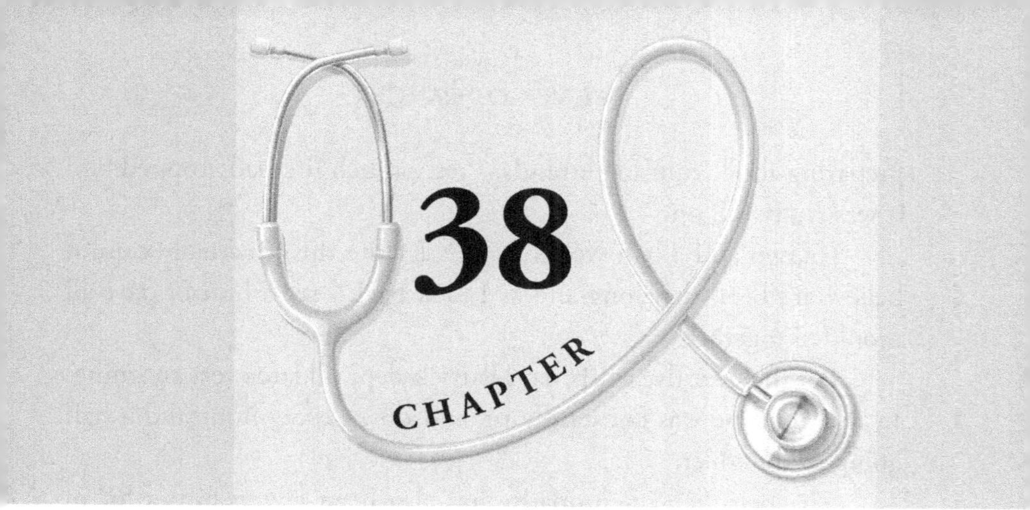

Home after Stem Cell Transplant

"Life requires movement."
- Aristotle -

Home again, home again, clippity clop!

I want to say how 'lovely' it was having Patrick home again, but quite frankly it wasn't. It was actually full on!

A day after checking out of hospital, we returned for a Doctor's check-up which included blood tests; being a provision of his early release. His body was still holding up and his platelets had risen, although his immune system had dropped. The doctor told us not to worry, that this apparently was common. Hmm, I did worry though.

The trip back to hospital wiped him out for the next two days and I was pretty much left to do everything around the house… walking the dog, getting in whatever food Patrick felt like eating, doing his washing regularly and keeping his area clean and bug free, preparing food, running errands. Pretty much life had stopped and it was really full on.

It's two and a half weeks later as I write this. I actually cannot believe it's been that long and as I look back I see a blur of days all moulded together.

For the next five or six days Patrick slept till late every morning. In the night he was constantly up and down every hour and a half going to the toilet.

The peripheral neuropathy has also been giving him a lot of grief. At night it is worse causing heat in his lower legs and feet. It keeps him awake, and though not as bad as it was while having his five months of induction chemotherapy, it still causes him grief. He groans a lot and says his legs feel like lead.

His nausea is still a problem so he is eating only small amounts regularly. Bananas are being eaten faster than I can keep up with buying them, and Edam cheese on crackers is a staple. I am constantly off to the supermarket or vege store to get what he will feel like that morning, or afternoon, or evening. He never knows through the day what he can eat so planning is out the door.

Energy is probably the most difficult thing. When he can finally muster the energy in the morning he gets up for a shower, and then collapses back in bed exhausted from the effort for the rest of the day. After a few days he managed to get up to have dinner with us, but then would leave as soon as we were finished and go back to bed.

I started getting concerned as he was nowhere near as good as he had seemed in hospital. All his joy was sucked out of him and he was just plain exhausted. It was becoming a worry. Around this time I wasn't sure if I'd preferred he was in hospital, it may have been the better of the two evils… except Patrick loved being in his own bed.

By day six of his release from the Motutapu Ward I was pretty exhausted and getting really stressed as my own 'to do' list was piling up on top of me. It was not only the physical assistance that was exhausting, but also the emotional support; keeping him positive, nurturing him, encouraging him. Then there was the underlying stress of hoping he was going to be OK, checking his temperature, looking for signs of anything going wrong together with knowing my own life was falling apart as I didn't have the energy, time or space to follow up my clients or catch up on my to do lists, exercise etc.

On this particular day we had been back at the hospital for three quarters of the day just for more routine blood tests. Our duty nurse was running really late so we sat around for an hour and a half just waiting to get the bloods taken… then we had to wait another hour and a half for the results to come through… then we had to wait for Susan to come and check on him, advise the results, and book new appointments, write up a script etc. We had left home at 8.30am and didn't get back until 3.00pm. I had thought it was only going to take the morning. I had my own list of urgent tasks for that day and it was very distressing it had not even begun.

I got home even more exhausted and now really frustrated. Patrick himself looked unusually quite good so maybe that's what made me feel I had a license to let go on how I was feeling. All of a sudden I let him have it, telling him of all this stress and strain on me. I felt guilty here, but it was what it was, and I couldn't hide it any longer.

It's funny how it works out though, he was so lovely and kind and tried to ease my strain. "Don't worry, he said, I'm feeling better, honestly. I haven't had a chance to tell you that I've had a real shift today. My waterworks seem to have come back to an even flow, and I am pooping properly now. It seems to be helping me to feel so much better, and I think I will be able to do more for myself now."

Bless him. I felt terrible. I rambled on saying "Oh no, I don't mean I don't want to help you, or that you have to do that. Honestly, I want to help and take care of you. I just need some time for myself too, it's too hard with it being so constant."

Part of my frustration I knew was because I was doing it alone. Where was everyone? Everyone else gets on with their lives and I'm left to do it all. Frustration, sadness, disappointment and anger, all there in layers building up on top of my to do list!

However Patrick was right, he had experienced a real shift in his well being that day. It was quite fascinating really, we had no idea this toilet problem was affecting his wellbeing so much. As soon as his bowels and waterworks started working properly, woohoo, it took him to a new level of healing.

The next day I was delighted to get a cup of tea in bed, the first time in three weeks! Patrick had woken, felt good, got up early and here he was… teapot, cup and my thyroid tablet at my bedside. He spent most of the day out of bed! His laptop was out all day as he punched away doing affidavits, responding to clients, organizing serves… he was on a roll. I kept reminding him not to overdo it, but he even went out and did a serve later that afternoon, driving himself the twenty minutes there and back!

The next day I expected him to crash but no, another cup of tea in bed and he continued to work that day, albeit a little slower and with not so much zeal. By the third day he slowed right down, and Friday he was pretty much in bed for the day with low energy and a migraine, but hey, well done Patrick.

He had his bloods done again at the end of the week and now his platelets had lifted to 65. Woohoo! A big jump. Still in the zone of needing to be very careful but a very impressive leap. His immune system had improved and he was now out of the real danger zone.

And I was starting to get a life back!

So the first week was pretty tough when he got home… really, when I look at it now, poor bugger, it was pretty awful for him. He was so low in energy and had so many underlying problems going on.

The next week was a lot better. I no longer had to prepare food for him during the day and though I didn't feel I could leave him a lot, I went out for a couple of coffees with friends, and managed to get my end of year accounts done. I also managed a few clients. At least there was some progress for me too.

Then it was the Queen's birthday - 1 June 2018. This meant a long weekend holiday was coming. Patrick had been out of hospital for just 17 days, that's two and a half weeks.

We had planned a couple of months earlier to book that weekend for ourselves at my place in Warkworth and had invited friends to stay. The antenatal group again! We had planned this when we thought Patrick was not going to do the stem cell transplant. I really didn't know if he was going to even make it until pretty much the day we left, I however was going regardless. We had already decided this long ago, that no matter what, we wouldn't let this stem cell transplant get in the way of this weekend happening.

I was so looking forward to the weekend with my friends. It had been 26 years since we all met and we'd got through thick and thin with our babies and supported each other through it all. They have been such wonderful friends to me as well with all this going on now. My four WhatsApp buddies, constantly in touch seeing how I was doing, offering emotional support every step of the way. Unfortunately in the end one of the couples wasn't coming to stay the whole weekend and one of the men couldn't make it at all, but we had the crux of our group together and I was looking forward to some fun.

I spent the day before grocery shopping at a few different stores getting what we needed for the weekend. Patrick had a good day that day too, he actually spent half of it out working. He'd had a meeting with lawyers and drove around Auckland doing a couple of serves… this is two weeks after getting out of hospital! He was so exhausted that night though I wasn't sure he would have the energy to come to Warkworth the next day. I cooked us all dinner and crashed myself too as it had been a full on day getting ready.

Come the morning to leave, Patrick was fatigued, but he was determined to come and I was delighted. It was hard to believe really that just two weeks out of hospital, just over one month after stem cell transplant, and we are getting out of town!

It was Friday. Our friends were arriving Friday afternoon and we had intended to leave home by 9.00am. We had a couple of stops to make on the way up and I wanted to be in Warkworth by 10.30am. I'd had guests staying during the week and needed to change beds and clean bathrooms before my friends arrived. This however ended up way too ambitious with Patrick coming. He was so tired from his busy day the day before that the effort for him to even shower that morning was tough. Just in packing his bag he needed lots of rest in between.

I was then left to pack not only for myself but all the groceries and everything we needed for our time away. So it was 11.00am before we left. We had a couple of stops to make on the way as well so it was after 12.00pm when we arrived. I'm very house proud and had worked so hard the day before to be really organized so I could get up there early and have everything ready. The others we're coming early afternoon and now I would still be cleaning and unpacking!

These are the sort of things I really should have taken care of better. Over this last month I should have insisted on more help somehow. I was taking on so much more with Patrick being ill; Patrick would have carried the groceries to the car, done the copious trips up and down stairs, and packed the car. When we arrived at Warkworth early we would have both got stuck in and had the place sorted in no time.

I was staggered when we pulled up to the house to see my Airbnb cleaning lady sitting in her car outside my house. She had the window down and was having a cigarette. It's one of the moments I'll never forget which shows how much I needed support and should have asked for it more! My heart gave a leap as my mind tried to grapple with why she was here. Did I get it mixed up? Was she booked to clean today? Did I make a mistake booking her when we have no guests? Or do we have guests and I'd missed it? Honestly, the way things were I could have done that yet I knew she usually could not clean for me on a Friday as she is booked up in advance with other clients.

I pulled up alongside her and wound down the window and exclaimed, "Are you cleaning for me today?" "Oh no," she casually replied. "I clean the house across the road and am just waiting for her to go out." Whew, I took a sigh of relief that I hadn't screwed up with a booking. She then continued. "I do have a bit of time though if you want me to come and do some cleaning."

There she was. My next guardian angel. I was delighted and she ended up giving me an hour. She changed the beds and did the bathrooms while I unpacked, cleaned the kitchen and put the washing on, and we had pretty much finished just as the first friend arrived. Another couple arrived soon after and though I wasn't dressed and looked like shit, the house was ready! Patrick had got in and just relaxed so he felt quite ready to receive everyone while I changed and we had the most wonderful couple of days together.

I was so amazed at how well Patrick kept up. OK so he didn't do the walks with us, or come to the markets early in the morning, or in fact help out physically entertaining wise, but he kept up socially. He managed to come out for lunch with us all on the Saturday and stayed up most of the day, and for dinners. It really was a fun time that I know I desperately needed. By Sunday though we were both pretty exhausted. One friend was staying on till Monday but we had a quiet afternoon and night. On Monday Patrick was still exhausted and was unenthusiastic about doing anything, eating anything or saying anything but I managed to get him out for a coffee and a wee walk.

Tuesday was pretty much the same. I had to pack up the house myself and do all the cleaning. Patrick was exhausted just from dressing and packing again. However by the next day, Wednesday, Patrick woke up feeling great and for the next two days he worked pretty much all day. For two days he worked and then Friday he came to a halt again. Friday and Saturday he did very little and by Sunday he was good again.

So here is the new cycle for now. A couple of good days, a couple of bad days, as we are now halfway through week four home from the hospital after stem cell transplant. **So that's approximately six weeks after the actual stem cell transplant began.**

The best thing is Patrick is now completely out of the woods. His blood results that came in at the end of the week show his platelets are now in normal range and his white blood cell count was at a level that means he is now not vulnerable to colds, infection, or bleeding out any more meaning he won't be back in hospital any time soon.

Meaning he's the record boy for stem cell transplants. Meaning, yay!! We've got through the worst of it. Meaning some form of normal life coming up for us in the near future. Meaning he is well on the road to recovery and meaning I can breathe again! It's now time to talk about things other than cancer again. It's time to talk about things other than how Patrick is… it's time to get a life!

Seriously you wonder what's worse at times, the cancer or the treatment. It certainly takes away so much quality of life. When you're in it, you are so absorbed in it all and it's not until you start coming up for air you realise how debilitating it all is, and how tough a ride it is.

I realise now that I was too accepting of putting my life on hold, too accepting of getting shattered, too accepting of getting chronic fatigue, too accepting of getting behind in myself, too accepting of the stress of trying to keep up, too accepting of caring for Patrick on my own. I've said it before, it was my own fault.

It wasn't until the end of all of Patrick's treatment on the Kiwi Trial that I could look back and see the neglect I had enforced on myself. At this stage here for example, I hadn't done my yoga practice once over the past eight months. I was too worn out to floss my teeth at night and I noticed at this point my gums starting to bleed and I'd put on weight comfort eating. Feeling I had the space to meditate was a joke, let alone ever having my nails done. I couldn't shake the early morning wakeups of 5.30am so I was tired before I started the day. Coffee with friends was rare, and if I did I felt like a prisoner that has escaped. It was even hard to rest during the day when I needed it as Patrick was in bed most of the afternoon.

I noticed how, even on the weeks off when we did go away or catch up on things, I still was not able to drop into my life. My normal life, my normal way and routine of life… that went by the by until treatment was finally over.

I should have put a plan in place. Even having help with the small things would have made a difference. Perhaps things like each of the children one night a week could have come with food and cooked a meal. Each of them could have had a weekly job to do as well. One could have been to mow the lawns, another get the main groceries for the week, that sort of thing. The children could have had turns each month having a day with Patrick on the weekend so I could do my thing.

I could have asked for help from friends. With all the friends I have, I could have set up a roster helping with my house in Warkworth. It probably would have only meant them giving a day each to me over this eight month period. I had a general cleaner for the bookings, but there were always the bigger jobs that needed regularly doing. The garden, the windows, the decks, extra cleaning, getting in supplies, etc. For Airbnb you have to have the place tip top at all times. Sometimes the cleaner couldn't make it to get the place ready for a booking, and I'd have to go up and do it myself at whatever cost to me, no matter what was going on with Patrick, I just had to go. That was enough for me to deal with without all the extras. Gosh, what a difference that would have made if I had done that. The money I was getting from this was helping me be available to support him, it had to keep going!

This is one of the reasons I am writing this whole story. There is not enough said about how difficult it is for the carer as well as the patient in these situations. It may sound selfish, which could be why it is not spoken of much out there but if you are a carer, you know what I'm talking about and it needs to be said. The primary carer needs support from family and friends. Full stop! They should be entitled to their own lives to be able to continue, but first you have to own that knowing yourself so you can ask!!

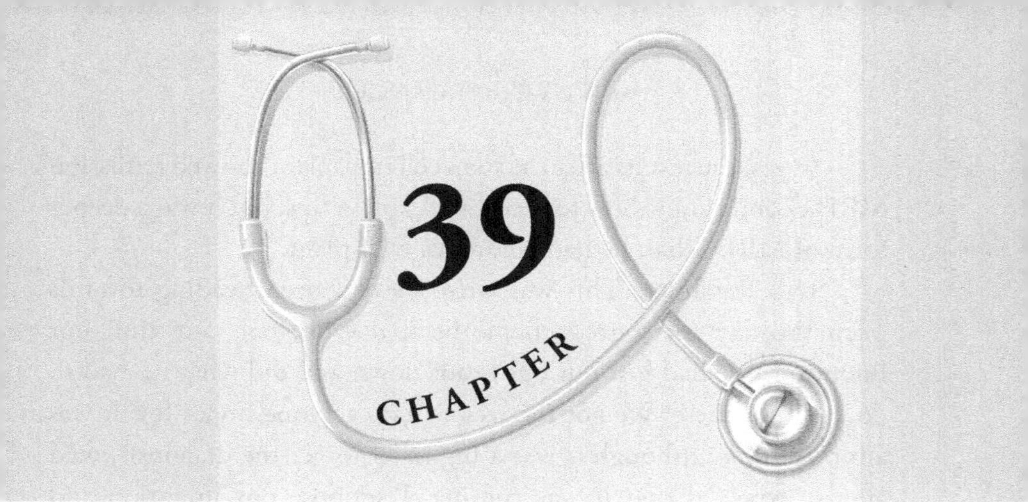

Life After Stem Cell Transplant

"There are only two ways to live your life.
One is as though nothing is a miracle.
The other is as though everything is a Miracle."
- Albert Einstein -

It stopped there… my writing that is. As Patrick gained more energy with his good and bad days I started to get a 'bit' of a life back and just didn't want to write any more. I just wanted to get on with life without hospital visits, treatments, and the reminder of cancer every day. Even once Patrick started his consolidation therapy I didn't feel like writing.

I realise, in coming back and writing this section now, that it was just such a relief to have gotten through the five months of induction therapy and then the stem cell transplant. But exciting news… Patrick is now free of the 80-90% saturation of cancer in his body and is now MRD-!!! It no longer feels life threatening and insecure with so much unknown ahead of us.

So yes, the results after the stem cell transplant showed remission MRD- I don't know how to medically explain this, but it was a deeper form of MRD- than he had before his transplant.

This was huge. This was what we had been heading towards from the day we started chemotherapy. Our goal, our aim, our intention. We had just put our heads down and did what we had to do, and got there! We got the result that everyone hopes for. It was a bit weird, as although it was a big relief to get the diagnosis, we'd almost expected that it was coming. I suppose our intention and purpose had been so strong, we didn't really think it wouldn't come through. Maybe it was because he had been progressing so well all the way along as well that encouraged us to expect this.

I think, throughout the treatments of chemotherapy and stem cell transplant, my biggest concern was Patrick surviving the treatments. Having a heart attack through chemotherapy was always an underlying concern no matter how much I'd let go. Patrick's white blood count returning to normal after the stem cell transplant was of course a concern, then of course recovering from the stem cell transplant, what would he be like!

I don't think either of us ever deep down actually questioned if Patrick would achieve MRD-, we just expected he would. It was just surviving to get there! What a lesson in the law of attraction and also the need to be present with just what's here today and meeting the need.

Patrick on the other hand had not been stressed about whether he survived or didn't through treatment. He was very philosophical about it all, that's not saying he didn't care if he died, because you know that's not true. He just knew he was doing his best in getting on with the treatments and whatever would be, would be. So, so, so present!! He had his goal in mind of MRD- and just focused on achieving that!

We were absolutely delighted to get the results of 'Remission MRD-' after the stem cell transplant of course, and the word 'relief' comes to mind. We'd got through the worst of it, achieved what we needed to and the pressure was off.

And I just didn't need to write. Didn't want to write. So I'm going back now filling in the gap.

After stem cell transplant we had ahead of us three months break from any further treatments, while Patrick recovered. That alone brought such a relief. We both felt we had got through the worst of it and that he was no longer in immediate life threatening danger. All those scary words we had faced at the beginning… multiple myeloma, paraprotein, light chains, bone marrow tests, chemotherapy, Dexamethasone, Carfilzomib, steroids, trial programs, stem cell transplants, neutrophils, of course to name a few… all the googling and researching…. we knew them all now.

We were past the worry of how Patrick would cope with chemotherapy and a stem cell transplant… would he get through it? How would he be affected? Would he have permanent disabilities as a consequence? Could he still work? How would we cope financially? He'd got through it OK and right now his body was cancer free.

And then we had a three month break from having to go near a hospital. All I can say is, boy we needed that!! Although he was still recovering and needed to rest a lot it was such a great break that I switched off from writing too and it took some time before I needed to get back to it. Not until it got unbearable watching Patrick at the end of consolidation therapy, struggling so much with the chemotherapy.

But let's backtrack and keep some order here!

I'll start with the picture following, of Patrick six weeks after stem cell transplant began. Bald but looking great! Having a morning cuppa at our favourite beachfront cafe with our dog Indi. My son Taylor bought Patrick this beanie when travelling through South America, knowing he was going to lose his hair through treatment.

Patrick's nephew Ryan, from London, arrived to stay on 13 June for three weeks. He arrived the week following our return from the Warkworth weekend away with the antenatal group of friends. At 20 years old he was travelling, doing a bit of an OE, and his final stop was NZ before meeting up with his family in the States for a wedding. It was Patrick's brother's son's wedding in Los Angeles but unfortunately we would not be able to go as Patrick was not well enough to travel overseas at this stage.

However Patrick, despite having his bad as well as good days now, was determined to try and make his nephew's visit memorable. Ryan had his list of what he wanted to do while visiting, and Patrick was determined to be a part of that.

So blow me down on 20 June 2018, just five weeks after coming home from his stem cell transplant, seven weeks after starting stem cell transplant, he booked for Ryan and him to go black water rafting at Waitomo Caves! I thought he was mad, but there was no stopping him. The drive there alone was over two hours each way, let alone the energy needed to go rafting, but he was determined to give Ryan an experience of a lifetime.

I got it, of course I did. Patrick didn't know when he would see Ryan again. Nothing was clearer to us now that moments in life are precious and if we don't grab them they are gone… and we just may not get them back again. So just seven weeks after receiving a stem cell transplant he's going black water rafting with his nephew from England!

They had a ball and it was an experience of a lifetime for them both. I was thrilled for him but he came back white and really exhausted. He rested most of the next day and the next… but he did it. Most importantly they had that special quality time and adventure together but wow, what was also clear was that he was really recovering from his stem cell transplant. Never in a million years would we have imagined he would have been doing something like this so soon after, in fact I had wondered if he ever would.

This left me with a new hope. Life may get relatively back to normal eventually.

A week after this, six weeks after leaving hospital, eight weeks after his actual stem cell transplant, Patrick started back at squash. He lasted only 45 minutes and he had to come off the court twice as he was feeling faint, but he persevered and got his game in. That gradually increased over the next six weeks to one and a half hour games. Not bad huh? In fact it's brilliant!!

Then to top it all off we went on a ski trip! Yep, right there 13 July - Auckland to Queenstown. Departing 10.20am arriving 12.15pm. Just over eight weeks after leaving hospital, ten weeks after his stem cell transplant. We even bussed to the airport. That might seem small but it takes a lot more effort to catch a bus than an Uber. Life was still measured in energy levels at this stage, so catching a bus was a big deal.

Patrick's best friend, Mark, who lives in Palmerston North, had offered for us to stay with them at their timeshare in Wanaka for a week. (The same good friend that helped come clean up the section when Patrick had just started treatment.) We had not been able to confirm we could go until the last minute as we had no idea if he would be up for it. But, bless Mark, he kept the room free for us. Right there, that sort of kindness and care was worth millions to us. Patrick loved skiing so this was one holiday he was keen for!

We all met at Queenstown airport, arriving at similar times then we travelled by car to Wanaka. Mark, his wife, their son and us were in one apartment and Mark's brother and his family in another.

We wasted no time. The very next day on 14 July 2018 we were skiing Cardrona ski fields, precisely two months after leaving hospital! I'll never forget getting on that chairlift for our first ride up the mountain. It was such a stunning day and the snow conditions were perfect. I really just couldn't believe we were there doing this.

To be honest, I hadn't been sure if we would ever go skiing again together. I of course didn't know what Patrick's 'new norm' was going to look like. You have no idea how many hundreds of times that phrase 'new norm' has played out in my head!

Yet here we were, gear on, skis and poles set, ready to jump on the chair and go for it! Woohoo. It was a very emotional ride and I cried most of the way up as we revelled in how miraculous it felt that we were doing this. Crying and grinning almost simultaneously all the way to the top.

OK, so we didn't ski all day as Patrick tired, and actually I did too just from not being ski fit, but we did a good few solid hours before we stopped. It was amazing and I felt so grateful. My heart was swollen with joy all day.

The next day Patrick was pretty exhausted, so we had a rest day while the others went skiing. The following day they all went off on a road trip to have a game of curling. I didn't feel like going but Patrick went. It was about a two hour drive each way, so again he did really well mustering the energy to go.

It took its toll on him so we then took a few rest days. I wasn't sure if we'd get up the mountain again, but I wasn't concerned, I was amazed we had even got there in the first place. In fact, I was amazed that we'd even got away! Wanaka is one of the most picturesque towns in the world so it was no hardship going for strolls by the lake, drinking copious amounts of cuppas in the cafes, and we even managed a bike ride along the lakefront one day.

However, 19 July we woke and Patrick felt energized enough to ski again and thankfully it was another stunning day. This time we managed to ski for most of the day and had so much fun. Patrick and I had just stuck together and let the others go on so we could ski at our own pace, as we had done the first day. We'd just taken off our skis at the end of the day when Mark and his brother came down the mountain. We hailed out to them but they signalled they were going up for one more run. To my great surprise, Patrick grabbed his skis and raced after them to the ski lift, just managing to get his skis on in time to join them and jumping on the chair for a final run.

I waited at the bottom to see him, in no time at all, come hurtling down the mountain… it appeared the race was on. Typical boys, and he loved it! I was so delighted for him and I felt in that moment a glimmer of light that maybe everything was going to be really OK.

Over the next month Patrick grew stronger and stronger and he went back to working part time. He still needed naps in the afternoon occasionally but was generally getting through the day OK.

His hair started to grow back; just a tiny bit poking through. Just a note, by the time his hair grew back fully, it was really curly and really grey. I'd like to say peppery but probably with a bit more salt! The photo you will see was taken in November so he had a full head of hair within six months of the stem cell transplant.

It was like this only for a relatively short time though. A year later it straightened and darkened to almost back to how it was originally, weird huh? It's well known that chemotherapy can do that, maybe the curling of the hair, but I'm putting the greying down to the stress and shock his body has gone through.

So it was three months after stem cell transplant and Patrick was now feeling the best he's felt in years, even better than he felt just before stem cell transplant, which we'd thought was awesome enough then. No more day sleeps, he looked well and felt great. I was feeling so much better too and I had my life back. I had more focus for work, more time for friends and leisure, and I found myself laughing on occasions, surprising myself again when I did. However a dread was hanging over us as Patrick was expected to begin chemotherapy again. The first week in August was looming, three months after stem cell transplant. Time for consolidation chemotherapy.

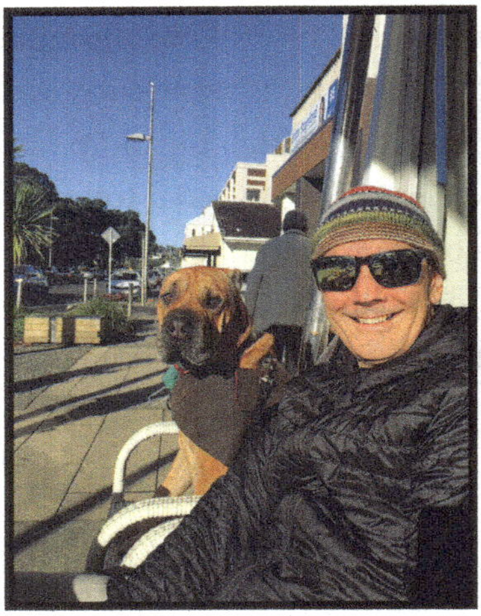

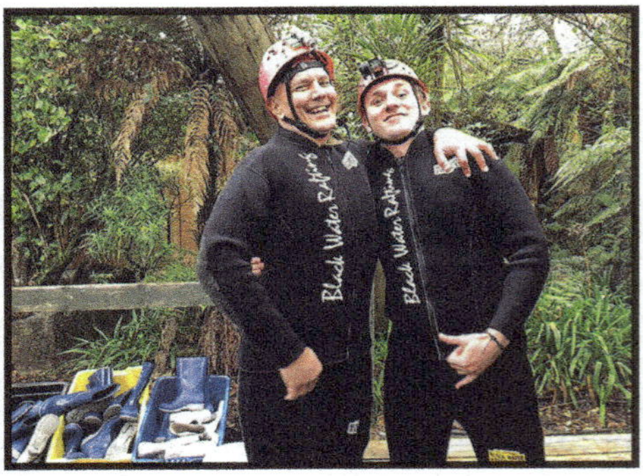
Black Water Rafting
Black Water Rafting

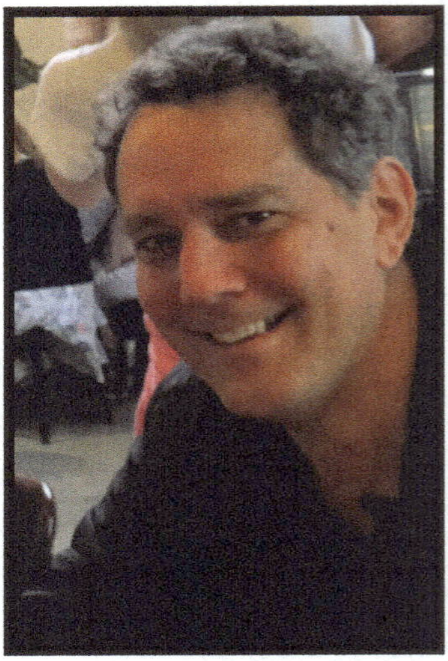

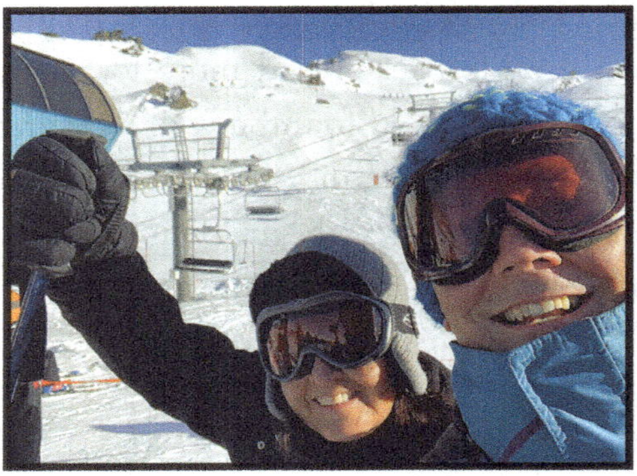

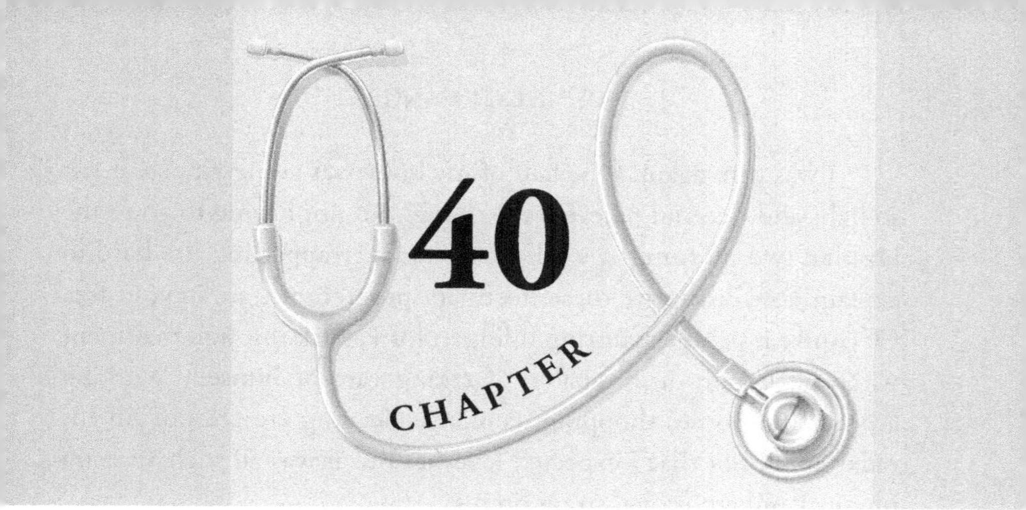

Consolidation therapy

"Promise me you'll always remember:
You're braver than you believe,
and stronger than you seem,
and smarter than you think."
Christopher Robin to Pooh.
- A.A.Milne -

Patrick started talking a new language. He didn't want to do the consolidation therapy. I mean he really didn't want to do it! It was like the stem cell transplant decision all over again.

He started discussing with me that he didn't see the need to, he was in remission MRD- already. His last bone marrow test had shown he was now in 'complete remission'. Why put himself through more treatment, more hammering. Going back to feeling so tired and unwell with all the visits to the hospital, the time off work and the financial toll. He just wanted to get back to a normal life. He was also worried about the effects of peripheral neuropathy. It bothered him so much that he could end up with permanent damage.

I was torn again. One half of my body was going yippee! It felt so light and free and relieved; the thought of not having to go to the hospital two mornings a week alone was very appealing. It's hard to explain how disruptive these treatment programmes are in your life. Of course it's also exhausting filling in for Patrick through treatment while he is only just capable of taking care of himself. Working around the house, shopping, cooking, cleaning etc are not on his radar at all, not that I expected it to be. But it was all such an extra physical and emotional strain on me.

Over these last three months off treatment I'd caught up with myself in many ways. Work was getting back on track and I had caught up with most of my friends. I'd started up yoga again and managed to get to a couple of philosophy meets. My energy levels had improved and Patrick was able to help out more now so I didn't have the weight of doing everything to run two households on my own.

Most significantly, Patrick was well. I wasn't having to watch him exhausted, flat out lying in bed every day needing rest. I didn't have to put up with his moodiness from the drugs, or the lows each week he was on treatment, nor bear witness to his foggy brain and lack of concentration that frustrated him and left it difficult for him to cope. The financial cost of him not working a full day had also been such a worry for us both.

The thought of being thrown back into the cycle of chemotherapy was grueling in more ways than one! I wasn't sure if even I had the energy to do it all again. I knew where he was coming from and didn't blame him at all for his thoughts to not continue. We were getting a taste now of quality of life and didn't want to give that up!

The other half of me though, well, that felt a sense of dread. Like we were playing Russian roulette. Without the treatment, how would this affect his time span of progression free survival? How would it affect his overall survival? Scary questions that no one could ever really answer unless you had a crystal ball. I was literally torn in two.

Then of course this wasn't my decision. The decision impacted me significantly, but it had to be Patrick's decision. Once again I was on board to support him in whatever path he chose. Once again I insisted he was well informed before making any decisions, and held off any decision until he'd met with the specialist.

I went along to the appointment with Patrick, as I always did. I wanted to know the options and the consequences as much as Patrick did.

The poor specialist. It was Dr David Simpson we were seeing, the head of the Kiwi Trial program. He's such a lovely patient man who was well accustomed now to Patrick's enquiries. It appears not many patients are of this mind, most of them just do as they are told. So the long and short of it is that by the end of the appointment David managed to convince Patrick to proceed with consolidation therapy. I suppose the convincing factor out of it all was funnily enough, the unknown. Not what we knew, or the doctors knew or what the results did show, but what we didn't know. I'll try to explain!

David drew a picture. I wish I had taken a shot of it to show you now. It was a simple but significant few lines.

He drew a line, being the surface of Patrick's body, then he drew another line about an inch below that signifying the depth of his body that the MRD testing reached. In the not too distant past that line would only have been at say a quarter of an inch. MRD testing didn't go very deep testing only 1 in 10,000 cells. NZ only recently, in February 2017, got the new technology which now tests 1 in 1,000,000 cells!

David then drew another line much further down, say another two inches further down, signifying the depth of Patrick's body. He explained that this gap here below the inch line is the unknown and this unknown area is a very vast space. We don't know if there are cancer cells there or not and the purpose of the consolidation therapy is to keep on blasting any possible cancer cells that we don't know about, that we can't know about and to continue treatment to blast as deep as we can. So in all truth we won't really know if it was necessary at the end of the treatments but we will know we gave it the best shot.

David then went on to explain again to us how important the 'best shot' is! He's told us before, but he told us again. Honestly, this guy is a legend with his patience and perseverance. and commitment to ensuring that Patrick gets the best possible outcome.

David explained in layman terms, the more cancer cells you can kill off, the deeper your positive results. The deeper your positive results, the longer your remission. The longer your remission the better chance you have of fighting it again when it comes back.

So of all the assessment of medical blood results, bone marrow tests, past historical statistical analysis, it all came down to this one sketch David drew on this day that convinced Patrick to proceed with consolidation therapy.

There were two good reasons. One, you'll possibly get a longer remission. Well that's pretty bloody important. Secondly, the longer the remission, the better chance you have of fighting it second time around, to get another good remission… and then a third benefit that David came forward with. Words that we had heard in our very first appointment with Dr Ross Henderson and numerous times since. The key is to keep you going as long as possible as new technology is coming out all the time for multiple myeloma, exponentially fast, that can give better and better results.

So although quality of life is important for now, when you hear that, hanging in there with treatment that'll extend your life seemed exponentially more important. New treatments may in the end have the possibility to extend your life significantly, so this is a critical factor. With Patrick's chromosome deletion 1p32 and the statistical medium overall survival period of just over two years, it was clear to us both that persevering through more treatment with the hope of extending his remission period, and possibly life span with new treatments in the future, was a priority.

We walked out of that appointment with the decision made. It was a no brainer. Patrick was going back in for more!

As we left the hospital we were both silent all the way to the car. We now both knew what we were in for, it was no mystery. No research was needed, there was nothing we needed to do, or could do, but go for the ride... again. It was clear neither of us were looking forward to it, but neither of us said it. It was a long ride home.

I sank into a bit of a low for a few days. It was very much like when Patrick finally decided to do the stem cell transplant, I hadn't realised then how secretly I was looking forward to not going through it if he decided that path, and it had been such a downer at first when he decided he would go ahead.

Don't get me wrong. I was also so pleased Patrick was going ahead with the consolidation therapy, I knew it was the only right way to go, but man, I was not looking forward to it. I hadn't realised how much that half of me that was elated to not have any more treatments, was hoping for that. I saw now it had been a bit of a high, and now I was coming down... with a crash. Treatment was starting in a week!

I didn't really know how I was going to do it. Whenever I went there I hit a brick wall. I didn't want to go backwards again. I didn't want to lose the life I had started restoring and I didn't want to be exhausted all the time. I didn't want to feel his pain or watch him suffer again. Aarrgh!! After a few days I made a very difficult decision, I had to do it a bit differently this time as my own health and wellbeing was too important not to. I decided I needed to put myself first a little, finally!

The consolidation therapy period was for another four months and I had to find a way to get through this better than before, so I decided I wouldn't attend all the hospital chemotherapy treatments, I would go only once a week!

This broke my heart to let go. I had from the start wanted to be with Patrick for every step of the journey as I didn't want him to do this alone, not one inch of it, but I just couldn't keep up, I had to admit defeat. The crazy thing is, in letting go I realised it had really been all about me in this regard. I wanted to be there 100% as I knew if I was him, this is the sort of support I would have wanted, actually not just wanted, but needed. It would have meant so much to me to have someone always by my side and I had been transferring this on to Patrick's situation.

Patrick had, right from the start, insisted he didn't need me with him all the time, that he was fine to go on his own, that I really didn't need to be there, etc, etc. I had heard this probably a dozen times over his first five months of treatment. However it was too important to me, I'd had to support him 100%.

I realised now I could let some of that go. Patrick knew what he was doing now and he was comfortable with going to the hospital. He knew all the nurses, they are all so lovely and make him, in fact us, always so welcome. He knew what he was in for with each visit so I didn't need to always be there anymore.

Well what a difference it made to me immediately on making the decision, it started to feel manageable and that we would get through it so much better now. I'm not sure if it was the extra time I would now have or the drop in responsibility, either way it helped. I would still go to all of the specialists' appointments of course, and the first day of chemotherapy each week… just one day less a week at the hospital.

So consolidation therapy began. I went the first day with Patrick and the nurses welcomed us as warmly as they always had; it was actually lovely to see them again. It staggers me that they can maintain such wonderful dispositions day after day, week after week, month after month, and even year after year for a lot of them.

It was around this time the nurses were starting to protest for higher salaries and better working conditions. One day there was actually a full on national strike. Good on them, they sure deserved it. I know I've said it before, but I want to say it again, the nurses at

North Shore haematology day stay helped us significantly to cope with all we were going through just by being so kind and caring every time we went in, and their extreme professionalism always left us feeling in safe hands. Indirectly it helped us feel part of a team and not alone in our desire to have Patrick reach his goal of MRD-! It made all the difference in the world.

With Patrick's veins so fed up with being poked and prodded and with their now extreme aversion to needles it had become increasingly tough on him, with the nurses trying here, there and everywhere, digging into his arms and hands trying to get veins each week. Patrick had therefore asked for a port to be put in this time around for the four month consolidation therapy period. The specialist had agreed, but he was on the waitlist to have it put in and in the end it was nearly three weeks into treatment I think before it was done. To have a port put in requires a small operation with a local anaesthetic. This needed to be done in the surgery ward so hence the wait. In the meantime, with it being very difficult to get Patrick's line in at the beginning of each week to administer the chemotherapy, it was quite taxing on him.

Though it's nothing in the whole scheme of things, we highly recommend it if you are starting long periods of chemotherapy to get a port put in at the start. You may have good veins now, as Patrick did at the start, but they certainly only seemed to have so much tolerance for being jabbed! Two of our dear chemotherapy friends had it done from the outset and they never looked back.

It wasn't long before we were back pretty much into the old routine and the cycle became all too familiar again. One of the drugs had changed now for consolidation therapy. The induction therapy for the first five months included treatment with Cyclophosphamide, Dexamethasone, and Carfilzomib. For the next four months of consolidation therapy Cyclophosphamide was to be replaced with Thalidomide, and Dexamethasone and Carfilzomib remained the same.

Over the three month break after stem cell transplant the problems Patrick had been having with peripheral neuropathy had been slightly improving as the weeks went by. As mentioned this was one of the key reasons Patrick had not wanted to undergo consolidation therapy. He hated this condition and he had heard that the new drug, Thalidomide, was even worse for it.

Sure enough, by the end of the first month of consolidation therapy Patrick worsened again with peripheral neuropathy. It upset him greatly as not only was this condition extremely painful and uncomfortable but it could have dire consequences on Patrick's ability to perform his magic shows - and who knew for how long this would last!

All the other side effects were back in full force as well of course and, utterly exhausted, Patrick spent many hours just lying in bed over the three weeks of treatment period. Again, towards the end of the week off chemotherapy he would feel relatively good again… then back in again!

The brain fog and memory recall didn't lift though over the week off nor did the constant need to urinate. These had become quite difficult side effects for him to live with.

As with induction therapy, we always saw the specialist in between each month's treatment. After the first month Patrick expressed his grave concerns again about the increase in peripheral neuropathy already. Basically he wanted to go off the Thalidomide. The specialist on duty sensibly suggested instead of just stopping, how about we reduce the dose of Thalidomide to 50mg to start with, and see how he was with that and he reluctantly agreed.

The benefit of writing this as I look back now is that I can inform you straight away that this helped significantly. Patrick's condition didn't worsen too much each month from then on. He then was able to adjust his mindset knowing psychologically that at least it seemed it wasn't going to get too bad. He now felt comfortable staying on Thalidomide for the duration at the reduced dosage, even with the current discomfort he had, as he felt confident it wasn't going to get any worse.

The next three months of consolidation therapy were as we were expecting, a very similar experience to the initial five months of induction therapy. The chemotherapy treatments weren't much better or worse than the time before.

Giving myself only one day a week going to the hospital for treatments, however, did give me some reprieve in the first month… though really just more time to run the household at Patricks for him and my Airbnb in Warkworth as well as more time for work with less stress. All in all we were managing a bit better than through the past treatments.

I'll just say here, looking back, I don't think Patrick cooked one meal through his whole treatment time. He still did very little in the way of housework, shopping, maintenance etc. He did continue to manage to wash his own clothes regularly though. He insisted on this as he still didn't want me handling his 'chemo clothes', as he called them. He was continuously very aware of the chemotherapy being pumped and released through his body. He hated it. He was back again to scrubbing his body rigorously for days after treatment to help the chemotherapy release from his body, and drinking copious beer glasses of water a day.

Oh yes, and he still managed to mow the lawns the first month on his week off chemotherapy. However over the next few months of consolidation treatment the lawns grew to a new length as Patrick struggled to be able to do these too…

Pneumonia

"Dig within. There lies the wellspring of good;
ever dig, and it will ever flow."
- Marcus Aurelius -

So the consolidation therapy over the four months, as I said, went pretty much as before with induction therapy, however an extra side effect of the chemotherapy hit Patrick hard during this four months of treatment, he got pneumonia.

He first got it just after his first month of consolidation therapy. He had developed a constant dry cough and was coughing up yellow sputum. He had intermittent chest pain too and we started to get a little worried. On 28 August 2018 we decided he really should go to A&E to get checked out.

I had a doctor's appointment of my own that morning, and then a client. Patrick said he was feeling OK enough to go by himself so I decided to not put too much pressure on myself and stick to what I had on that morning rather than cancel to take him to the hospital. Yes, I was getting better at taking care of me too.

When I finished work at 3.30pm I phoned him and was very surprised to find out he had been admitted. They had taken a lot of tests and wanted to put him on an IV of Cefuroxime and Roxithromycin, antibiotics for viral infections and respiratory infection, and he was to stay in hospital overnight.

This was one of those many times I felt blessed my office was just across the road from the hospital. I raced over and spent the rest of the day and evening with him. Being a recent stem cell transplant patient, Patrick's immune system was still compromised, enough that he had been given his own room due to his susceptibility to infection. That was such a treat for him.

Just noting here, you also get admitted immediately into A&E as a chemotherapy patient. This was a blessing for Patrick on the day, instead of having to wait what appears to be the customary minimum couple of hours! To be honest, I think as a cancer patient you certainly earn that right. You go through enough and are at the hospital enough though it's really because you can't sit in a waiting room with sick people due to being exposed with your low immune system.

The following morning he was showing signs of improvement so the doctor decided to release him with oral antibiotics Cefaclor and Roxithromycin and they put it down to a virus. Although chest X-rays had been taken, they did not show pneumonia at this stage. He was released with 'an impression of likely viral illness and possible mild LRTI (lower respiratory tract infection).'

This however created a difficult situation. The day he was released 29 August 2018, was the day Patrick, myself and Patrick's daughter Katelyn were supposed to fly to Wellington for 4 nights. This was his week off chemotherapy which had fortunately coincided with the Open Day at Victoria University, which we were to attend with Katelyn. We had booked a trip to check out the University, see all the halls of residence and help Katelyn get familiar with Wellington.

We had all been really looking forward to it and had rented a nice Airbnb on the outskirts of town for our stay.

There was no way Patrick was well enough to make it. You know it's one of those life moments that you won't forget as this trip was to be a special time taking time out for Katelyn, his youngest child who was now fleeing the nest; to be there to encourage and support her to feel comfortable when entering into the next stage of her life. Patrick had wanted to visit the halls so he knew the nicest places for Katelyn to ask for accommodation. He wanted to walk the campus with her, help her firm up her subjects while there, and basically help her get to know Wellington with him at her side.

It was with great disappointment that he had to admit defeat and that he couldn't get on that plane, and I know Katelyn was sad also. She was a casualty of a Dad with cancer and was now stuck with just me, the Stepmum… not even close to the Dad she adored. I vowed to try and make it a great trip for her all the same but unfortunately I got the most awful flu which started coming on the night we left Auckland. I managed the first day visiting the halls and arranging Katelyn's subjects then I crashed. Temperatures, horrid coughing, nose like a tap and managing just an orange a day. I hadn't had a flu like this for years but it wasn't surprising I suppose. With all we had been through, the stress, the extra load etc, my immune system would also have been low.

Bless Katelyn, she still managed on her own, going to lectures, a tour of Parliament, and a visit to Te Papa museum and she had a fabulous time.

Patrick felt a lot better over the next week on the antibiotics, although he hadn't fully recovered before the next month of chemotherapy, Cycle 2 of consolidation therapy. Unfortunately as he continued with the chemotherapy he got worse again.

This time, when he went to A&E the chest x-rays definitely showed pneumonia. He was admitted immediately into hospital and spent 3 nights there on IV antibiotics. Once again he had his own room and he was relatively comfortable through it all. Once he was showing signs of improvement he was discharged again with further antibiotics. I felt sorry for him, as if he wasn't taking enough drugs already and now having to take antibiotics for so long.

At this stage this is the list of drugs Patrick was taking, not including the 2 antibiotics:

Synthroid, Cilazapril, Allopurinol, Aspirin, Dexamethasone, Carfilzomib, Felodipine, Trimethoprim, Thalidomide, Valaciclovir, Zopiclone, and Viscotears for his eyes which were still very dry.

We had been hoping the specialist would agree to postpone Patrick's next chemotherapy treatment and push it out a week to give his body a break to recover from this bout of pneumonia. Patrick even requested this however there was no rest for the wicked. It was deemed by the specialists it was better to continue with the second cycle on time rather than break up the cycle. This worried me as I really felt his body needed a break, but the powers that be said soldier on which Patrick did, only to find himself deteriorate again, this time even further. He had finished the antibiotics and still felt unwell. He knew he hadn't fully recovered and he felt worse as each day went on. By the time he had finished his second round of consolidation therapy he was very ill again.

Here we were now into our break from chemotherapy after Cycle 2. It should be a break for Patrick from needing to rest all the time, a break for him from feeling so awful with all the side effects from his treatment, and a time to catch our breath… a time to catch up on things, even have a bit of time away, a wee holiday as we'd promised ourselves previously.

On the last month's break we were going to Wellington with Katelyn, instead Patrick was really ill with pneumonia and I got the flu. For this month's break we hadn't planned anything as we didn't know how Patrick would be feeling. Just as well.

A few days after completion of the second cycle of consolidation therapy, we woke up to Patrick having a very high temperature. The thermometer showed 39.5C and he felt terrible. I insisted we go to the hospital and get him checked but he thought I was overreacting. I think Patrick had gotten so used to feeling lousy that he didn't realise how bad he was. I was very concerned. A high temperature is not good for a person on chemotherapy who's body is already run down and in the end it took the threat that I was calling an ambulance right away if he didn't get up and get dressed so I could take him in. He told me I was being ridiculous, but once he saw how serious I was, he got up.

Thank goodness we did as I'm not sure what story I would be telling today otherwise. We were admitted immediately into the A&E upon my telling them of Patrick's symptoms. The doctor arrived quickly, took his temperature and assessed his condition. The next minute it was all go. The defibrillator arrived on the bed and the tests started to roll. Patrick's temperature was now 41C and they were obviously very concerned about a cardiac arrest.

Patrick was wheeled off for X-rays but not before a specific cardiac assistant was assigned to go with him with the defibrillator. Yep, it was all pretty scary as Patrick was really unwell.

I'll never forget, after he had the tests all done and we were waiting in the A&E room. Despite medication his temperature had not come down and he was feeling worse and worse, he looked absolutely dreadful. He needed to go to the toilet; it was only around the corner, say twenty steps away, but they wouldn't let him go without me with him. We hobbled along and on the way back Patrick stopped for a breather. I'll never forget what he said. He looked at me, seeming so frail and looking so forlorn and said "This is all pretty shitty isn't it?"

I caught my breath and took a big pause. Seriously, with all this guy had been through, this is the first time he had actually complained, the first time he had stopped to feel sorry for himself. It really hit me in that moment how amazing he has been. Here Patrick was, for the first time complaining, that this was all actually 'pretty shitty'.

It showed how awful he was feeling. Gosh, with all he went through with stem cell transplant he never complained, not once. Through all the months of chemotherapy, he never complained. Oh sure he would say what he was experiencing or how bad it was affecting him, but he never actually complained that he was having to go through it, never felt sorry for himself. It was quite staggering really, and this was very apparent to me at that moment. It also made me realise how truly awful he must be feeling, and how truly sick he was. I was worried. Really worried.

Of course I didn't want to alarm him further so I decided to be honest, but light, and replied with a light laugh "Patrick, that's an understatement. It's been REALLY BLOODY SHITTY." and with a light whiff of a smile I carried on walking slowly with him back to the bed. There was nothing else I could do, we just had to keep soldiering on.

I can still see myself sitting at the side of the bed for what seemed an eternity in A&E, so consciously aware of the defibrillator. As you know, I know first hand how cancer can cause a heart attack and it's been one of my biggest worries through all of Patrick's treatment. So here was fear literally staring me in the face.

Patrick was admitted into a ward this time, no private room. Apparently his immune system had recovered enough now that it was safe to be in a standard ward. There were four beds in the room, though he was past caring about that, he was so unwell he was almost oblivious to it all. The tests had come back confirming pneumonia, an IV of antibiotics had been administered, and now we had to just wait.

Patrick spent five nights in hospital and I gotta say I was concerned. The first night when I got home, I ensured all of his family were notified, I felt they needed to know as soon as possible. He hadn't been able to shake this pneumonia, which in itself was a worry but now, with his temperature so high and it having worsened, I knew it was serious.

It's not uncommon to hear of people passing away in the hospital of pneumonia, right? That was ringing in my ear all night and I hardly slept and I was keen to get back to the hospital the next day. It took a good few days to get Patrick's temperature down and when it did I finally started to breathe again.

Six days after checking in, Patrick came home. He was still unwell and was sent home with antibiotics, but with nearly six days of intravenous antibiotics now as well, we were hopeful this time he would get on top of it.

So our week off chemotherapy this month was unfortunately spent in hospital. For me it consisted of daily visits, getting food for him to eat, (no offense but hospital food really needs a shake up) and when others visited I took that opportunity to go home to walk the dog, eat, and sleep. Nothing else got done which at the time didn't matter, the rest of life could go on hold. Nothing was as important as getting Patrick through this but in the same breath, it was exhausting.

Fortunately this time the specialists did decide to delay the next round of the consolidation therapy for a week. They pretty much had to as there was no way Patrick was up for it or would have agreed to do it. He was wiped out! So once out of hospital, he had a further week and a half to recover, and he needed every bit of it.

Patrick was feeling a lot better by the time he started the third cycle, however, by the end of the third month, he really wanted to stop… everything! He was really struggling with the effects of the chemotherapy. He was so over feeling lousy, really over it. I know some people just cannot continue through with the full treatment of chemotherapy because they can't tolerate the side effects anymore and I was concerned he was becoming one of 'those' people.

As I said earlier, Patrick wasn't even sure initially if it was necessary to even have the consolidation therapy. The still unknown factor was whether it was really going to help, or whether it was really needed now, which was difficult for him when he was struggling so much. You can understand where he was coming from. He was seriously questioning whether he should continue, however in the end he decided he could push through another month and give it the 'absolute best shot', as the specialist said. We just had to try and remain present with what is now, what we need to do now, today only, not think of tomorrow, and move forward one day at a time.

We are now coming into the last week of the last month of chemotherapy…

Tough Last Month of Consolidation therapy

"Even a happy life cannot be
without a measure of darkness,
and the word 'happy' would lose
its meaning if it were not
balanced by sadness."
- Carl Jung -

One week to go!

It's Friday morning and Patrick is always at his worst at this stage of treatment. This month chemotherapy treatment has been on Tuesday and Wednesday. By Friday he was almost beside himself with a feeling he often found hard to describe. He said, his whole body felt like a heavy leaden weight with a poisonous feeling running throughout…

Patrick was to come up to Warkworth with me for the weekend; We had a small party to go to on the Saturday night and there was work on the house I needed to do also, so it was to be a weekend for me of work and pleasure.

However, Patrick was feeling pretty rotten. He was also very stressed. He had so much to do as he had been ineffective this week. The chemo fog affects him terribly and it's difficult for him to to apply himself to get things done especially when added to the tiredness that leaves him lacking in energy. Again, the peripheral neuropathy has him going to bed with ice packs strapped to his feet to help the intense heat. Agitation is always high at this point too with the steroids affecting him, and heightened emotion is at its worst at this time. On top of it all this, the strange feelings in his body that he tries so hard to describe, overwhelm him. He had reports to write, invoicing to do… all overdue, and this morning he was quite clearly overwhelmed.

Basically he just felt horrid! Trying to explain it to me, he got very emotional. "It's like my whole body has been taken over with something awful," he cried. "It's so hard to explain how it feels, but it's just so awful." His face was crumpled in such dismay as he went on, "I can feel all these drugs in my body. I took 25 pills in one day alone this week, and, well you added it up, what was it? About 60 pills I take a week and on top of that lot, the Carfilzomib chemotherapy twice a week!" He went on. "And I have this weird sensation of pins and needles throughout my body, I can't think straight, and I just feel terrible. I can't describe it, I just feel terrible!"

Oh bless him. I just stood there, tears welling myself, looking at what looks like a normal person, beside himself with angst, imagining the hell he must be going through.

I don't think I could have done it. Truly I don't. I'm so bad with drugs as it is. I have such utter respect for Patrick that he has gone through with it all. The fact he is in remission and MRD- yet still puts his body and himself through all of this shows his supreme devotion to getting as well as he can. I suppose the end goal of the promise of a longer life is all the incentive you need, although if I was honest, we both know there is no real promise… not for him with this del1p32 lurking in the background.

What could I do as I stood there watching this grown man cry. Do I reach out and hug him, cry with him, or tell him to pull his socks up? I opted for the latter. "Patrick, Friday is always your worst day. Seriously, you forget this. Tomorrow will be a better day. Just take it easy today and hey, only one more week to go!!!" In that moment I felt there was no point dwelling in the sadness of it all, the despair. We have to just keep going to get through this. The road is so short now, we can muster and keep going.

Have I got harsh? Have I got immune to the destruction this cancer has caused? Not at all. I'm heart broken. Distraught. Grief stricken. Lost. Overwhelmed. Exhausted. Yes, terribly exhausted, however it feels the only way to get through this now is to just put one foot in front of the other and keep going. Keep going forward to get to what I imagined would be the light at the end of the tunnel. One that would stay lit this time!

How do I describe how it feels that we are almost there? Over 14 months with 11 of them in treatment. The tears well as I write this now, I can't quite believe it will all be over.

Our lives have changed so drastically. We hardly plan anything these days as I don't know if Patrick will be up to it, or if he is, he's not himself so it's still difficult. I am always exhausted doing more than my usual fair share, and trying to keep up. I am in bed by 8.30pm or 9.00pm as I'm so tired at the end of the day. We're pretty much broke after 14 months of both struggling to work through it all. This last month I decided to go to each appointment at the hospital with him again, to be there for the home stretch. His pneumonia dragged me back into feeling the need to be there all the way, so with two days in hospital a week, time again became my enemy as I am on the mouse wheel constantly trying to get ahead.

Patrick is almost always tired now and huffing and puffing around me. It has become an irritation. Eek, can I say that?

My heart feels permanently broken watching him go through this discomfort and pain, knowing he has an incurable disease, not knowing what our future is together, going through such a tough time. We are both feeling pretty sorry for ourselves right now!

I had thought these last months of treatment would be more of a breeze. Only four months of chemotherapy left, then we're done. We're used to it now, we know the routine. Just four months left to go of what had initially, dauntingly, sounded like forever. So while I hadn't looked forward to it, I had thought it would be easier... but it wasn't. Patrick had felt so good before the start of the consolidation therapy, the best he'd felt in years, and now he's been trashed for four months. It's stupid I know, but it feels so nasty and unfair. I know it's extending his life, and I try to go there often, but wow, at such a cost to him right now.

Today turned into a particularly bad day and Patrick worsened as the day wore on. He even went into hospital to get his bloods checked before we went to Warkworth as he was getting worried about how he felt... but they were all normal; his normal. It's just a really bad day so I had to leave him and go to Warkworth on my own. Patrick was not at all up to the 40 minute car trip and just wanted to be in his own bed. It was rare for me to have time to be at the house while it's free, and the weather was good to paint! So I decided to go on my own. I felt bad leaving him, but I had to accept that I had priorities too.

Driving up to Warkworth today I had been talking to my mum on the phone. I updated her on how Patrick was today and how I was heading to Warkworth on my own now. I didn't want to be as negative as I sounded on the phone so I started to talk about the positives. I spoke of how grateful I was of people who had offered their homes to us for the small breaks we have had through this, that it had been so valuable to be able to get away and rejuvenate, and how we have managed to get through this financially, even if in debt, we have made it.

When I hung up though, the biggest gratitude of all came to me. Patrick had been diagnosed with only six to ten months to live without treatment and now more than a year later we are looking forward to Christmas. Lest We Forget! We have so much to be grateful for which we will take with us into our healing. We've just got to get through this last week. How do I feel it's almost over? Well I just can't believe it.

I had such a productive weekend at Warkworth and had now returned to Patrick's for week three of the last month of consolidation therapy; four months of consolidation therapy almost complete.

It was Tuesday and we woke early to a glorious morning. No wind, sunny, a beautiful spring day in Auckland.

Patrick was now feeling and looking much better than he was on Friday. Finally feeling a bit better, then back into the slaughter house for more treatment! Sorry but that is how it feels right now!

As the months of treatment have passed the weeks felt more drastic to deal with and hence my terminology has strengthened over time. Slaughter house sounds so severe and I'm being melodramatic of course. But it's literally how it feels. Heading into treatment knowing that the joy of life is about to be sucked out of us again. Like a lamb to slaughter. Of course today was different, it was our last week for hopefully a very, very, very long time!

We decided to walk Indi together this morning and go early to enjoy the stillness of the morning. It must have been about 7.30am when we hit the sands of Browns Bay. Indi was ecstatic and was roaring around, swimming, and chasing the tennis ball.

It was so weird. I really wanted to feel joy, exhilaration, fun, laughter with it being our last week of treatment. I kept digging deep in myself to find some elation, or even just a glimmer of lightness, but it just couldn't be accessed. Instead, all that kept rising was the past months of treatment and all we had been through. As we walked and I was feeling into it, significant memories of the last 14 months kept coming to my mind one after the other. As each memory rose, my emotions rose with it, and my body reacted feeling the sadness or the grief, or the loss, fear, or worry. It would start in the pit of my stomach, rising up into my heart, my throat, my mind, and emotions. As each memory came it compounded until it was overwhelming me with sadness, grief, resentment, helplessness all bundled in one.

I decided to surrender to it. I trusted that this was to be the natural and right way for me to move through this, not to fight it, push it aside, cover it up, but allow it. It felt each memory needed to be acknowledged, needed to be felt, needed to be heard and needed to be understood, that wow, this was tough. This has been a hard road.

I realized my whole being was saying to me, you are almost there and you don't need to be brave anymore! You are coming to the end of the road, you don't need to hold yourself together anymore. It was time to surrender to all that has been and allow it to just be what it was. Acknowledge that, so you can move on.

As we neared the end of our walk on the beach I knew that the memories still weren't over. I seemed to be going through all the shock, the grief, the worry, the stress, the strain of events from the moment the warning signs went out that Patrick was sick, to now. This was clearly going to take some time. I knew I had to stay open and I could feel I needed to keep giving the layers upon layers of memories permission to be seen, and allow their effects to be felt, and in doing so, allow them to release. It was impossible for this to happen all at once as it would have been too much, too overwhelming. What was happening, although difficult, was healthy. I knew this through my training. I was purging… and it would take some time to do this in a healthy, safe way. A deep sense of me knew this was also an honoring. As hard as it was, it was like an honoring to all we had been through.

It feels like we've been in treatment forever. Some friends and family comment that in some ways it's flown by… but not for us. So much has happened in these last 14 months. We could never have imagined our lives just over a year ago, going through this and doing what we have done.

Chemotherapy that day was nothing unusual. We left knowing just one more day to go, and Patrick and I started planning a nice wee 'something' for the staff as a thank you for the next day, our last day.

The loveliest thing happened that night. I woke with a quite typical 4.00am wake up. As I lay there willing myself back to sleep I noticed how I was feeling. I was so relaxed and calm. Often at this time of night there will be some anxiety, or something to worry about, some dread I would feel so I was pleasantly surprised to feel nothing. I went back to sleep after a bit and slept until 9.30am!! Unheard of. I woke with a start realising we had to leave in an hour to the hospital. We needed to pick up cupcakes on the way for the staff so I quickly got dressed.

Patrick hadn't slept with me last night. He was too restless from the chemotherapy and constantly up and down to the toilet so he'd decided to sleep in the spare room which was unusual for him. Now that it's almost over I suppose he thought he might as well since it won't be for too much longer.

By the time we were leaving the house we were rushed and quickly jumped in the car. I was driving. Hands on the wheel, we headed up our steep drive and I'll never forget the feeling. It was like we were driving up into the sky, about to leave behind this difficult time and I realised then the lightness in my body. Wow. It was gone. The anxiety. Without even realizing it, I had been carrying around with me, right at the core of my being, anxiety, through all we were going through. I could feel now how it had been there every day through every moment and now, on our last day of chemotherapy it had lifted just like that. Until this moment I had no idea how much I had been holding on and how much I had been affected with worry and strain. With the end here, I am finally free.

We picked up the cupcakes and arrived at the hospital. As we walked through the corridors to the ward for Patrick's last day of chemotherapy, we were both silent. The memories of the past year were still rising and falling, and I remembered when we first walked these corridors to our first specialist appointment, unsure of what the future was to hold. Then, when we first walked these corridors to our first chemotherapy treatment. How naive, scared and worried we were. How overwhelmed we were, and how long the road seemed ahead… but how full of intention we were that the treatments would work for Patrick, and that he was going to be OK!

We delivered our cupcakes, greeting the nurses in the haematology day stay for the last time, for hopefully a very very long time.

As I sat down next to Patrick another memory came flashing up of our first week on chemotherapy. I remembered it was the second day and we were next to a lady who was also receiving treatment, she commented on my shoes. Jude was a dashing lady herself, with a fantastically wrapped scarf disguising her bald head. Jude and her husband John became two of our 'chemo friends' ever since that day, but what she went on to say has stuck with me all through Patrick's treatments. She threw her head over towards the staff and said to me "They're fantastic you know. All the nurses here, everywhere actually. Auckland hospital too. They are all really lovely. You're in good hands." It was reassuring to hear at the time, but as I sat down some 14 months later I reflected on how right she was, I could hear Jude's exact words in my ear as if no time had gone by, loud and clear. She was so totally right through and through.

Everywhere we went we had received respect, dignity, care and consideration, on top of totally professional service. It was flawless. And truly, it made all the difference. Undergoing treatment in a bid to save your life, treatments that make you ill and exhausted leaves you feeling vulnerable. Really vulnerable! To have nurses greet you with a smile, remember your name, listen to your woes and share in each other's lives actually gave us something to look forward to at these appointments… And we never had to worry, we always knew we were getting the very best of care. It was flawless every time no matter which nurse was on duty that day… totally flawless. I have such admiration and respect for the nurses helping in this constant manner every day. In my opinion, it cannot be discarded how important this is to the healing process of the patients.

The ward was relatively quiet today. We had some lovely chats with the nurses as they worked around Patrick. I was on my phone a lot sending a picture of Patrick with the cup cakes to all those friends and families who had sent supportive messages over the last year, letting them know it's our last day.

Before we knew it, it was over. Patrick was already looking a bit rough and his face was swollen with all the drugs in his system. His cheeks swell up and go red. His curly, smokey grey hair was getting long, and he looked so different to the man he was before he started chemotherapy, but he's survived!

How is that? One minute life is ticking along, and then wammo! It turns completely upside down and inside out. You have no say, no control. All you can do is go along for the ride… which we did. And we did it well, considering!! Full remission, MRD-, last chemotherapy treatment over, and we said our farewells. We're not stupid. We know we'll be back one day… but again, hopefully not for a very very long time!

As we left the ward and started down the corridors we high fived for the last time. Nailed it!!

Even as I write this now, Wednesday evening, and there are no more treatments ahead, but I am still overwhelmed. Tears are forming as I still naturally go to reflection on the past 14 months. It's been tough. Really tough. Self indulging actually feels pretty bloody good right now to sit back and honour this.

Celebration, excitement, well it's just not here. It will come, but right now Patrick doesn't feel great. We went into town for a celebration lunch after the treatment today and had a lovely lunch on the waterfront with celebratory virgin cocktails. We could have invited people but it just wasn't right, it needed to be just us. We started this together, we went through this together, we finished it together. In our toast Patrick was quite emotional thanking me for going on this ride with him. It was a touching moment.

Through lunch we started talking about Europe. When we would like to go next year, what we would do; happy thoughts and seeds getting planted for moving on.

In the car on the way home he was falling asleep on and off. As we neared home he woke. "You know," he said. "I just want to take this moment to thank the chemotherapy for all it has done for me." I said "Oh gosh yes, thank you chemotherapy. You have saved Patrick's life!" Lately we had been so mean to the chemotherapy. Bloody chemo upsetting our lives and Patrick's body so much. What were we thinking? We had forgotten to be thankful.

Another emotional moment not to be forgotten as we paused together to do just that, give thanks to the drugs that had saved the life of this great man. Tears were in both of our eyes as I reached out to Patrick and held his hand as we drove home.

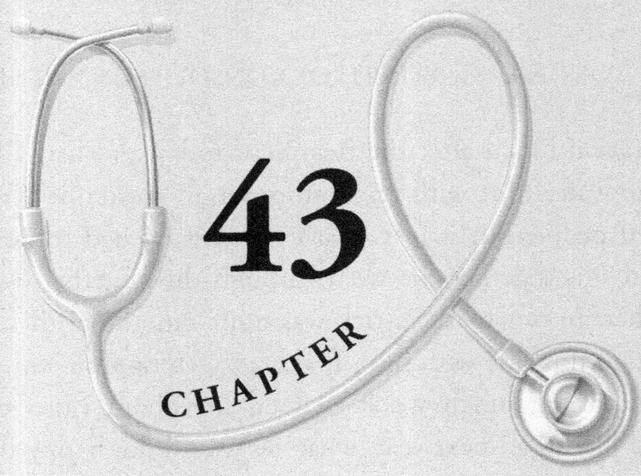

Financially Coping with Cancer

"Life is like a bicycle,
to keep your balance you must
keep on moving."
- Albert Einstein -

The day after Patrick's final chemotherapy session I woke feeling laden with heightened emotion, and this remained for the rest of the week.

When I spoke to friends I would cry. I didn't know how I was going to cope with work. I should have taken this week off, but I'd not had any idea that the completion of Patrick's treatments was going to put me here.

Yes, put me here. It felt like I had been dumped. Dumped in a pit of past trauma and I couldn't get out. The memories and emotions of the past 14 months now, instead of lessening, were becoming stronger and more frequent. While I still felt that I needed to go through this, to allow it, it was really tough… and annoying. I wanted to be elated, joyous, laughing, but the flashbacks kept coming, the emotions too, of the past year all surfacing in my mind and my body reacting. What should have been some of my happiest days became some of my worst.

Somehow knowing the future for us held no more chemotherapy, no more regular hospital visits, no more Patrick feeling sick or exhausted, seemed to create the space for an uprising of all we had been through. I know more than anyone that to be free and let go we need to really allow ourselves these feelings.

So I continued to allow it all. With each memory I allowed the pain, the suffering, the trauma, the fear, the sadness, the loss, whatever was here, all to rise, as they did, overtaking my body with such heightened emotion. The waves came and fell away, one thought, one feeling, one memory, one emotion at a time.

I used a simple process that seemed to be working. As each wave came I opened into it, literally dived into it, and although I noticed the story around it, I opened into the feelings as I dived through. And welcomed them. Embraced them. Told them I was sorry, surrounded them in my love and care. Let them know it's over now. That it's going to be OK. That they can let go, it's safe to let go. It's over and a new beginning can start to come through now. The feeling that always then arose was a feeling of calm and a space for freedom… immediately. As the wave subsided and the heightened emotion was washed away, a period of calm rested, and freedom was here.

It wasn't easy in one way but in another it was powerful. It was an acknowledgment of how serious, tough and traumatic this past 14 months was, and an honouring of what we have been through together.

We had been so busy just getting the job done there had been little time for true self indulgence of emotions of what it was like getting through these past 14 months. Sure it was there at diagnosis, we were very open and raw to how we felt, but once we got on with treatment… well perhaps only on the surface level. The times I'd bitch and moan writing in my diary that it was too exhausting, there was not enough time and I was overwhelmed with the 'to do list', feeling sorry for Patrick etc. It was all things that were captured in the present of what we were experiencing whereas now it was like I'd stepped well back and I was looking over the whole experience, what we'd endured and what it had cost us at a much deeper level.

There were no celebration drinks with anyone that it was over. No parties or toasts. Just between the two of us, the knowing, 'we nailed it' was enough and all we were up for. A week later the memories were still coming. Their intensity had lessened now though and were slowly starting to come less often. Interestingly, the anxiety I had noticed had definitely completely left me. I was sleeping through the night now to a reasonable time in the morning. That part was over!

I'd had to refinance my house. The 14 months of supporting Patrick through his treatments had financially taken its toll on me also. My credit cards were at their limit and I could see no way of recovering without refinancing my home in Warkworth. Thankfully I was able to. The money had just come through in the last week of chemotherapy and my debts were all paid. What a relief. Hmm maybe that helped the anxiety and early morning wake ups also.

I had asked for a little extra from the bank so I could landscape the front garden. It had never been landscaped and it had been put off this last 14 months with Patrick in treatment, but now it really needed doing. We had decided that we would bite the bullet and do the landscaping in a week's time. Patrick felt if I could just give him the next week to recover he would 'hopefully' feel up to some planting.

The weather was forecast to be perfect over the next week. The window was there and we needed to open it! I knew there was no way for Patrick to do it all on his own, and I certainly couldn't do it on my own. I broke it down into stages and when we looked at it we decided that together we could handle it and would go for it!

So I spent the week after chemotherapy driving around all the garden centres in Auckland buying and delivering to the house all the plants we needed. I would have the garden centre load them into my car filling every space possible, from the front passenger seat to the small hatchback boot filled to the brim, then I'd drive each load to Warkworth unloading them myself as Patrick didn't have it in him to help at this point, he was still weak and prone to exhaustion.

A week later, my courtyard was filled with potted plants and looked like a garden centre itself. There was no stopping now, it had to be done. At the beginning of the second week after Patricks final chemotherapy session, we were now ready to plant.

A kind friend of mine managed to find a couple of guys I could hire to help dig the holes on the Monday, and Patrick's daughter Katelyn was coming to help too. There was no way he could have done that on his own and with chronic fatigue I would have been mad to have taken on any digging myself.

Patrick, who had been feeling better and better each day, now arrived at the house feeling ready to get into it. By the time everyone arrived on Monday to dig the holes, we had measured and marked with paint the exact placements. 125 trees and plants to be dug and planted this week!

After everyone arrived I left to head south to Clevedon, which was miles away, to get the last load of boundary trees. Returning approximately three hours later, I was delighted at the number of holes that'd been dug already even though it had been raining on and off. The truck with the garden mix had arrived and there was Patrick on the back of the truck, soaking wet, in the pouring rain shovelling, at a rate of knots, the garden mix off the truck. He looked like a machine! Wow I was so surprised and he said later himself that he didn't know he had it in him.

All the holes were dug that day and even some plants planted; it was much more than I'd expected we'd achieve. The boys were only booked for one day but I felt we could now manage, especially after seeing this new found energy in Patrick. Stage two done.

The next morning he was exhausted, for sure. He was really had it actually. We hadn't scheduled to do the garden today, thankfully, knowing he would need a break. As the morning went on Patrick managed to pick himself up going to an appointment with his new client, and an appointment with the specialist. I went to work and we gave our bodies a modicum of physical rest, ready for the next stage.

So for timeline, it's now nine days after Patrick's last chemotherapy session and he is about to have his post chemotherapy specialist appointment. Unfortunately he had forgotten it was booked until he was reminded the day before (chemo fog still present!), and I had a client booked so I couldn't attend. Patrick told me not to worry, he considered it just a routine checkup and that I wouldn't be missing anything. The big appointment was in a couple of weeks with the head specialist of the Kiwi Trial program Dr David Simpson, and I ensured I had that in my diary,

When I came out of my session that day there was a missed call from Patrick. I rang him and was somewhat surprised at the heightened tone in his voice after I asked how the appointment was. "I have got such good news to tell you!" he burst out. "It's really good news darling. Such good news, but I haven't got time to tell you right now." "What!? Wait, what!?" I retorted. "You can't do that to me! You can't leave me hanging! What is it??"

Patrick carried on in a high I hadn't heard in his voice for a very long time "I can't," he said "I just can't tell you now, I've got this meeting in a few minutes, and I don't want to over the phone. I want to tell you in person, it's too huge! Let's wait till we're home tonight!"

Every word he said was punctuated and accentuated. He was getting me excited though I didn't know what about. I respected his opinion and let go. "OK! OK!" I said, "we'll wait until tonight", actually enjoying the anticipation of this news. Now that's a nice feeling for a change, enjoying anticipation of good news to come. A future of tonight bringing something great… something really positive by the sounds of it, something to look forward to. I realised it's been a while since I've had that feeling.

I thought about this as the day went on, wondering what the news could be. I felt I was cheating a little, trying to guess before Patrick had the chance to tell me. Curiosity is one of my best friends and I couldn't help myself.

I rang him later in the day to see how his next appointment had gone. He was working on obtaining a new client which he hoped would bring a lot of business. Already Patrick was feeling well enough to start thinking about progressing his business again.

There is something that is so worth mentioning right here, as it is such an important part of being diagnosed with cancer.

In New Zealand we have two main types of Government support for illness. One is called ACC - Accident Compensation. The other is called the sickness benefit.

Accident Compensation is for when you have an injury or illness due to an accident. They pay 80% of your most recently completed financial years taxable income and it's a payment most people can pretty much get by on.

The sickness benefit is for those who are sick or injured, but not by accident, so it's not covered under ACC. It provides a set amount of money that is slightly dependent on your circumstances. For example you receive a little more if you are deserving of an accommodation allowance or have dependents. However there is always a lot of canvassing in New Zealand around poverty for those who are on any type of benefit as the payments are not enough to cover basic needs in normal circumstances. If you earn the average income and fall ill, unable to earn, the Government subsidy is not usually enough to cover even just your rent or mortgage. How awful is that on top of fighting to stay alive. On top of the emotional trauma you are going through. On top of how ill you feel, to have that worry.

So here is a big hole in the system. I recently heard this on a popular talkback station in Auckland. People calling in, telling of how they and their families even ended up sleeping in cars on the street when they became ill as they couldn't afford to keep their rental homes as the sickness benefit was not enough to cover food, living expenses and a roof over their head. Heart breaking stuff!

Patrick's monthly living costs were high. Even when you just consider the basics, such as food, rent, power, phone, petrol and insurances. His expenses reflected his lifestyle pre-cancer which of course reflected his pre-cancer income. If Patrick had to live on a benefit he would have had to move house in the middle of his treatments into a one bedroom flat. He would have had to get rid of the furniture etc in his two lounge, four bedroom home as he wouldn't have been able to afford storage. He would have had to scrimp on food and caught buses to the hospital as he wouldn't have been able to afford the car or insurance and would have had a meagre existence while going through cancer treatment.

There needs to be a better benefit type in place for these circumstances. I seriously don't know how people cope financially, how they get by when faced with these chronic illnesses.

I can only say here, if you can afford it, get trauma insurance! I've just signed up myself. Whatever you can afford, do it. If you are diagnosed seriously ill or injured, you get a lump sum payout to get you through. It really hit home for us how incredibly helpful that would have been. What a weight it would have lifted off of our shoulders.

If someone you care about gets cancer and needs treatment, I urge you to pass the hat around if you think they're going to need it. It's the kindest most helpful thing friends and family can do. If you are reading this and have recently been diagnosed or going through these financial difficulties, consider asking friends and family for financial support. Maybe ask a friend to create a Give A Little page for you. If everyone just gave a little it can add up to a whole lot to get you through. Just saying. Don't be too proud to ask for help. This is a common problem, you are not alone, and you shouldn't feel shame you have been put in this financial position.

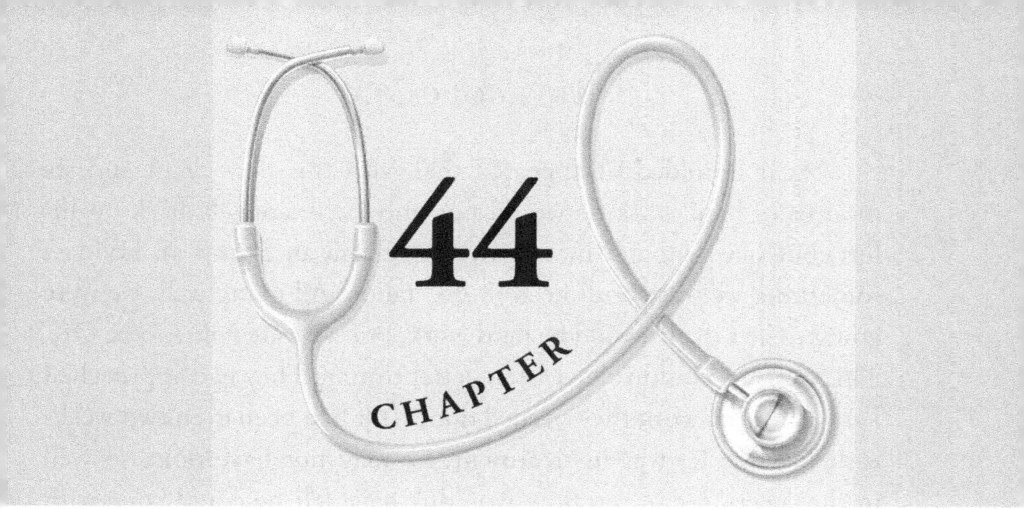

Stringent Complete Response - No Deletion!

"However difficult life may seem,
there is always something you can do
and succeed at"
- Stephen Hawking -

Now back to the good news story Patrick was coming home with. We both got home at about the same time and put together a quick dinner. Patrick was on a definite high. The appointment with his potential client had gone well and he had secured their business. We mainly talked in fits and starts about that while preparing and eating dinner. Purposely neither of us spoke about the 'other' good news, we unspokenly knew it needed no distractions like being busy in the kitchen. Complete attention was required.

When we finally sat down after dinner to really talk, Patrick started by launching more into the detail about his new client. Saving the best until last I suppose... like dessert!

As it unfolded, it appeared that with this new client and six months of hard work he would not only be financially back on his feet, but have enough money to venture on an European holiday; something we were both keen to do. Yahoo! All going well, we were going to be OK. It would be hard work, but we were going to be OK. This contract couldn't have been better timing. They had approached Patrick for the work they needed done. If it had been even two weeks earlier, while he was in treatment, he may not have done so well in the meeting. He certainly wouldn't have felt he could cope with the job either so we felt very blessed and grateful that the stars had aligned!

The stillness was finally here. There was nothing left to talk about but Patrick's 'exciting news' from his specialist appointment. Sitting together on the couch I insisted he start at the beginning of the appointment as I didn't want to miss a thing. Initially he spoke of all the standard procedures so I hurried him along. I couldn't wait any longer. He said first of all "Actually I've got a video. Maybe it's better I play that first as it explains everything."

My mind went all confused at this. What on earth is he on about? I just wanted to hear what the specialist said, not watch some video so "No!" I quickly replied. "Just tell me what she said from the beginning about all this. What is it Patrick?!"

"OK, OK" he finally went on. "Anna (who was the specialist he saw today) has given me some information today that has blown me away. Literally blown me out of the park. It was so huge I was emotional in the meeting. Me. Emotional in a meeting!" he laughed.

Patrick was dragging this news out in true Patrick style, but I stayed silent watching his every move. His face, his eyes, his body movement, for signs of what was to come. All I could see and tell and sense was that it meant an awful lot to him and I wanted to respect that and give him the space he needed to share it.

He continued. "So we already know that I am MRD- and we know I am in full remission. So we know out of about a million cells no cancer was detected right?" He looked at me to check I was clear on this. Wanting an answer. "Right." I responded, nodding my head. Obviously this was going to be important to what he had to say.

"Well what I didn't know is that the deleted gene I have, this del 1p32, is only present in the multiple myeloma cancer cells." Right here Patrick already started getting emotional. His voice started to crack as he continued. **"So this means if there are no cancer cells detected, there are no cells with the chromosome deletion."** He stopped for a moment then continued "So do you get what this means? **At this moment there is no 1p32 deletion present in my body** as it cannot exist in healthy cells and I only have healthy cells now out of the one million detected."

My mind tried to grapple with this news. What this means, it's significance and consequence. Why didn't we already know this?

It hit me how confused I was. Here we had been sitting up night after night after night when we first discovered Patrick had this deletion, googling and googling what this chromosome deletion was. Talking to every specialist under the sun about how to get the best help and treatment for it, thinking we knew it all. But we didn't know this. How is that? What is this? Gosh it has all been so complicated!

Patrick went on, as it was the obvious question in the room without me even voicing it. "I found it hard to believe because my original understanding from the FISH test right at the start of being diagnosed, that identified the gene, showed 171 cells out of the 200 tested had the deleted gene. When we asked the specialist about this he said you cannot do anything about getting the deleted genes back or repaired. So in my mind, I had only an average of 29 cells out of every 200 that had the gene intact".

I had been in the appointment with Patrick at the time of this discussion and I had heard him many times over the following months explaining his perception of this news. He had 29 cells intact without the chromosome deletion, out of 200 sampled. This was one of the reasons he felt he could be a good candidate for the Car-T trial when it came to NZ because he had this estimated 29 cells intact, per 200 cells, that they could use… so this had been his logic passed on to me. Having the detrimental chromosome deletion of 1p32 apparently put Patrick as a good candidate to benefit from Car-T therapy.

Patrick continued. I wasn't saying a word, just listening. "This is why I wanted to repeat the FISH test along with the bone marrow test that I'm doing next week, to find out whether more cells had now been affected with the chromosome deletion. For future reference, for possible Car-T treatment."

I just nodded that I understood. I knew this too as I'd been at the last specialist appointment, with the same specialist he saw today, the lovely Dr Anna Elinder Camburn, when he requested the FISH test for this very reason. It all made sense at the time, and she had agreed to ask the Kiwi Trial specialist Dr David Simpson, to request the FISH test for us.

This was important to Patrick as he wanted to be sure that his cells weren't all affected with the deletion, so he would become a candidate for Car-T when it became approved for treatment and financially more available… or even better, if it became a funded treatment in New Zealand… though we weren't holding our breath on that one.

Patrick continued, "Anna, however, has come back today saying actually that I do not presently even have a chromosome deletion because the chromosome deletion is only in the cancer cells! When there are no cancer cells present, there is no chromosome deletion! **Meaning in essence I am free of cancer and free of the chromosome deletion right here and now. FREE OF IT ALL!"**

By now Patrick had broken into tears as he spoke. Another moment I will never forget. My mind however, was still grappling to get a grip on what this meant. It was confusing and all I could say was, "but I thought that once you have this deletion, you have it. There is nothing you can do about it."

We both sat there, and I could see he was grappling with this himself. He went on "Yes you do, but it is such a huge relief to know that for now all my cells are intact and are normal and healthy. My cells do not have this deletion. Possibly 100% of them as currently all my cells are cancer free and the deletion is only in cancerous cells. The deletion is not only absent now, but I have a plentiful supply of healthy cells for Car-T if that opportunity ever arises!"

He paused to allow us both to absorb this, then he went on. "When we take the bone marrow test next week there is no point doing the FISH test. It tests 200 cells. When we did this test initially it showed I had 80-90% blood plasma saturation of cancer cells so there was plenty to test for the deletion, as it exists in the cancerous cells. While I have no cancer cells, there won't be any point doing a FISH test basically because there is nothing to sample. Do you get it?" he asked. Patrick was very keen to know I got the significance of what he was saying. No cancer cells, no chromosome deletion.

Here watch this video. He proceeded to pull out his phone. "I knew you would be upset you had missed this appointment," he said laughingly now, "so I asked Anna if I could record her giving you the good news! Straight from the horse's mouth" and he proceeded to play the video. There she was, the specialist sitting in the same room as the first day we went in to see Dr Ross Henderson and had received the news Patrick had multiple myeloma. The day we received that shocking news, some 14 months earlier.

Anna was sitting in the same chair, large as life, addressing me personally on video. "Hello Kushla," she said with a beaming smile. Just right here… how beautiful is this? This top Auckland specialist being so humane as to take the time in such a busy, full on schedule, to entertain making Patrick's video to share this good news with me. She went on to explain all that Patrick had said in such a warm happy manner showing her own delight at the news, and even through the video I could feel how truly thrilled she was for us. At the end Patrick and I hugged and cried. Quiet tears.

There is no cancer. No deletion. At present his body was free.

Patrick then broke away and continued, "BUT THERE IS MORE." He rushed on, "Anna said the latest results show her that I am not only in full remission, I have achieved what is called **Stringent Complete Response, which is even better, in fact the best there is!"**

Oh my God. I really didn't, right there, fully understand the implications of that, but it sounded fantastic! Really fantastic. The best of the best news. I knew I'd be googling this later but could now just go with Patrick's exultation.

The word stringent I knew was about to take on a whole new meaning to me, more than what it had before now. However unlike when he was diagnosed and we were facing so many words we had never heard of before, and spending sleepless nights, in fact weeks awake googling to get some sense, with such a heavy foreboding feeling learning about his diagnosis, our time had finally come to be googling with excitement and joy of the incredible outcome from it all.

What a day!

We poured a bottle of non-alcoholic bubbly into wine glasses and raised them "You did it Patrick," I toasted. "you bloody did it!"

We were thrilled of course, it was everything we had aimed for since the first day of chemotherapy. We talked about celebrating with friends but neither of us had it in us. We were too exhausted to want to plan it or entertain it. I don't want to sound too negative here but we had found it such a huge road to get to the end that we still felt bruised by it all. In a way I wish we had found out months after we had recovered from it all so we would have felt like celebrating!

I was so proud of Patrick though. What a man. He had gone through so much without complaint and achieved amazing results. The goal had been put out there and he just headed straight for it. That was all he was living for and all that mattered. Although that had been hard on me, I certainly am thankful he did. I've complained to you, dear reader, along the way. I know I've bitched and moaned but I wouldn't have had it any other way for Patrick.

Patrick in fact taught me a lot. We really do have to take care of ourselves, do whatever we need to do to be OK. No one else is going to do that for you. It's a great lesson for life in general. Looking back and seeing how Patrick did this and the end result is quite enlightening. Looking back and seeing how I didn't for myself has been enlightening too!

The following day we went back to Warkworth and planted the rest of the plants. Patrick actually managed relatively easily… 125 trees now planted! Stage three done! We went back to Patrick's that night to be on the North Shore for his bone marrow test the next morning.

The next day, Thursday, the bark was delivered. I took Patrick up late that afternoon for us to 'bark' the garden the next day. He had just of course had his bone marrow test done this morning, so he was feeling quite sore and delicate. The test was standard as part of the Kiwi Trial program, to assess him after the full treatment plan. This time the bone marrow test went beautifully. Just one attempt, one hole, and quickly in and out of hospital for it!

We pulled up at the house to see wow, two huge mounds of bark on the front lawn. I was all of a sudden filled with great trepidation on how on earth we were going to do this by tomorrow, when Airbnb guests were arriving at 3.00pm. Patrick was sore from his bone marrow test and I had little energy… but it had to be done!

Patrick, in his true style, woke up the next morning without a complaint and got himself ready to get stuck in, which is exactly what we had to do. Patrick's other daughter Jasmine arrived early and helped for a few hours. I had no choice but to have to get into it also, or it would never have got done. Shoveling, tipping, spreading.

We were tearing through it working so hard with hardly a break. Murphy's Law saw the guests show up an hour early, and we had to send them away for a cup of coffee. We were still in chaos. We stepped it up another notch and managed to completely finish it, bar moving the rocks which we saved for another day… fifteen minutes before 3.00pm. The sweat was pouring off us. We were completely shattered, our bodies aching and my back felt like it could break in a dozen places, but we did it. Stage four done!

Wow. We were both so surprised that we had managed it; so pleasantly surprised that we both had it in us.

"Not bad." said Patrick, as we sat in the car about to leave, looking at our great achievement from the car window. "Just the rocks left to move, otherwise done." I patted his back and said "Not bad for someone who is only two weeks out of chemo. Amazing Patrick. Amazing." We had a brief moment between us where we both knew he was truly on the mend and hope formed of possibly a bright future ahead for him.

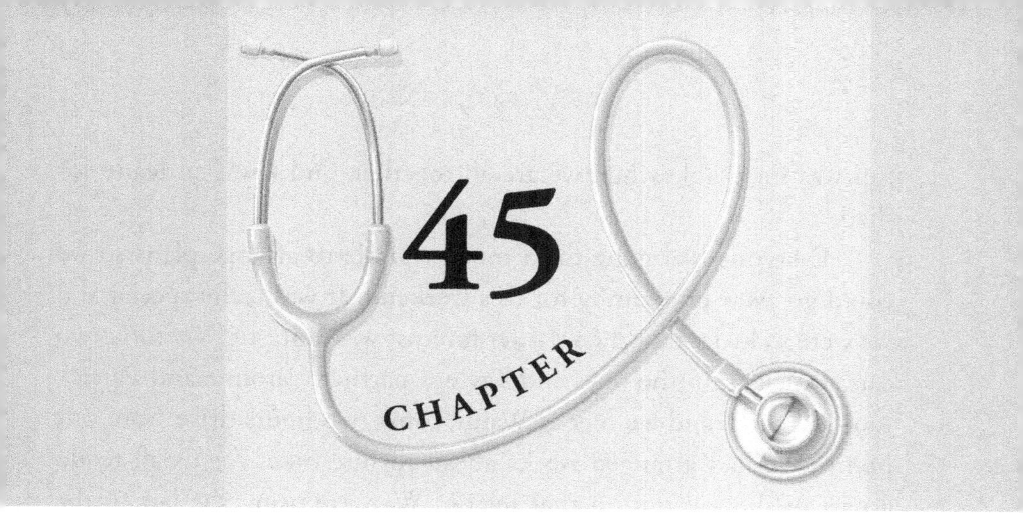

113 Hospital Visits in 14 Months

""It always seems impossible
until it's done."
- Nelson Mandela -

Saturday morning I woke with such delight. We were both still very exhausted from gardening but raring to go on an adventure weekend with our babies. Following on from when we had all gone away when Patrick was first diagnosed, we had now decided to make this a yearly family event!

Last year it was to bring us together to commiserate and support each other through the devastating news, now, three weeks after Patrick's very last chemotherapy session, this trip was to be a joyous one. We were coming together and celebrating not only the end of treatment, but also celebrating, unbeknown to the kids yet, such an incredibly successful outcome. I was so looking forward to it. Having fun was inevitable when we are all together, and I was so ready for that!

Everyone had gone to so much trouble to arrange plans so we could go away as a family for this weekend. It was really special and we were so lucky that the weather forecast was fantastic. We took two cars; I picked up the boys and Taylor's partner Caroline and Patrick took the girls, and we met at Waihi, some two hours drive from our home. We had arranged weeks ahead to hire bikes for us all to do a part of the rail trail in that region. We were using the last of the money Patrick's brother had given us at the beginning of his diagnosis - the money we had put aside for holidays. It was a perfect finale for it!

What a stunning ride it was between Waihi and Paeroa, it took us all along the gorge and river. The scenery was so kiwiana with native trees and birds, the fresh clear stream bubbling along with us as we took to the trail. Everyone went at their own pace and we all caught up with each other somewhere along the way for chats as we rode side by side.

Patrick was in great form, both of us were. The ride was pretty easy which was a huge bonus, but getting out of Auckland on an adventure was the best part of it all. We came across a tunnel that went for what seemed miles as we biked through. People riding or walking in the opposite direction would appear before us suddenly out of the darkness. The area was an old gold mining town in the 1800s where old relics had been left behind and old ruins were seen along the way.

It was such a stunning picturesque trip that had us come into the small town of Paeroa, the town where the Lemon and Paeroa soft drink was created. We were to stop for lunch and then continue to Te Aroha where we were to stay the night.

Patrick and I were both pretty tired by the time we got to Paeroa. The trail was only 16km so far but the week had caught up with us so we decided to finish biking here. Apparently, when Patrick phoned the bike people to collect the bikes, they said we had biked the best part of the trip so we didn't feel we were missing much. The kids were pleased too as the cafe we'd been recommended to go to was really funky, and had great food and drinks so they were happy to settle in!

We had a really lovely late lunch at The Refinery, taking our time, enjoying the rest, refreshment and quality time together. We then wandered around the town looking through its quirky second hand stores. I found a gong I had been searching for online, would you believe it… in little old Paeroa.

Once we had been picked up by the rental bike company and collected the cars we then drove to Te Aroha where we had a relaxing hot soak in the mineral spas which I'd pre-booked. We then checked into our Airbnb accommodation and went for dinner in the local town of Te Aroha.

It was here that Patrick gave the children the great news. He had held off telling them, looking for the right time… just as he had done when he gave them the shocking diagnosis some 14 months earlier. He made it a speech and he was sometimes emotional, especially when he got to the part about the deletion no longer being present. This still was sitting with him deeply as a gift he couldn't quite still believe. He told them of his results. Not just a 'full remission', but what we recently found out from his last specialist appointment with Dr Anna Elinder Camburn - Stringent Complete Response. The children were so quiet listening, taking it all in. The girls had tears and all the children congratulated Patrick.

Generally though the news just sat there. I felt a stiffness in the air of unasked questions. I felt that everyone was too afraid to voice them, or perhaps didn't want to crash down on the good news. I wished I could have piped up and answered them all, alleviating their concerns, fears and worries. But I couldn't because I didn't know the answers. "What does this mean really? Are you cured? When will it come back? Does this good result mean it won't come back for a long time? Does this mean the deletion is gone for good? How long will you live for now then?…."

I didn't know the answers. Patrick didn't know the answers. In fact no one knows the answers although I must say I was hoping, after we saw the specialist in two weeks time, we may get some more clarity as to what 'stringent complete response' means considering Patrick's initial diagnosis of the chromosome deletion.

I'd by now had time to google 'stringent complete response' (the correct terminology). These are some of the explanations:

'Patients able to receive stringent complete response after undergoing autologous stem-cell transplantation (ASCT) for multiple myeloma, achieved improved long-term outcomes, including overall survival and time to progression, compared with patients who achieved lesser levels of response.'

'Patients achieving stringent response had a 5-year overall survival rate of 80% compared with 53% for complete response and 47% for near complete response.'

'Results showed that achieving a stringent complete response was an independent prognostic factor for survival.'

Sounds pretty positive huh, and shows just how important these different categories are, so we're running with that for now. Although we both know the big question is still, what about the deletion? Will it resurface and bring the cancer back quicker even with such a good response?

I finally decided to speak of the elephant in the room and said as much as I could; it was weird not to. "We don't really know what this means," I said, "except that this result is the best possible result we could have hoped for, and that's a fantastic thing. The best result now is the best opportunity, so well done Patrick. After all you've been through such a great outcome deserves a toast." We all raised our glasses and toasted this incredible man. I then had a moment to say my own thing.

I had the week before added up all the visits to the hospital Patrick had made over the past 14 months. Wow I had got such a fright; I worked out it was 113, which took me by complete surprise! No wonder it was such a rough year.

Approximately 113 Hospital Visits:

12 specialist appointments at North Shore hospital over 14 months

- diagnoses
- treatment plan
- monthly checkups

4 specialist appointments at Auckland hospital

- stem cell transplant review
- stem cell transplant confirmation
- stem cell transplant post appointments

30 Monthly induction chemotherapy treatments

1 Port put in for consolidation therapy

5 Stem cell collection

- pre-stem cell collection checkups
- Intense chemotherapy
- Stem cell production check, port put in for stem cell collection
- Stem cell collection
- Port removed

19 days Stem cell

- Introduction morning on stem cell transplant, see ward etc
- Hospital day of tests and new port put in
- Stem cell transplant two weeks
- Two follow up trips to hospital after stem cell transplant for blood tests
- Port removed

4 Bone marrow tests throughout the 14 months

24 Consolidation chemotherapy treatments.

Pneumonia

- 2 days including 1 night overstay
- 4 days including 3 nights overstay
- 6 days including 5 nights overstay

2 Post Treatment

- MRI
- Port removed

Approximately 113 days of hospital visits in 14 months of which only 12 I had not been to with Patrick. Some were just specialist appointments, some half days having tests or short admissions for ports etc, chemotherapy days were pretty much a half day, and others were full days and nights in hospital. Sitting with him through each visit through thick and thin, when you add it all up you can appreciate how that volume of appointments impacts your life.

Anyhow that exercise was useful. It really helped me to have the full picture on why I have been so pressured this year. Not only had I been through so much helping Patrick through feeling ill, taking care of the family, houses, and working when I could, but wow, also 101 days of hospital visits!

With this load I was always trying to catch up, I was stressed actually. No wonder I'd felt such trauma at the end of Patrick's treatments, that seemed to have been trapped, needing release. It had been a really tough time in more ways than one so I decided I would let the kids know the sheer volume of hospital visits. I felt it was important for them to have an opportunity to acknowledge what Patrick had done, what he had been through to achieve this amazing result, just in the time commitment alone, let alone acknowledging how much treatment he actually went through. If I hadn't realised how often it was, they obviously wouldn't have either…

When I told the kids they were all surprised, except Katelyn who I had already cited it to earlier. Chase spoke up stating "Wow, good on you Patrick." The others chimed in, and we toasted again to Patrick for his commitment and resolve to get through his treatments.

We had such a gorgeous rest of the weekend. We had no other discussion on Patrick or cancer. We all knew this was a weekend of celebration and for a good time, so we went for it.

The next day, Sunday, again brought great weather and the day to do the beautiful waterfall walk at Wairere Falls. I was elated to be taking the kids and feel their enjoyment of one of NZ's great bush walks and highest waterfalls.

Patrick felt tired today after the bike ride, and decided not to do the walk. It was time for him to take a break. When we'd woken this morning, he had told me about this decision but went on to say "You know I'm so impressed with myself. I can't believe I have done so much this week and coped. The week before I never would have imagined I could have done all that I have. I'm really getting better already darling. I'm coming through this!"

He spoke with pride, a bewilderment, hope and lightness, that just filled me with joy. The consolidation therapy had been so difficult for him to get through. MRD-, full remission, and still back for more. 14 months of coping with the constant hospital visits, and him being unwell. But now we have really pulled through with a stringent complete response to top it all off! How dare I have complained! Ever!

It was mid afternoon before we arrived back in Paeroa for lunch. We'd had such a fantastic walk, so picturesque and adventurous. The kids even had a swim in the freezing cold waters when they found water holes. It was all a lot of fun.

By now the cafe's were all closed so it was a stop at McDonalds takeaways and leftover cheese and bread for a picnic at a local park, then it was time to head home. Patrick and I were going in separate cars; he was taking the girls and I was taking the boys and Caroline.

Before heading off, we stopped for a hug and kiss and it was then that it hit me. Oh my gosh, I could smell him… Patrick. His smell was back, and, as I kissed his neck with delight I could feel under my lips the touch of his skin. His skin! I don't know how to describe this, but Patrick was back. I knew at that moment that the chemotherapy had left his body. The steroids too. He was free of the drugs that had been taking over his body and really was literally coming back to his old self again.

Funny I hadn't realised until then that he'd lost his 'smell'. How could I have been so oblivious? I gave him the biggest longest hug in such appreciation. It really was over.

In the car on the way down with the boys and Caroline, we had all talked and talked, catching up on news and each other, now on the way back it was time for music and we had it blaring. Chase as usual was in charge, mixing it up and playing music we all wanted to hear.

We were on the home stretch on the southern motorway into Auckland when I noticed how much I was smiling. Really smiling. I had my hands on the steering wheel and was singing away as I followed the traffic into the city. I could almost see my smile… like I was observing myself, which made me smile even more. Wow you're happy. Really happy. When I felt into it my body was so light, so free of any dredge. Nothing was weighing me down. I realised that no past memories had risen all weekend. Here I was driving home free in myself and when I looked ahead I saw a future.

I don't know if it was realising Patrick was back physically or if it was getting away for the weekend having fun. If it was putting distance between us and Auckland. If it was all the releasing of emotion over the last couple of weeks. If it was just time. Or if it was the lightness and joy at the prospect we now had a life to look forward to, a future.

Heading home, I knew we had work to go back to. Money would be coming in and there were no more drugs for Patrick to endure. No more sick Patrick. No more tired Patrick. We can make plans. We can have fun. We would be able to afford to do nice things again and plan on catching up with friends. Get into some kayaking again and take long walks, Travel! The world was opening up in front of me as we took that long straight stretch of highway. I smiled and smiled and haven't stopped since. Life is here. Wow, I had finally let go and now we could celebrate. The trauma of the past was left behind and my vision and energy was only moving forward. You couldn't wipe the grin off my face if you'd tried! For the first time in 14 months I was looking forward to going home.

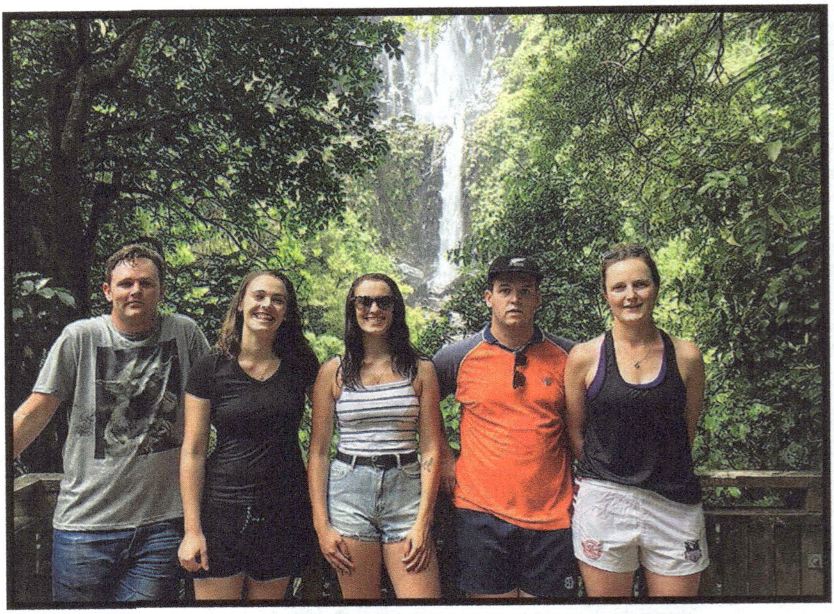

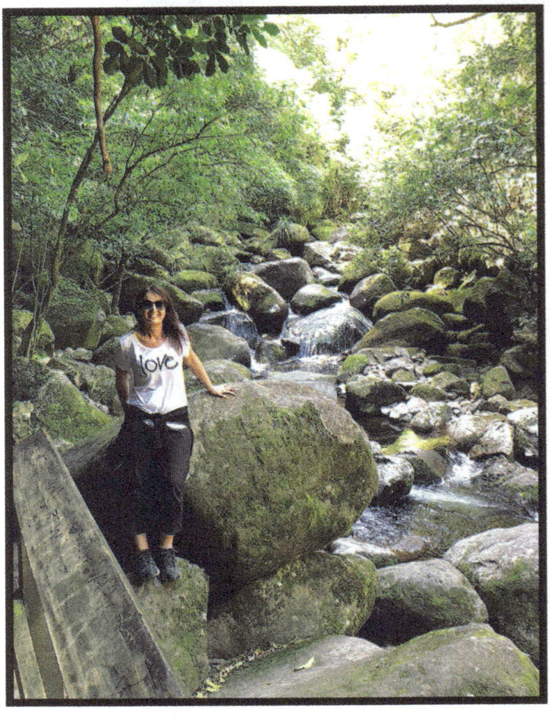
love

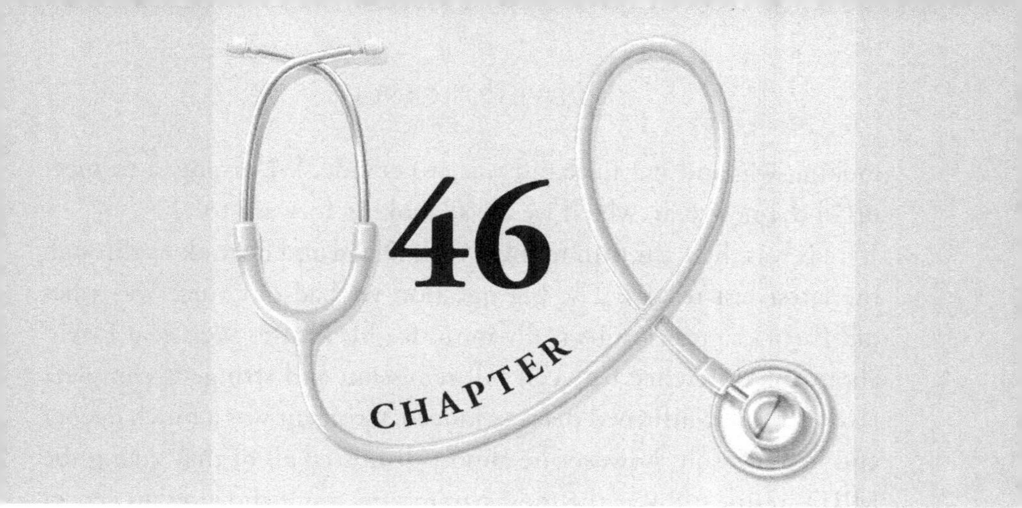

Possibly a Cure for Multiple Myeloma

"The lesson that I have learned and
follow all my life is that
we should try and try and try again -
but never give up!"
- Richard Branson -

So it's four weeks after consolidation chemotherapy and our last hospital appointment to see Kiwi Trial specialist, Dr David Simpson. The grand finale.

It was so hectic in the waiting room that day that they had run out of chairs for those waiting. Understandably everyone had scheduled their end of year appointments before Christmas.

One of our dear 'chemo friends', came out of David's consulting room. What a pleasure to see her. She had been through exactly the same Kiwi Trial as Patrick, but started a few weeks before him, and today was looking so happy and well. She was still sporting her great-looking wig and her husband was at her side. We arranged to meet up in the new year, which we are so looking forward to.

It was then our turn to meet with David and he took us through the latest test results. The big question we had of course was what did Patrick's great results really mean for his future. We asked David about the difference between full remission and stringent complete response. He confirmed that yes indeed, stringent was a much deeper and better result, however he almost dismissed all of that saying the MRD- result still was the most paramount result showing no cancer detected at all. Although he went on, combined, it was the best possible result that could be expected or needed. Patrick definitely had done amazingly well!

We asked about the deletion and what impact it could have now, considering he was in stringent complete response and MRD-. He said he really couldn't answer that question, as it was unknown. However what he did say was quite incredible, I'll never forget it. "You know," he said, "we are working towards curing multiple myeloma. The new treatments, everything we are doing, is towards finding a cure as much as increasing the longevity of life. With these new treatments we actually don't know exactly how effective they are long-term as they haven't been out long enough. We don't really know what they are capable of."

Stop right there. I grabbed that, I really felt he was trying to say, 'This could even be a cure, don't lose sight of that guys. Don't get caught up in this deletion as it only exists in cancer, and for all we know, with your results it may not come back, or at worst possibly not for a long time.'

I heard those words even though they were not spoken at all. I held my breath for a time as it sank in. Wow, wouldn't that be just incredible. There is a possibility. Who would have thought? We had always considered it was definite that this cancer was not curable and we had considered that Patrick would not have a long life. But now with Patrick's great results, it's…'who knows' and that felt pretty damn good.

We went on to talk about maintenance treatment with Lenalidomide being the only topic for discussion. Pharmac in New Zealand are still not funding this treatment until a patient is in their third round of recurrence. Unbelievable when it has been proven overseas to keep cancer at bay, improving quality and longevity of life!

David was strongly recommending Lenalidomide to Patrick. He said that as Patrick has done so well, he should do as much as he can to ensure that continues and cover all the bases, all odds… particularly considering his 1p32 chromosome deletion and his body's vulnerability around that!

Patrick was reluctant due to the potential side effects of Lenalidomide, and gosh, quite frankly he was just over drugs. You can hardly blame him for being hesitant but luckily he had time on his side to decide. They agreed that Patrick would hold off on Lenalidomide for now, continue having his bloods taken every six weeks and David would assess him after three months.

We both thanked David profusely for all he had done for Patrick. We knew he hadn't been his easiest patient, with all the research and questions he'd raised! David, and indeed all the specialists, had remained solid, patient and constant through it all, guiding us into what ultimately was the absolute right direction for the absolute best result. Of that we would both be forever thankful.

We left the consulting room that morning in quiet contemplation of the incredible effort and result that had been achieved and the possibilities this may bring. We found ourselves high fiving again but this time it felt like more of a high five for the future; for potentially a great future, a long future.

As we walked out of the hospital, through the main doors and started down the outside steps, I looked back at the building. Patrick had achieved this for sure but not on his own. This big solid concrete building behind us with its wonderful nurses, doctors, and specialists, the drugs that were drip fed into him, and his friends and family supporting him in different ways, all contributed to making this journey what it was. Successful!!

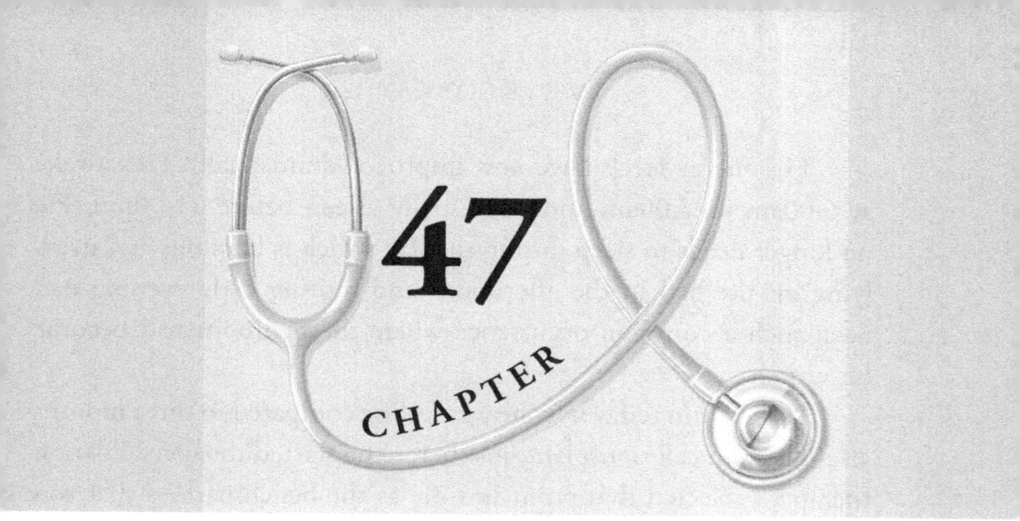

It's Over

"I can't understand why a person will take a year to write a novel when he can easily buy one for a few dollars."
- Fred Allen -

It's now two weeks after Christmas and six weeks after Patrick's last chemotherapy session. Finally summer has arrived and we have glorious weather to bask in. It's been a lazy couple of weeks with both of us just taking time to recover.

Just after Christmas Patrick got his first haircut. He had allowed his hair to grow long when it grew back however it had grown back so curly, grey and was almost frizzy, so he decided to cut it right back. It's a lot darker now and you can't notice the curls. He's looking distinguished and it's a nice look.

Patrick now has a lot more freckles than when he started treatment. These had continued to sprout over his body since starting chemotherapy and I look at them affectionately as such a small side effect of something that so amazingly saved his life.

His energy levels have now improved dramatically. He's awake at 6.00am or 7.00am and not usually asleep before 11.00pm. He no longer needs to sleep during the day which is fabulous as Patrick lying on the bed in the afternoons and retiring early evening had been such a common occurrence where the bedroom had become his crutch.

I asked him today how he was feeling compared to three months after his stem cell transplant, just before he started the consolidation therapy. I selected that point in time as the benchmark as that was when he'd said he was feeling truly better than he had in years. He considered this for a bit, felt into his body and said "My body still aches. It's weird, but it still aches. I feel so much better but not yet back to where I was three months after the stem cell transplant. My mind can still be foggy, and I find it hard sometimes to take things in, but it's definitely better than it was."

After thinking a little more he continued, "The peripheral neuropathy is still there but a lot less, like a deadness at the base of my feet and the tips of my fingers, but it's definitely much better than it was." Then more positively he commented "It's great I have so much more energy now. I feel so much better handling a day and don't need the rest like I used to, that's pretty fantastic!"

That chemotherapy takes a toll on the body, there is no denying that and six weeks later he is still recovering from the four months of consolidation therapy. Patrick went on to say that if he measured how he was now by percentage, he put himself as 75% on the way to feeling better.

Just a mention as well, he's horny as a jack rabbit with no problems in that department. Something we were both very relieved about!

But how's that? Seriously, we wondered if he would ever be the same again going into stem cell transplant and if he would have to find that new norm. During consolidation therapy we worried again what permanent side effects it would have. Even if it was only three quarters of his old self back we would have been delighted but knowing how good he felt now we realised that subconsciously we are quietly expecting a full recovery.

These two weeks of holiday were certainly helping. Patrick is not usually the sort to seek adventure. He's happy moseying around, which for once suited me as I got myself back together. We had stayed at my home in Warkworth for a few days at the end of the first week, and the weather has been so beautiful we are having early morning swims at the beach, breakfast out, then just relaxing for the day.

It's the first week in January and my skin is almost white; I'm usually sporting a lovely all over tan by now. I loved to torture myself by lying in the sun deliberately for the purpose of getting that gorgeous tan. Cancer is too real to me now and I realised my subconscious has got it and I shouldn't do that. It has not even been on my radar. BTW it's a lot more pleasant not needing to lie in the hot baking sun. It gave me headaches and it's uncomfortable! All for a tan.

I found after two weeks I was finally really relaxed. And it felt good! I knew that this year I'm going to need to work extra hard as financially we need to recoup but I just wasn't ready to go back. So I didn't, I took an extra week off. It's Saturday now, the end of my holiday and I feel I've made it. Today I truly, deep down feel that we got through cancer.

24 January 2019

There really is not much left to tell. There are a couple of loose ends to tie up in regards to hospital visits, and other than that we are now getting on with normal life.

Unexpectedly a week ago Patrick was phoned out of the blue to do an MRI. We were surprised but were told it's part of the Kiwi Trial program. When we started the program he needed to do an MRI so we supposed it made sense to do another at the end as well.

His first MRI showed 80-90% saturation of cancer in his plasma cells in his bone marrow. To be honest, right now it's causing me a little anxiety. I feel I've gone back to the beginning, wondering and concerned what the results will show up. The bloods have shown there is no trace of cancer, and we are so, so happy to go with that. The MRI bloody better not show up anything other than that!

We met up with a friend for coffee today who is part of our cancer family, our whānau, just before going to have Patrick's port removed. She had been on the same Kiwi Trial as Patrick. It was such a treat for all of us to share stories, to celebrate how well they had both done, look back on what a year it's been, share results and discuss future treatments and life going forward.

For both Patrick and our friend, their outlook on their lives has changed significantly. As we talked at the cafe, I could feel emanating from them both the desire to live life to their fullest. It showed in so many ways from the big things they wanted to do this year like holidays to smaller things like helping family and prioritising fun times with friends.

It was such a lovely catch up. I can't recommend highly enough finding like-minded people that are undergoing similar treatments, to touch base with occasionally. Both Patrick and I found it very supportive to have friends going through this same journey, chewing the fat on side effects, treatments, feelings etc, so you know that a) you are not going crazy and b) you are not alone. It has been such a special part of the journey for us. A heartwarming treasure of what I hope will now be lifelong friends.

Like Patrick, our friend hadn't yet had her port removed. For both of them, it's been two months since their ports were needed for chemotherapy, and over two months since they put in the request to have them taken out. They spoke of how they both felt ready to rip the blimming thing out themselves, they really hated it still being in. Funny, when it was in for its purpose it was not bothering them so much. I recall our friend saying that herself. We'd asked her what it was like to have the port when Patrick first considered getting his done and she had said it was no bother at all… yet here we are today, it's no longer needed and she wants it out, she can no longer stand this foreign thing in her body! Her body, her emotions, her awareness, all know it's no longer needed, so it's foreign, it needs to go. I know for Patrick it was really affecting him emotionally having it still in. Not just that it was uncomfortable, not just that it was a constant daily reminder of what he's been through, when he wants to just move on now, but it's foreign. It shouldn't be there now.

So it's been a real shame that this one last leg of the journey has been a difficult one to complete however I'm pleased to say that today we are going to go to the hospital to have it removed. After numerous phone calls and follow ups and pleas, it's happening. One last trip for medical care, then it's over… for now. Sure Patrick needs to take blood tests every six weeks. He will have, for now, three monthly follow up specialist appointments to check how he is doing but otherwise we're done.

Other than that, around the house I still see a few reminders. The huge extra large beer glasses in the cupboard to carry the large amounts of water Patrick needed to flush out the chemotherapy. The scrubbing brush tucked away in the shower that he always used after chemotherapy to scrub the excreting fluids off his body. He loved that brush. All abandoned now, and I really want to throw them out, to get rid of the reminders after today, and move on.

Next week Patrick is off on holiday. One of his gorgeous brothers offered to shout him a trip to Australia for a week's motorbike ride through Tasmania, an area Patrick has always wanted to explore. His brother is flying over from England especially to do this with him… how special is that! And Patrick is up for it.

So here we are. Two months after the very last treatment and Patrick is now back working. He's back playing squash for an hour and a half on the weekends. And he feels fit enough to do a full week of motorbike riding! It far exceeds anything we could have possibly hoped for so soon. I remind myself of the thought Patrick had after he did so well through his stem cell transplant. A thought that he has said a number of times since then to me, that maybe he wasn't supposed to have this cancer. That God, or the universe has made some mistake and they are correcting it for him now.

I'm coming to the end of the story. The days of needing to write are coming to an end and I thank my iPad for giving me this opportunity. It's been healing for me to write. This story has been my friend, my outlet and my savior in so many ways. To record events has helped me clear my mind, ready to take on the next thing. Writing has helped me to express my feelings, dumping them onto paper, allowing me to get them off my chest. To sing Patrick's praises has helped my heart swell for him. To write of medical results and processes has given us the history and to write of Patrick's pain and difficulties has allowed me to share his suffering. It really has been such a wonderful gift of which I am eternally grateful. I hope that for anyone who has cared to read this that, even in some small way, it may help you along your own journey.

Sincerely
Kushla and Patrick

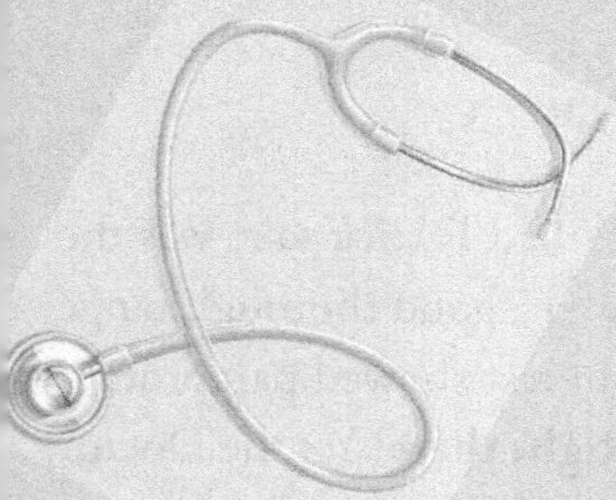

APPENDIX

- Warning Signs

"Seeing is easy,
Predicting is difficult."
- Benjamin Franklin -

Patrick was recalling a few nights ago the two times when he really noticed himself feeling different, not realizing of course at those times that the myeloma was developing in his body. He talked about the first time which was not long after his 49th birthday, when he just felt 'something wasn't right'. I remembered it well. It has prompted me to add this to the book as I think it is so important as a symbol of how important it is to take charge of your own health.

Patrick decided to go and see the holistic Dr Y a couple of months later. His birthday is in July and he went to the doctor in September, 2013, to a doctor that I had started to see. He was the initial doctor I'd seen that had uncovered that I had adrenal problems and told me I was on the brink of chronic fatigue at that stage. He told me to stop doing everything and rest, and to take certain vitamins to help me get my body built back up. I wish I had listened to him now!

Anyhow, we had been impressed with him at the time and so Patrick decided to see him for a full check up. Patrick really felt something wasn't right. He wasn't feeling his 'norm', and still had this feeling like he was aging since his birthday. We both thought a thorough once over would be good.

One of the many blood tests the Dr Y had Patrick take was the Total Protein test. He certainly had requested a good thorough range of blood tests to be done. The Total Protein test showed paraprotein quantification: <1.0 g/L. **That's MGUS! Right there!** Yet the Doctor let it slide! He focused on the fact that glandular fever had shown up in the bloods, and all he said about the paraprotein level was casually, we need to keep an eye on that.

Patrick had no idea what the meaning of this result was. It could have been as insignificant as your iron being a little low to him. It was combined with at least a dozen other blood tests he'd had done at the same time and a number of them were for things he'd not heard of before. Well he's not a doctor right!

I still can't believe this even now as I write this. Knowing what I know now a sense of guilt washes over me when I look at these results from back then. I should have dissected Patrick's results as I do my own. Patrick should have dissected his own results too, in fact I had expected he had, but we were so caught up in the glandular fever diagnosis that we presumed, I think, that it was all tied in to how he had been feeling, and hadn't looked into it further.

We had never heard of paraprotein. It sounded like some protein food type of thing that didn't seem important at all. We had no idea what it meant if it was elevated. Even 1 point above 0 is highly significant. It is called smouldering multiple myeloma (MGUS) and needs to be seriously monitored.

The actual paraprotein test result (looking into it properly now, as we should have then!) stated 'suggest 4 monthly follow ups in the first year (clinical review, serum electrophoresis, immunoglobulins, blood count, calcium and creatinine). If stable, annual follow up is recommended.'

Patrick was not sent for any of those further tests and it was never explained to him that he had MGUS, which can potentially turn into full blown multiple myeloma! **We relied on the doctor reading our results to inform us and act appropriately. Don't!!**

Take charge of your own health. Dr Y went to live overseas two months later and Patrick's results were filed and forgotten.

Remember I mentioned earlier about the misdiagnosis when Patrick's blood results showed his paraprotein level at 42 indicating something was seriously wrong, and the doctor laughing off our concerns saying 'There's nothing seriously wrong with you. You'll live to get your pension ha ha.' Just saying it again. Take charge of your own health. Don't rely completely on doctors!

Patrick went on to describe the second time he noticed he was feeling different. "The other sign of when I noticed I felt different was when I turned 52. Do you remember?" He continued "I felt like I was really in my 50's all of a sudden, as opposed to the year before I felt like I was in my early 40's".

I remembered that day also very well, funny isn't it that it had stuck with me? On that day he'd repeatedly said "I'm feeling old darling. I'm getting old." I'd just hushed him. "Don't be silly." I'd said. I was shocked actually, as it wasn't like him to talk like that and I wanted to dismiss it. It was silly. He looked ten years younger than his age and everyone thought he was my toy boy. (Well he is actually, but just by a year!) To hear him talking like this though, what was he talking about?

But I should have listened more soundly. We should have listened to these feelings or intuition or thoughts. Whatever they are, we should sit up, take notice and get checked out. Fully. And I mean fully.

It takes me back to my dear friend Nikki's partner Darryl. When he was diagnosed with cancer the only symptom he had for some time was that he was more tired than usual. Then he started losing weight which set the alarm bells off. It just makes me want to point out, don't underestimate being out of the norm tired. Don't just put it down to aging or slowing down. Get it checked out. Thoroughly!!

Patrick then, some six months or so later, decided to go to a new holistic doctor as he was concerned at how much more unusually tired, lethargic and aged he was feeling. This was six months before his actual diagnosis. He did a series of thorough tests but paraprotein wasn't one of them. Of course we hadn't thought to request this as we hadn't picked up its significance those years earlier. The doctor requested white and red cell count etc and that was all fine. As there were no alarm bells showing, no further tests were done. The Total Protein test is not routine. Multiple myeloma is not a common condition so it is not routinely tested for.

So my points here are:

1. Listen to what your body is telling you. Take it seriously and get thoroughly checked out. Better a false alarm than leaving it too late.
2. Learn to read your blood results yourself. Don't rely on your doctor alone.
3. Ask for a Total Protein test as part of a thorough check up. In fact, from our past experience, I'd say demand it if you feel you have cause for concern.
4. Take your blood results seriously. Don't skim what they are telling you.

Take charge and accountability of your own health. Lucky for us, Patrick has managed to rid himself of this cancer before irreparable damage could be done to his organs or bones. He has come through this remarkably well; exponentially well. All thanks to eventually, his lovely GP going the extra mile in testing Patrick and this same lovely GP reading Patrick's results accurately, and then testing further. I bless the ground he walks on. We were lucky but don't rely on luck. Take charge and control of your own health, is all I'm saying!

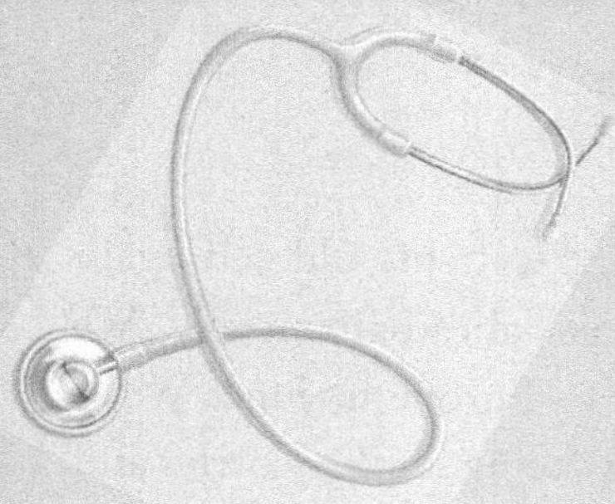

ADDENDA 1

Latest Research - A Cure for Multiple Myeloma

"I intend to live forever.
So far, so good."
- Steven Wright -

I couldn't help myself. Just when I thought I had finished, new information has come to light that I felt I must include.

The significance or MRD-. We knew it was a great result, but we still weren't sure exactly how great it was for Patrick considering his del 1p32.

It's now 31 March 2019. I am at the stage that when someone asks how Patrick is doing I have to stop and take five to remember that, yes, that's right, he had cancer and we've been through all that. It's a bit weird. For a brief moment I wonder if I am a fraud. Cancer? Oh gosh yes we did go through all that, almost psychologically having to pinch myself to remind myself. Yes of course we did! This just goes to show how much we have moved on since then!

Notice I'm saying Patrick HAD cancer! Because that's how it feels. And I suppose it is the reality. Right now there is currently no cancer showing up in his body.

Patrick seems to be recovering well. He is his old self again and we are both working really hard to get ahead financially. We are taking nearly six weeks off and going to Europe in June. We've moved on. Hospitals, treatments, tiredness, being ill, the worries and fears, it's now all behind us and is just a memory.

I am so proud of him. He has been so fortunate to have not only done so well but recovered so quickly in such a short time. I honestly didn't think he would be the same person ever again when we started treatments. But here he is larger than life cracking the same old Dad jokes, and choosing to live life to the full.

So exactly how far removed are we from cancer now?

We have just been to a talk at the hospital. It was by a top cancer specialist from the USA, Dr Munshi, who particularly specialises in multiple myeloma. His talk was specifically on the importance of MRD- for multiple myeloma patients. This was personally our biggest question which was still hanging around. What was the meaning of MRD- as a diagnosis for Patrick, considering his high risk factor of the 1p32 chromosome deletion? How much can the impact of this chromosome deletion have on a long remission for him even though he is MRD-? So of course we both were keen to hear Dr Munshi's talk.

It was weird going back to the hospital. The talk was held in a lecture room separate to the hospital just a stone's throw away from the main hospital building. We'd been there before to other talks. It's a new modern building with blinds that go up and down at the push of a button with good acoustics and tiered seating.

As we walked in we were met by the cancer support team. Donal, who has been such a wonderful support to us, came and greeted us with a shake of the hand to Patrick and a hug for me. Always such a lovely smile on his face, making you feel welcome and inclusive.

So here we are back with our cancer family, our whānau. Dr David Simpson, bless him, was running the talk through Myeloma NZ. One thing I have definitely come to know over the last year of being under his wing is that he really cares, about the people I mean. He's the one who initiates these speakers, because he wants us to be informed. He's the one on the board of Pharmac trying to encourage new life saving drugs to be introduced to NZ. There's no skin off his nose if these events didn't happen, he simply puts in his own time, for us!

He quickly introduced Dr Munshi, who proceeded to talk about the latest findings around MRD- launching with a power point presentation. I soon realised I needed to take pictures of the slides as the information was fabulous. The following is what Dr Munshi had to say, in my layman terminology!

He first explained that MRD testing is done as it can reach much deeper to see if there is any cancer, than other normal blood testing. The first slide that he showed, **'Why assess MRD in Myeloma?'** indicates clearly how much MRD testing matters and how significant it is. Myeloma can sit deep below the surface and not be detected with standard testing. MRD testing at this deep level is relatively new, and its findings and benefits of its findings is the basis of this talk.

The results of MRD testing, and surveys done since, show the success of being MRD-. If you view the following chart headed **'Superior PFS with Deeper Response'**, you will see the PFS (Progression Free Survival) rate with MRD- outcome is by far greater than without. PFS is the length of time during and after treatment that a patient lives with the disease but it does not get worse.

The red line at the top is the outcome when MRD- that Patrick obtained. As you go down the chart through the MRD testing levels you see the different progression free survival rates as a consequence of your results. The red level of MRD- showing it has such a better outcome we presume because out of 1,000,000 cells there was no cancer present. The yellow line for example shows that cancer presented in 1 in 10,000 cells with the MRD test. You can clearly see the different progression free survival periods relevant to the success of your result!

The next slide **'The effect of MRD status on PFS and OS'** shows the OS (Overall Survival) difference when MRD-, again significantly improved. It indicated the studies showing you have more chance of living longer when achieving MRD-!

Considering Patrick is MRD- it was fantastic to see what the latest findings are and what this actually potentially means. The chart was showing approximately a 50% chance of overall survival reaching eight years. This is a far better outcome than studies have shown in the past where overall survival was just five years without HR (high risk) factors.

Dr Munshi then went on to discuss whether different forms of treatment would have an impact on PFS (progression free survival) with MRD-. No matter what treatment path you took to get there, it seems the resulting longevity is the same, as it shows in the following chart headed **'MRD Negative Patients Has Improved Outcome Irrespective of Therapy Used'.**

For those fortunate like Patrick, who are MRD-, whether you have had a stem cell transplant or not, doesn't seem to affect the outcome too much up to four years. Either way **over 75 % of MRD- patients survive over four years in remission.**

Dr Munshi then talked of High-dose Therapy combined with stem cell transplant, and the benefit of its assistance in achieving MRD-, refer the following slide **'Higher MRD Negativity with High-dose Therapy'.** The High-dose therapy that Patrick had was the strong chemotherapy he received just prior to the stem cell transplant. Melphalan. The slide shows that with a stem cell transplant 29.8% achieved MRD- as opposed to without stem cell transplant only 20.5% achieved MRD-. This result really helped doubly confirm for Patrick that he had made the right decision going ahead with his stem cell transplant. Also doubly confirming the specialists were absolutely right in recommending that Patrick have it too.

In the next slide following, you will see HDT which is High-dose Therapy which Patrick received, and Transplant, achieved much better results for progression free survival, compared to RVD alone which is just induction therapy. **'HDT and Transplant Provides Superior PFS compared to RVD alone'.** Look at the bottom line that shows the difference from 65% to 80% achieving MRD- with HDT and Transplant. In medical reference that is a significant increase.

If you can recall before Patrick had his stem cell transplant he had contemplated not going ahead with it considering he was MRD-. Only to find, when discussing this with David, that he wasn't in complete remission, so it would still be very beneficial for him to proceed with the transplant. Patrick had trusted David's and all the other specialist's recommendations and went ahead.

To come out of it with MRD- and complete remission was fantastic only to find from David yet again that an even deeper response rate could be achieved with Consolidation Therapy. David at the time couldn't stress enough, as he had over and over again throughout Patrick's treatment, your best outcome is to get as deep a response as possible for the best outcome long term. The picture David drew the day Patrick decided to go ahead with consolidation therapy was very much like the first slide in this chapter, with the iceberg showing the depth of measure MRD testing can go to. This also shows how deep the multiple myeloma can be. Now I get even more the meaning of a 'deep response'. Deep really being the operative word!

So by the end of the consolidation therapy, Patrick did indeed have a deeper response and had achieved 'stringent complete response'. It doesn't get any better, he had done and achieved all he could.

Dr Munshi also talked about the significance of multiple therapies being used at once. He said multiple concurrent therapies had been shown to produce a higher rate of MRD- results than the traditional two treatment approach which is still the standard treatment in New Zealand.

Patrick had been lucky enough to receive multiple therapies for both the induction and consolidation phases on the Kiwi Trial. His induction therapy involved Carfilizomib, Dexamethasone, and Cyclophosphamide and his consolidation therapy involved Carfilizomib, Dexamethasone, and Thalidomide. We couldn't be more thankful in that moment for Dr Ross Henderson putting us forward for the Kiwi Trial. I felt for others at the end of the talk at question time, asking why they weren't able to receive 'multiple treatments' when it was clearly so much more effective. It's a sad fact that patients in NZ aren't getting the best treatments available, which in fact can potentially be deadly, or at best shortening their lives. These talks are hard to hear when you learn of treatments that are delivering superior results but are unavailable in NZ due to a lack of government funding. Cruel don't you think!?

Dr Munshi next went on to talk about the most important part to us. The part I'd come from Warkworth for that day to hear about! HIGH RISK FACTORS!

Check out the following chart headed **'MRD- Patients Have Improved Outcomes Irrespective of Risk Category'**. This is Patrick. Risk factors are chromosome deletions which include del 1p32. Without a result of MRD-, the yellow line shown in this chart, only 25 percent of patients make it past two and a half years! With Patrick's high risk del 1p32 being one of the highest of all risk categories that forecast is not great as we had read in the reports on del 1p32 about a year ago!

Yet even with High Risk, with MRD- the red line is such a better prognosis… and not far off those without High Risk Factors!! A 75% chance of survival at two years is a lot more encouraging, right, and it looks about 60% chance of survival of up to four years.

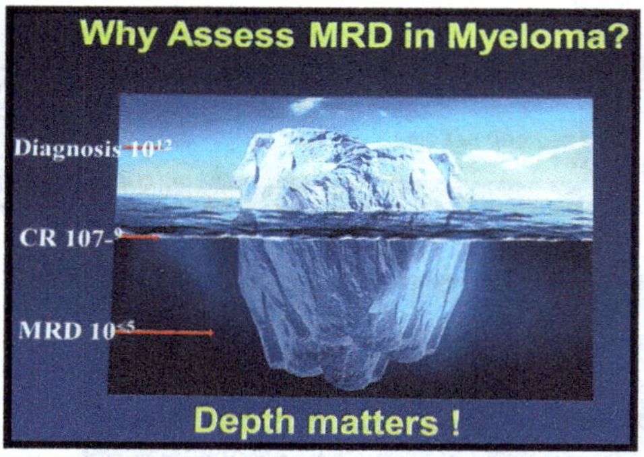
Why Assess MRD in Myeloma?
Diagnosis 10^12
CR 107-9
MRD 10-5
Depth matters !

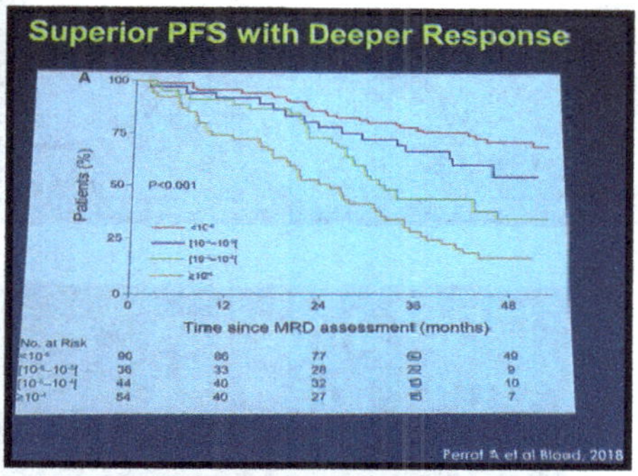
Superior PFS with Deeper Response
Patients (%)
P<0.001
Time since MRD assessment (months)
No. at Risk
Perrot A et al Blood, 2018

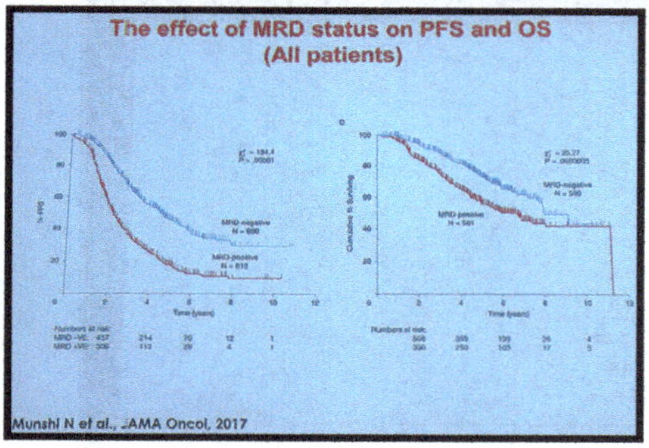
The effect of MRD status on PFS and OS
(All patients)
Munshi N et al., JAMA Oncol, 2017

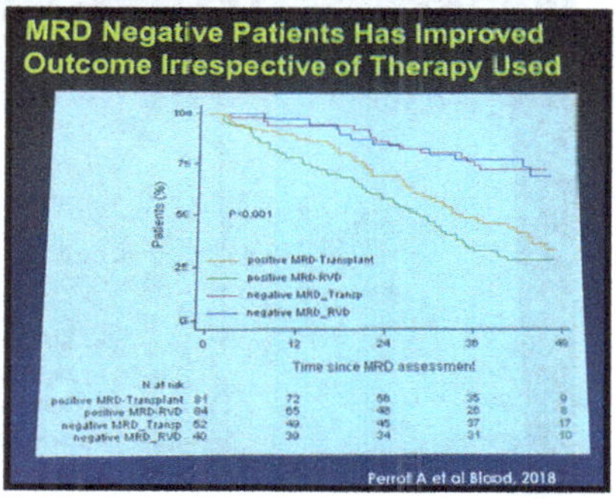
MRD Negative Patients Has Improved
Outcome Irrespective of Therapy Used
Patients (%)
P<0.001
positive MRD-Transplant
positive MRD-RVD
negative MRD_Transp
negative MRD_RVD
Time since MRD assessment
N at risk
Perrot A et al Blood, 2018

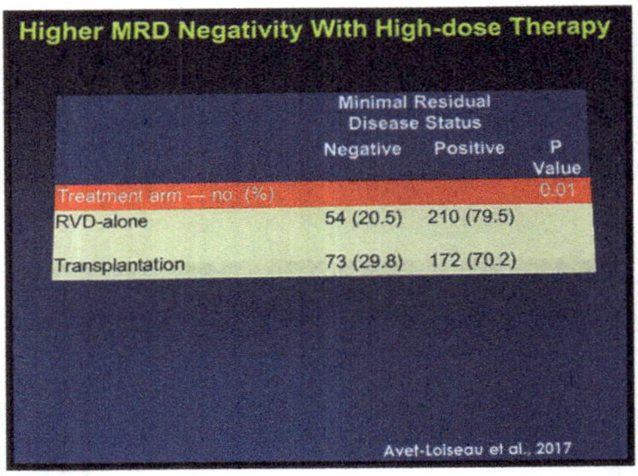

Higher MRD Negativity With High-dose Therapy

	Minimal Residual Disease Status		
	Negative	Positive	P Value
Treatment arm — no. (%)			0.01
RVD-alone	54 (20.5)	210 (79.5)	
Transplantation	73 (29.8)	172 (70.2)	

Avet-Loiseau et al., 2017

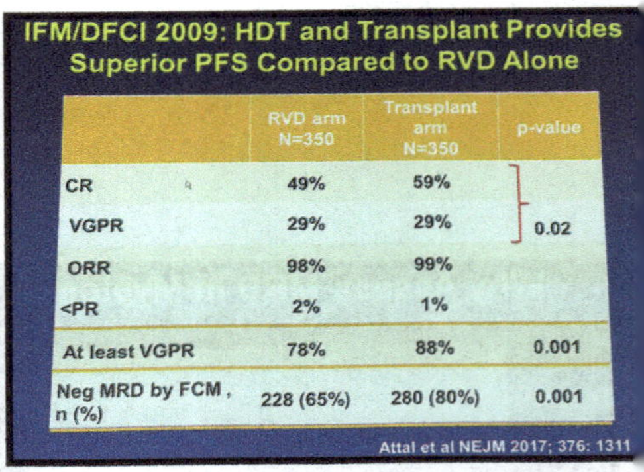

IFM/DFCI 2009: HDT and Transplant Provides Superior PFS Compared to RVD Alone

	RVD arm N=350	Transplant arm N=350	p-value
CR	49%	59%	0.02
VGPR	29%	29%	
ORR	98%	99%	
<PR	2%	1%	
At least VGPR	78%	88%	0.001
Neg MRD by FCM , n (%)	228 (65%)	280 (80%)	0.001

Attal et al NEJM 2017; 376: 1311

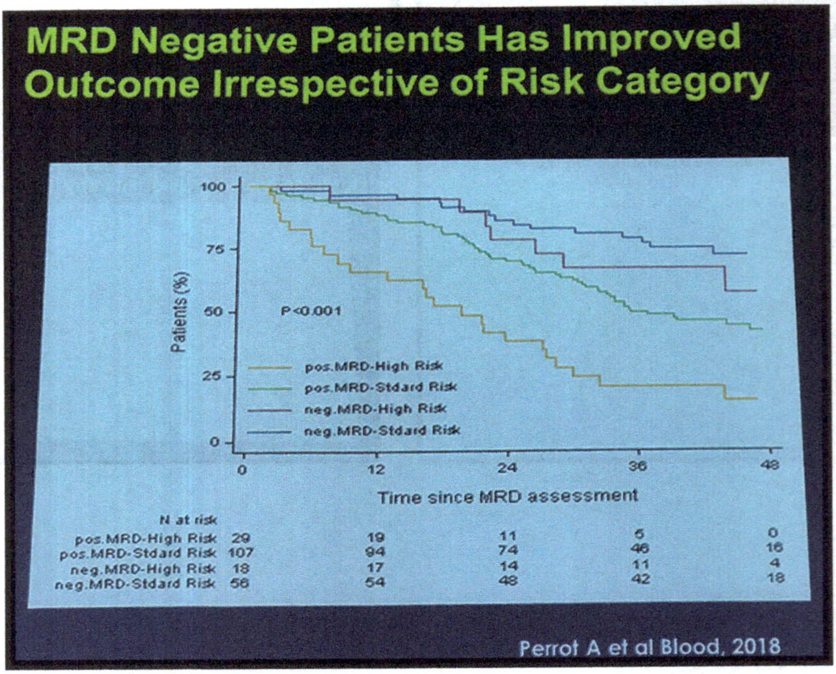

I asked, at question and answer time, about longer prognosis possibilities for those with High Risk Factor, past the four years shown on the chart, and also particularly for those with a chromosome deletion 1p32. Unfortunately it seems that testing at this depth is so recent that research data into the future is consequently limited, so there doesn't seem to be much more they can tell us. Assessments haven't been done past this four year period. Also Dr Munshi replied that no survey has been done specifically on del 1p32. In fact nothing was shown on any of the individual risk factors, they were all compiled into the one group.

In the past MRD testing only tested for 1 in 10,000 cells. And with such limited testing, MRD- wasn't deemed as a significant indicator of longevity. However, now that testing is expanded to 1 in 1,000,000 cells, specialists have been able to get a greater understanding of the importance of MRD-.

So if you can imagine, when only considering 1 in 10,000 cells the iceberg beneath the surface wasn't tested anywhere near as deep. Many people would show as MRD- due to the minor level it was tested at, but could still well have had a lot of cancer cells residing at the deeper level, that were not able to be tested, therefore the longevity of those who were deemed MRD- was not showing as significantly longer.

Now they can test for 1 in 1,000,000 cells, and this new bar is required now to be characterized as MRD-. The bar has shifted along with its significance and the outcome associated with it. Assessments that have been done to date now show a definitive improvement in overall survival with this category.

As much as assessments have not been done specifically for del 1p32, Dr Munshi did reiterate when answering my question, that the graph clearly shows already significant improvement on longevity for high risk factors and it suggests this will continue to show better prognosis with MRD- than without, over time. Good news huh? Better than the very dismal prognosis we had seen right at the start, whereby Patrick would be lucky to make it to two years. Woohoo! Go Patrick!

You know at the beginning we knew it was important to get as good a result from treatment as possible. Patrick had done enough research to know he had to do his best to get to MRD-. This was always the intention that was put out there but what we didn't know at the time was exactly what that would mean for him, particularly that he would fare so much better even with his del 1p32 condition.

This information provided at this talk was new information that was about to be released at a medical conference in NZ. The conference is the reason Dr Munshi was here in NZ. His coming to speak today was a gift from him to us, organized by David and Myeloma NZ. It was cutting edge information that we were extremely grateful to have had shared with us.

What does it really mean for Patrick? Firstly the overall prognosis for survival is obviously so much better now that Patrick has achieved MRD-, stringent complete response. I recall getting such a shock last Christmas reading one of Patrick's brother's general Christmas letter that he wrote to family and friends. In it he wrote of how his brother was having treatment and was 'fighting for his life'. Even as I write this now it makes me emotional. Reading that was a real reality check, that yes, that is exactly what he was doing… and he survived. Not only did he survive the treatments, and the year, but has given himself extended time by doing so well.

Secondly, it also means we don't know how long it will be before he relapses and what his overall survival could be. Like we really don't know. Statistically there is nothing to show how well a patient with multiple myeloma with the High Risk Factor of del 1p32 will fare having received the multiple chemotherapy treatments, HDT, and stem cell transplant, and achieving this new level of MRD-. No one knows so it sort of feels like we are pioneers paving the way to better results. It's a good feeling and positive intention for the next part of the journey!

"Tēnā koutou e te whānau."
- Welcome to our family -

After the talk, due to the question I had asked, and in mentioning Patrick was MRD-, we had a couple of people come up to us discussing their situation.

One was a woman who was now considering conventional treatment, including a stem cell transplant. She was diagnosed ten years ago with multiple myeloma and had turned down chemotherapy and stem cell transplant. She had opted it seemed, in our brief discussion, to go for steroids and alternative/holistic therapies.

Another couple spoke about how they live quite a way out of town and travel to Auckland to be under care here to get the best treatment. How difficult for them on top of everything else, to have to do that.

Then there was the man who said he had no idea if he had a 'High Risk Factor'. At the time I was talking with him and Donal, from the Leukaemia and Blood Cancer NZ. At first they figured in the discussion that if he hadn't been told, he probably didn't. Until I piped in that this was not necessarily true.

It took me back to when we just happened to notice the comment on the letter from the specialist for the insurance company. 'FISH analysis from his bone marrow has shown 1p32 which is a recognized finding in myeloma associated with a less favourable prognosis.' This was the first we had heard about it. I presume that if we had not asked for that letter we may never have known about it as we hadn't seen the FISH test results ourselves.

I went on saying that it is a patient's right to know their full medical condition, and this diagnosis could well affect the decisions you make around your treatment, and what you decide to do with your life knowing a possibly different prognosis. I told them that the prognosis we found at the time for Patrick with this del 1p32 was overall survival two years. I had a very strong opinion around this and they got it!

I suggested to the man enquiring that he go back and ask for his initial FISH test results, presuming he had it done with his first bone marrow biopsy. The FISH test would advise if they had found any chromosome deletions. In fact I highly recommended it. Gosh, it makes me horrified to think there may be patients out there who are unaware of their full diagnosis.

In regards to the FISH test though, just a note, it is not performed for all cancer types. Leukemia, prostate, lung, melanoma and of course multiple myeloma, are key types it is used for. I highly recommend that if you are in any of these categories, to insist on the FISH test, and to request the results of course to view personally yourself. It's such an important thing to know.

When we were finally out of the conference and in the foyer I was surprised to see there were still many people remaining, milling and chatting. It was so lovely to see this conference acting unexpectedly as an opportunity for us all to connect. We spoke to a man who was diagnosed three years ago and had been through exactly what Patrick had. His wife was with him and I started chatting to her telling her that I was documenting Patrick's experience, and also what it was like for me. I opened the floor to how it's not easy on us as the main supporters either!

You know what she said, "Well actually I had a heart attack towards the end of it all."

I stopped in my tracks. Oh my God!

She continued "I can't say for sure it was because of that, of course, I can't absolutely blame it, but that's what happened."

I asked her, "Were you under stress at the time because of the treatments and what you and your husband were going through?" and of course the answer was a definite yes. Her husband had been very ill before he started treatment and had really struggled to get through. She said it took two years after the treatment for them to even start going out again.

So my point is, wow, everyone has a story. What we go through, how we cope, how we don't cope, the rights, the wrongs, the treatments, their effects, emotional drain, financial drain, physical drain, the list goes on. Everyone has a story, and each one is different, but they are all as important.

I was very thankful for that talk this day. Not just for the information we received from Dr Munshi, but for getting together with our cancer whānau, as we share and care about each other and our stories. It really helped Patrick and I to not feel so alone. I felt so much gratitude for that.

In looking for Dr Munshi's correct spelling when writing this Patrick and I came across a talk he did almost a year ago at the Cancer Institute in the USA on these latest findings. We decided to play a bit of it. Guess what he said at the end…:

'If you get to MRD- you do well, with or without transplant, it doesn't matter how you get there, with or without transplant, the same for patients with high risks, with MRD-, you do similarly well. What is happening is we have many more drugs where we are almost curing patients with MRD-. We are a little bit shy of saying they are cured, but I think they are cured'.

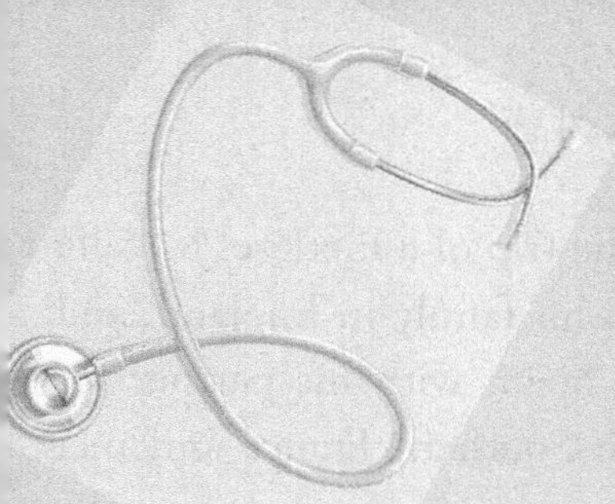

ADDENDA 2

- Lenalidomide and Pharmac

"Give the world the best you have,
even though it may often not be
sufficient."
- Mother Teresa -

We are now in October 2019 and it's almost a year after Patrick's last chemotherapy session. I thought you might like to hear how life without treatment has gone for us now.

Patrick has continued to take blood tests every six weeks and has had his three monthly follow up specialist appointments.

At each appointment Patrick has been advised to go on a maintenance drug called Lenalidomide but he had decided he was going to wait until after our overseas holiday. We planned to go to Europe for six weeks the coming June 2019 and he was over being drugged up, over feeling lousy on drugs, and desperately wanted a break.

I had to respect that. It's his body and his life, although I was worried again about playing Russian roulette. So many recent studies were showing that Lenalidomide, taken as maintenance therapy for multiple myeloma, was helping to keep patients in longer remission.

The first six months after treatment was spent working our butts off. We needed to recover financially, and we really wanted to get to Europe and have a well deserved holiday.

We got there in the end and had the trip of a lifetime. It really was fantastic. Patrick caught up with all his family in England, and his brother from the States met us in Spain with his partner for a week. We had a week with friends in Southern France and met friends in Paris for Bastille day, it was just what we needed to totally distance ourselves from life with cancer. There's something to be said about getting away for a long period of time to distance yourself from the past and come back for a new beginning. It really worked.

Just after our return from Europe, Patrick had an appointment booked with Kiwi Trial specialist Dr David Simpson for his regular three monthly check up. His bloods were all looking really good; no worries there, however David was concerned he still hadn't started taking Lenalidomide. He spoke again about the latest research and findings of how successful it has been to date and also mentioned that with Patrick's del 1p32, he is more at risk and therefore should start taking it!

Patrick spoke again about his concerns of the side effects but David pointed out that he would only be taking 10mg as maintenance therapy. That dosage was apparently very low and he should not expect much in the way of side effects. He also pointed out that if it's too much Patrick can always come off it, but he won't know until he tries!

Honestly, that guy has the patience of a saint. I piped up and told David not to worry, Patrick would be ordering it straight away. I told him how he had just wanted to wait until our holiday was over. He looked at me a little surprised that I had this force speaking for Patrick but I didn't care. Actually, he may have the patience of a saint, but I was no saint, I was done waiting.

As I said to Patrick afterwards, as we walked out of the hospital, "If you relapse as a result of not at least trying the maintenance therapy I will be so cross at you and never forgive you. This is your life we are dealing with here!"

He responded with the same response "I just don't want to live a poor quality of life if it makes me feel unwell." I stopped him right there "Blah blah Patrick, I'm sick of hearing it. Just go on the bloody drug. If it affects your quality of life fine, go off it then, but you don't know it will yet, so stop mucking around and find out!"

Honestly, I was done with it. We had held off until now, and I'd been quiet and said nothing. But the agreement was he would try it once we got back from holiday and I wasn't going to budge on that now. If he didn't want to do it for himself he could do it for me and his children, his family, and his friends.

It still took him a couple of weeks to put the order in. We had to get it from India, can you believe? Although Lenalidomide is now well proven to keep cancer at bay, and potentially help to possibly provide a cure for multiple myeloma patients, Pharmac, who provide funded access to the pharmaceuticals for New Zealanders, does not fund it as a maintenance treatment after your first line of treatment for multiple myeloma. It is only available on your THIRD relapse. Talk about the ambulance at the bottom of the cliff.

It took about six weeks by the time Patrick had ordered the Lenalidomide, transferred payment and received the product by courier from India. He had dragged the chain a bit, but it does take time. When the product finally arrived he had just caught the flu and he didn't want to start on it while he was sick.

It was actually on the day of his next follow up appointment that he finally took it so that was three months later again. Thankfully his blood results were still great and I'm hoping that means this delay hasn't cost him anything.

Patrick saw a new specialist, a lady who was filling in for a time as our dear Dr Simpson, head of the Kiwi Trial, had resigned. What a huge loss to the hospital and its patients is all I can say. This specialist also confirmed to Patrick that he really needed to get on Lenalidomide as soon as possible. She brought up an added reason that I hadn't realised before now.

Patrick's multiple myeloma was IgA related. There are two most common types of multiple myeloma, IgG and IgA. These Ig's are immunoglobulins. Immunoglobulins (also known as antibodies) are molecules produced by plasma cells (white blood cells) that act as a critical part of the immune response. The most common type of myeloma is IgG. Only about 15% of patients have IgA, what they call light chain myeloma. Patrick's IgA blood result at diagnosis was 40.7. Extremely high. The normal range is between .8 and 4.0.

What the specialist told Patrick today was that it has been found that people with IgA myeloma are more susceptible to relapse. We had no idea this was the case!! Actually that was quite a shock to hear that, why did we not know this before now? Gosh with all our research I am surprised we hadn't picked it up… or did we, and forget with all we were needing to absorb? On top of that the specialist went on to say that this combined with the del1p32, being in the High Risk group, further suggests they encourage patients to get on Lenalidomide for maintenance therapy.

That was all Patrick needed. Although it was a shock to hear this, thankfully it was just the extra spur he needed to come home and take it straight away!!

I was thrilled. Patrick now had full acceptance of taking Lenalidomide and he was happy to take it, the time was right for him all round. It's just a capsule. One capsule he takes himself at home once a day.

I must say I was thrown by this news about the higher chance of relapse with IgA Myeloma. My dear man has been through so much and really is still fighting for his life. It's not over and it seems it never will be. I decided to just hold on to Dr Munshi's conclusions about MRD- and its very positive results to date and let it go.

As a conclusion on this subject, I just wanted to pay tribute to a wonderful New Zealander that passed away recently. Blair Vining, a 39 year old father of two diagnosed with terminal bowel cancer in 2018.

Blair came forward in public speaking of how he had to wait eight weeks for an 'urgent' appointment with an oncologist after he was diagnosed. Blair lived in Southland, New Zealand. Southland is New Zealand's southernmost region and is home to snow-capped mountains and fjords. The famous and beautiful Milford Track and the Milford Sound is in this region.

Blair organized a petition throughout New Zealand requesting an independent party to authorize the decisions and distribution of drugs and health care in New Zealand. He raised approximately 140,000 signatures, which of course included our two as well. Blair was fighting for better cancer care for New Zealanders, even though he knew his time left on this planet was to be a short one.

In New Zealand, our pharmaceutical and medical product decisions are governed by Pharmac. Pharmac is responsible for deciding which medicines and medical equipment will be funded and therefore available for the treatment of New Zealanders. Pharmac's strategy as outlined on their website includes:

"Define three main outcomes for the medicine system":

Access: New Zealanders have access to the medicines they need, including equity of access to medicines.

Optimal use: medicines are used to their best effect.

Quality: medicines that are safe and effective.

I hardly see Pharmac fulfilling these three outcomes when it comes to not supplying Lenalidomide as a continued first line maintenance treatment for multiple myeloma.

I'm torn here. Patrick and I both feel so grateful that he got on the Kiwi Trial program and did actually receive the best care possible through Pharmac approving the Kiwi Trial program... but many others around us did not receive these latest drugs like Carfilzomib, nor did they receive 'multiple therapies' as Patrick did on the Kiwi Trial simply because it has not been authorized by Pharmac... even though this is now well documented to be the best and most successful form of treatment for multiple myeloma.

As I said earlier, it was pretty sad to hear from the Specialists of the wonderful and effective treatments that are now available, yet these are not available to every New Zealand patient who needs them. It's cruel and negligent if you ask me.

We are also torn in that, although through the Kiwi Trial program Patrick received the best available treatment plan, the maintenance drug Lenalidomide, that he now needs, is not funded. Fortunately this drug, Lenalidomide, can be bought from India otherwise we would need to find **$6,207 a month for 21 tablets, one month's supply** to access it in New Zealand. By purchasing offshore, Patrick paid just **NZ$865 TOTAL for 90 tablets…** As Patrick takes this medication three weeks on and one week break, that is in effect 4 months supply for $865. ($24,828 if we purchase the quantity in NZ).

Pharmac is apparently in the process of considering Lenalidomide to be funded for the stage Patrick is at. Goodness knows how long that will take. Latest research so obviously shows it's the right thing to administer, all the specialists are recommending it, but it all comes down to funding and in the meantime lives are being lost early unnecessarily… and I mean that. Lenalidomide is said to not only assist progression free survival and overall survival, but when combined with new treatments it could save lives with the progress that is happening with medicine in multiple myeloma.

But how's this? The Ministry of Health have announced they are working on a 'Therapeutic Products Bill' that will replace the Medicines Act and establish a new regulatory scheme for therapeutic products, **putting an end to personal importation of prescription medicines!!!!! That means Patrick will not be able to order Lenalidomide anymore when/if this comes into play.**

It is our specialists that are advising we obtain this medication overseas for Patrick's wellbeing! It is our specialists who give us scripts so we can purchase from overseas. It is our specialists who care about our wellbeing and our survival. Ordering from overseas has become a common practice that people have been forced to do, due to Pharmac not authorizing in New Zealand the best drugs required for our survival.

The Ministry of Health is claiming, as one of its key reasons it is looking at implementing this, is that it is because **people are being harmed by imported drugs.** No evidence of this has been provided to date to my knowledge, despite requests from cancer patients who have approached them asking for evidence of this. In fact requests appear to have been denied as it is apparently too costly administratively to answer these queries.

In fact, on my research, it seems that medicines that weren't publicly funded that come into the country have not even been tested by Medsafe (NZ's Medicines and Medical Devices Safety Authority). According to Medsafe manager of compliance management, Derek Fitzgerald, there has been no information recorded about their potential harms, they are just worried there **might** be a potential risk.

Whereas in fact, on my investigating this further, it seems they are not wanting to stop these medicines coming in, they are trying to regulate how they are obtained. Instead of purchasing directly we would need to go through the Special Clinical Needs Supply authority, or through a pharmacy who it seems would then obtain it from India. At what extra cost to the end user and who clicks the ticket along the way? Yep. Right there! I hate to ask it, but is it all about the money? You have to wonder right?

It has apparently been **well proven that Lenalidomide from India is manufactured appropriately and safe for use.** It is my understanding that the pharmaceutical company in the USA that own the rights to Lenalidomide have assessed India's manufacturing of Lenalidomide and they have officially given India approval to manufacture and sell Lenalidomide as long as they do not sell it into the USA.

With the progress shown on the latest drugs for multiple myeloma improving outcomes more and more, Pharmac should see the importance of approving Lenalidomide for funding as this could not only increase progression free survival, but it also seems to increase overall survival now, and possibly assist towards a cure. Doesn't this save them money in the long run and isn't this terribly short sighted? Personally I feel it's a crime to be so remiss that we are not supplying the most effective drugs to New Zealanders.

I come back to what the specialists have been telling Patrick. We want to keep you in remission as long as possible as with new treatments coming out in the future, there are possibilities of achieving a good life span with multiple myeloma. They all say get on Lenalidomide… but sorry we can't give it to you… unless you are wealthy of course. Or import, which may be stopped soon, sorry!

Blair's petition caused an uproar and created amazing awareness including the lack of funding and availability of the latest drugs in New Zealand for cancer patients. The Government had to stop and listen. Blair brought this problem right to the forefront of the political arena that eventually contributed to a decision from the Government in August 2019, to establish a **NZ Cancer Action Plan- 2019-2029.** Its aim is to ensure we work collaboratively to prevent cancer and improve detection. Its plan over the next ten years is stated:

★ New Zealanders have a system that delivers consistent and **modern** cancer care
★ New Zealanders experience **equitable** cancer outcomes
★ New Zealanders have **fewer** cancers
★ New Zealanders have **better cancer survival**

Cancer is the leading cause of death in New Zealand. Around 23,000 people are diagnosed with cancer every year and each year approximately 10,000 die. Our population is 4,800,912 as of 15 December 2019.

What a man Blair Vining was. It is something so special to leave in the hearts of not only his family and friends, but to all New Zealanders. Blair also had begun working on organizing a community charity hospital in Invercargill, to be focused on improving the region's poor bowel cancer screening rates. It became his personal mission to see reform to the way cancer is treated throughout New Zealand. Blair sadly passed away not two months after the NZ Action Plan was approved, on 11 October 2019. Apparently there were over 1000 people at his funeral. He has since been nominated for the 2020 Kiwibank New Zealander of the Year award.

NB. At this point of this story and about to be published, as of 1 April 2020 Pharmac in New Zealand have just approved Lenalidomide as a maintenance therapy for those who have been newly diagnosed with multiple myeloma who have undergone stem cell transplant.

Unfortunately though they have not stuck to their policy of '**equity of access to medicines**'. It is only available for those within six months post stem cell transplant, and even then only available for 6 months! As Patrick completed his treatment plan in 2018 he does not qualify. What's that all about?! We both individually wrote to Pharmac with submissions on this proposal, stating that no matter the length of time, if the patient is still in remission after stem cell transplant, they should be entitled to Lenalidomide i.e. if they have not regressed from their initial result after stem cell transplant, they should not be penalised on timing alone.

It fell on deaf ears, so I am happy for those coming up the ranks that Lenalidomide is now available for them, although considering it is recommended to stay on Lenalidomide indefinitely, within 6 months they will be needing to order it from overseas anyhow.

Patrick and I would like to take this opportunity to sincerely thank the Blair Vinning's in this world, the specialists who are constantly putting forward for better drugs, and the many other people out there trying to make a difference for others.

Kia Kaha
[Stay Strong]

Made in United States
Orlando, FL
04 November 2026

90207818R00233